Intelligent Medicine and Health Care

Intelligent Medicine and Health Care

Editors

**Chien-Hung Yeh
Xiaojuan Ban
Men-Tzung Lo
Wenbin Shi
Shenghong He**

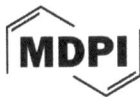

Basel • Beijing • Wuhan • Barcelona • Belgrade • Novi Sad • Cluj • Manchester

Editors

Chien-Hung Yeh
School of Information
and Electronics
Beijing Institute
of Technology
Beijing
China

Xiaojuan Ban
School of Computer &
Communication Engineering
University of Science and
Technology Beijing
Beijing
China

Men-Tzung Lo
Department of Biomedical
Sciences and Engineering
National Central University
Taoyuan
Taiwan

Wenbin Shi
School of Information
and Electronics
Beijing Institute
of Technology
Beijing
China

Shenghong He
Nuffield Department of
Clinical Neurosciences
University of Oxford
Oxford
UK

Editorial Office
MDPI
St. Alban-Anlage 66
4052 Basel, Switzerland

This is a reprint of articles from the Special Issue published online in the open access journal *Applied Sciences* (ISSN 2076-3417) (available at: https://www.mdpi.com/journal/applsci/special_issues/WW038E1NMQ).

For citation purposes, cite each article independently as indicated on the article page online and as indicated below:

Lastname, A.A.; Lastname, B.B. Article Title. *Journal Name* **Year**, *Volume Number*, Page Range.

ISBN 978-3-7258-0569-3 (Hbk)
ISBN 978-3-7258-0570-9 (PDF)
doi.org/10.3390/books978-3-7258-0570-9

© 2024 by the authors. Articles in this book are Open Access and distributed under the Creative Commons Attribution (CC BY) license. The book as a whole is distributed by MDPI under the terms and conditions of the Creative Commons Attribution-NonCommercial-NoDerivs (CC BY-NC-ND) license.

Contents

Nirmal Acharya, Padmaja Kar, Mustafa Ally and Jeffrey Soar
Predicting Co-Occurring Mental Health and Substance Use Disorders in Women:
An Automated Machine Learning Approach
Reprinted from: *Appl. Sci.* 2024, 14, 1630, doi:10.3390/app14041630 1

Shadi Eltanani, Tjeerd V. olde Scheper, Mireya Muñoz-Balbontin, Arantza Aldea, Jo Cossington, Sophie Lawrie, et al.
A Novel Criticality Analysis Method for Assessing Obesity Treatment Efficacy
Reprinted from: *Appl. Sci.* 2023, 13, 13225, doi:10.3390/app132413225 14

Basem Assiri
A Modified and Effective Blockchain Model for E-Healthcare Systems
Reprinted from: *Appl. Sci.* 2023, 13, 12630, doi:10.3390/app132312630 33

Guillaume Dessevre, Cléa Martinez, Liwen Zhang, Christophe Bortolaso and Franck Fontanili
The Centralization and Sharing of Information for Improving a Resilient Approach Based on
Decision-Making at a Local Home Health Care Center
Reprinted from: *Appl. Sci.* 2023, 13, 8576, doi:10.3390/app13158576 51

Rytis Maskeliunas, Robertas Damasevicius, Tomas Blazauskas, Kipras Pribuisis, Nora Ulozaite-Staniene and Virgilijus Uloza
Pareto-Optimized AVQI Assessment of Dysphonia: A Clinical Trial Using Various Smartphones
Reprinted from: *Appl. Sci.* 2023, 13, 5363, doi:10.3390/app13095363 63

Khalil Al-Hussaeni, Ioannis Karamitsos, Ezekiel Adewumi and Rema M. Amawi
CNN-Based Pill Image Recognition for Retrieval Systems
Reprinted from: *Appl. Sci.* 2023, 13, 5050, doi:10.3390/app13085050 92

Ming-Hung Chang, Yi-Chao Wu, Hsi-Yu Niu, Yi-Ting Chen and Shu-Han Juang
Cross-Platform Gait Analysis and Fall Detection Wearable Device
Reprinted from: *Appl. Sci.* 2023, 13, 3299, doi:10.3390/app13053299 108

Salaki Reynaldo Joshua, Wasim Abbas, Je-Hoon Lee and Seong Kun Kim
Trust Components: An Analysis in The Development of Type 2 Diabetic Mellitus Mobile
Application
Reprinted from: *Appl. Sci.* 2023, 13, 1251, doi:10.3390/app13031251 123

Salaki Reynaldo Joshua, Wasim Abbas and Je-Hoon Lee
M-Healthcare Model: An Architecture for a Type 2 Diabetes Mellitus Mobile Application
Reprinted from: *Appl. Sci.* 2023, 13, 8, doi:10.3390/app13010008 143

Elissaveta Zvetkova, Eugeni Koytchev, Ivan Ivanov, Sergey Ranchev and Antonio Antonov
Biomechanical, Healing and Therapeutic Effects of Stretching: A Comprehensive Review
Reprinted from: *Appl. Sci.* 2023, 13, 8596, doi:10.3390/app13158596 159

Article

Predicting Co-Occurring Mental Health and Substance Use Disorders in Women: An Automated Machine Learning Approach

Nirmal Acharya [1,*], Padmaja Kar [2], Mustafa Ally [3] and Jeffrey Soar [3]

1. Australian International Institute of Higher Education, Brisbane, QLD 4000, Australia
2. St Vincent's Care Services, Mitchelton, QLD 4053, Australia
3. School of Business, University of Southern Queensland, Toowoomba, QLD 4350, Australia; mustafa.ally@unisq.edu.au (M.A.); jeffrey.soar@usq.edu.au (J.S.)
* Correspondence: nirmal.acharya@aiihe.edu.au

Abstract: Significant clinical overlap exists between mental health and substance use disorders, especially among women. The purpose of this research is to leverage an AutoML (Automated Machine Learning) interface to predict and distinguish co-occurring mental health (MH) and substance use disorders (SUD) among women. By employing various modeling algorithms for binary classification, including Random Forest, Gradient Boosted Trees, XGBoost, Extra Trees, SGD, Deep Neural Network, Single-Layer Perceptron, K Nearest Neighbors (grid), and a super learning model (constructed by combining the predictions of a Random Forest model and an XGBoost model), the research aims to provide healthcare practitioners with a powerful tool for earlier identification, intervention, and personalised support for women at risk. The present research presents a machine learning (ML) methodology for more accurately predicting the co-occurrence of mental health (MH) and substance use disorders (SUD) in women, utilising the Treatment Episode Data Set Admissions (TEDS-A) from the year 2020 (n = 497,175). A super learning model was constructed by combining the predictions of a Random Forest model and an XGBoost model. The model demonstrated promising predictive performance in predicting co-occurring MH and SUD in women with an AUC = 0.817, Accuracy = 0.751, Precision = 0.743, Recall = 0.926 and F1 Score = 0.825. The use of accurate prediction models can substantially facilitate the prompt identification and implementation of intervention strategies.

Keywords: mental health; substance use disorder; machine learning; AutoML

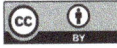

1. Introduction

An association between co-occurring substance use disorders (SUDs) and various mental health disorders is linked to substantial levels of sickness, death, and impairment [1]. Twenty-five percent of patients seeking medical care have at least one mental or behavioural issue; however, these conditions frequently remain undetected and untreated [2]. Substance addiction affects both genders, although there is evidence to suggest that women may face a more rapid progression toward addiction, encounter greater difficulties in sustaining abstinence, and have a higher susceptibility to relapse compared to men [3]. Women tend to resort to substance consumption as a response to negative emotions [4,5], and prior research has also revealed the distinctive mental health dimensions experienced by women who have substance-related issues [6]. These dimensions include higher levels of depression, traumatic stress, and borderline features in comparison to men [7]. The implications of these interconnected issues have broader consequences, as substance use disorders (SUDs) have been linked to increased risks of suicide and aggressiveness [7,8]. Women grappling with co-occurring disorders often navigate a multitude of hurdles, spanning familial conflicts, depression, educational barriers, economic hardships, past trauma, physical health concerns, reproductive health complications, infertility, early onset of menopause, and complications during pregnancy, breastfeeding, childbirth, unemployment, and more, highlighting the multifaceted nature of their challenges [1,9,10].

Machine learning (ML) has emerged as a promising tool for understanding and addressing these challenges. Previous studies have explored its application in identifying predictors for suicide, treatment success, and more. Acion, et al. [11] aimed to investigate disparities in substance use disorder treatment completion in the U.S. using 2017–2019 data from TEDS-D by SAMHSA. Employing a two-stage virtual twins model (random forest + decision tree), the research identified factors influencing completion probability (e.g., race/ethnicity, income source), revealing that those without co-occurring mental health conditions, with job-related income, and white non-Hispanics are more likely to complete treatment. Miranda, et al. [12] employed deep learning and natural language processing to develop DeepBiomarker2 that accurately predicts alcohol and substance use disorder risk in post-traumatic stress disorder patients and identifies medications and social determinants of health parameters that may reduce this risk. Adams, et al. [13] performed a study in Denmark that focused on individuals with substance use disorders (SUDs) and their elevated suicide risk. Using machine learning, the analysis identified key predictors for suicide in men and women with SUDs, highlighting specific factors such as antidepressant use, poisoning diagnoses, age, and comorbid psychiatric disorders. The findings suggest that individuals with prior incidents of poisoning and mental health disorders, especially women, are at increased risk of suicide among those with substance use disorders in Denmark. Aishwarya, et al. [14] investigated the use of machine learning, including AutoML and ensemble classifiers, to predict potential cardiovascular diseases by analysing real-time IoT-based healthcare data, highlighting improved accuracy and efficiency in data analytics for healthcare devices. Kundu, et al. [15] explored the application of machine learning (ML) in investigating mental health and substance use concerns within the LGBTQ2S+ population. Examining 11 recent studies, the findings suggested ML as a promising tool. A lack of studies evaluating substance use treatments in women with severe mental illness who differ in their needs and capacity has been noted [16], there are opportunities to explore the potential application to research in this field of Automated Machine Learning (AutoML) interfaces.

The current research utilises data from the Treatment Episode Data Set Admissions (TEDS-A) for the year 2020 and utilises an AutoML interface to predict co-occurring mental health and substance use disorders among women. The rationale behind leveraging AutoML stems from its growing significance in healthcare analysis [17–19], particularly within the domain of mental health and substance use disorders [20–22], where it often leads to enhanced precision and accuracy [23].

The opportunity for AutoML arises from the need to provide a more user-friendly method for anyone to generate and implement machine learning, offering a more intuitive approach for creating and deploying models with minimal reliance on coding or complex ML infrastructure [24]. Given the limited financial resources allocated to clinical coding and the high wages of data scientists [25], it is imperative to identify a cost-effective approach that enables healthcare organisations to leverage machine learning capabilities without incurring substantial expenses. Several AutoML platforms are currently available. Certain platforms are open source whereas others are commercial. Many prominent organisations in the field of artificial intelligence, including Microsoft Azure, Google, Amazon, $H_2O.ai$, Dataiku, and RapidMiner, have undertaken the development and dissemination of advanced systems, such as the publicly accessible Cloud AutoML [26]. Platforms such as Dataiku exemplify this shift, providing a graphical interface empowering users to fine-tune computational settings effortlessly, enhancing accessibility. Instead of being tethered to specific algorithms or coding languages, researchers gain the flexibility to explore diverse methods within a unified space, encompassing languages such as Python, R, and more, fostering the full spectrum of ML tools. Within the AutoML framework, users leverage existing algorithms and ML frameworks. The process begins with inputting data onto the platform. Users can then opt to employ a specific method or request algorithm suggestions. Once chosen, an algorithm is set up to facilitate training, seamlessly leading into the automated testing phase. This yields immediate access to ML insights, including model predictions and performance metrics, enabling researchers to employ validated models for forecasting or analysing various phenomena. Typically, AutoML workflows initiate with basic ML algorithms known for their simplicity, user-friendliness, and rigorously evaluated models such as k-nearest neighbors and decision trees. As the analysis demands more intricate scrutiny, more complex alternatives like boosted trees or deep learning (e.g., XGBoost) come into play for analysis and evaluation. Diverse intricate models can be crafted, often formed as ensembles—a fusion of basic models leveraging the strengths of each component while mitigating individual weaknesses. The synergy within an ensemble of algorithms aims to enhance overall predictive power and model robustness. ML techniques, particularly AutoML have led to improved granularity and accuracy in various studies [11,22,27]. This research capitalises on the power of AutoML to automate the process of model selection, hyperparameter tuning, and feature engineering, streamlining the analytical process and enhancing the predictive accuracy of the models. the super learning (SL) model has the potential to distinguish women with co-occurring disorders from those without. The super learning algorithm is a supervised learning method that uses a loss-based approach to choose the best combination of prediction algorithms [28]. The method achieves asymptotic performance comparable to the optimal weighted combination of the basic learners, making it a highly effective strategy for addressing various issues using the same technique; it can reduce the probability of over-fitting during the training process, employing a modified version of cross-validation [29,30]. The area under the curve (AUC) value of 0.817 achieved by the super learning model attests to its efficacy in capturing intricate patterns within the data, underscoring its potential as a robust diagnostic tool.

This study serves as an illustration of advanced statistical methods and machine learning techniques harnessed through Dataiku, an AutoML interface, in a real-world healthcare setting. It showcases the platform's ability to automate essential operations such as selecting models, optimising hyperparameters, and engineering features. The super learning model, which combines Random Forest and XGBoost, has superior performance compared to separate algorithms. It serves as a diagnostic tool for early detection of co-occurring disorders in women. The study emphasises the potential advantages of these powerful predictive models. By leveraging these technological advancements, we aim to bridge the gap between data-driven innovation and clinical practice. SUDs are often inadequately addressed in women [31,32]. The insight of the study holds the potential to develop a tool for early identification of mental health and SUDs in women. The findings also offer valuable insights that can inform future research and collaborations with policymakers, medical associations, and patient advocacy groups to develop guidelines for responsible integration and optimise the model's potential advantages while ensuring patient well-being and privacy protection.

The structure of the paper is as follows. The next section presents the materials and methods, covering the description of the dataset, the machine learning models utilised, and the statistical method employed. This is followed by the Section 3, where the findings of the study are presented. The Section 4 then follows, which discusses the application, limitations, and future prospects of the study. Finally, the paper concludes with the implications, recommendations for further research, and conclusions.

2. Materials and Methods

2.1. Dataset

This study used publicly available Treatment Episode Data Set Admissions (TEDS-A) 2020 [33], maintained by the Center for Behavioral Health Statistics and Quality (CBHSQ) of the Substance Abuse and Mental Health Services Administration (SAMHSA) to illustrate the machine learning approach to predict co-occurring mental and substance use disorders in women. TEDS, encompassing the Admissions Data Set (TEDS-A) and the Discharges Data Set (TEDS-D), is a notable representation of a substantial administrative dataset that may captivate addiction researchers in practical situations [34,35]. TEDS provides comprehensive statistics regarding admissions and discharges from substance use disorder treatment programs across participating states. However, the analysis for the year 2020 had to exclude Oregon, North Dakota, Idaho, and Washington due to inadequate data reporting. Notably, some states contribute data that document multiple admissions for the same individual, shaping statistical analyses to accurately portray admissions rather than individual clients [36]. The dependent variable in this study was co-occurring mental health and substance use disorder which is coded as PSYPROB (1 = Yes, 2 = No) in the dataset. As we focused on women, we extracted the records where the client's biological sex was female (n = 497,175). We then conducted data pre-processing which consisted of three steps. First, we conducted listwise deletion for records with missing values at the dependent variable and thirty-seven relevant predictors that include PSYPROB, STFIPS, SERVICES, PREG, IDU, EMPLOY, EDUC, ETHNIC, LIVARAG, BARBFLG, MARFLG, DSMCRIT, AGE, MARSTAT, RACE, PSOURCE, AMPHFLG, ALCDRUG, STIMFLG, MTHAMFLG, ALCFLG, SEDHPFLG, INHFLG, OTCFLG, PCPFLG, HALLFLG, OPSYNFLG, BENZFLG, TRNQFLG, METHFLG, COKEFLG, HERFLG, OTHERFLG, METHUSE, FRSTUSE1, SUB1, SUB2, SUB3, NOPRIOR. Records with incomplete data in any of the predictors, the outcome, or characteristics used for defining inclusion in the study were excluded from the analysis. Second, outlier detection was performed using the analyse function in Dataiku at the dependent variable and all relevant predictors. The outliers were handled by performing listwise deletion, leaving us a final analytic sample (n = 132,128). Finally, each feature was processed using target encoding, in which its original value was substituted with a numerical value derived from the target values. Within the dataset, several features exhibit different units and scales. This trend could result in certain features having a more significant influence on the learning algorithm compared to others, thus potentially introducing bias. To tackle this issue, we employed the min–max normalisation technique to standardise all the features, consequently ensuring that they are within a consistent range, typically ranging from 0 to 1 [37]. This ensures that all features contribute equally to the model. The provided sample was then randomly split into two sets: a training set comprising 80% of the sample (n = 105,760), and a test set consisting of the remaining 20% (n = 26,368).

As the data utilised in this study were sourced from publicly available information without any subject identification, the research design and methodology were determined to be exempt from ethics review.

2.2. Statistical Methods

Multivariant analysis was performed using Dataiku v12 [38], an integrated coding-free platform for data science, machine learning, and analytics [24]. The modelling algorithms applied for binary classification modelling for the prediction of the probability of co-occurring mental health and substance use disorders in women were Random Forest, Gradient Boosted Trees, XGBoost, Extra Trees, SGD, Deep Neural Network, Single-Layer Perceptron, K Nearest Neighbors (grid) and a super learning model (constructed by combining the predictions of a Random Forest model and an XGBoost model) [39] (see Figure 1). In the discipline of predictive modelling, conventional techniques such as linear or logistic regression have historically been used. However, the advancement of machine learning has introduced Random Forests (RF) and XGBoost as robust alternatives in the field of health sciences [40–42]. The rationale behind incorporating a Random Forest model and an XGBoost model into a super learning framework is in their capacity to overcome the limitations of traditional regression approaches [11,43–45]. Random Forest, with its collection of decision trees, offers resistance against overfitting and excels in capturing intricate, non-linear relationships within data. Meanwhile, XGBoost utilises gradient boosting to repeatedly improve predictive accuracy by combining weak learners and tackling obstacles posed by heterogeneous data. The objective of this integrated strategy is to capitalise on the advantages of both algorithms, promoting a more robust and precise predictive model.

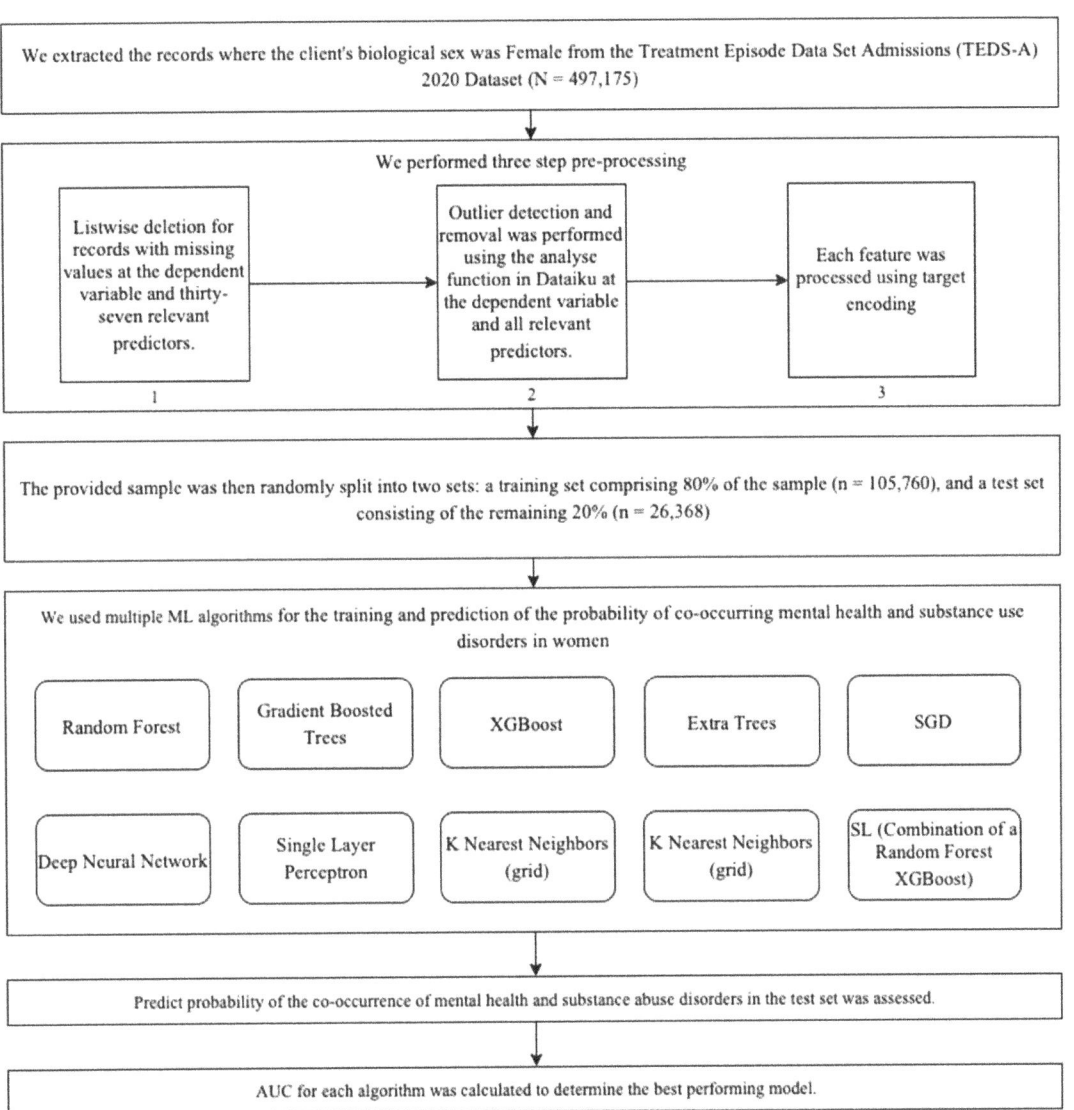

Figure 1. Analytic workflow.

The optimal analytic approach for forecasting the co-occurrence of mental health and substance abuse disorders was determined to be the model that maximises the Area Under the Curve (AUC) [46]. The AUC is a useful metric for evaluating prediction accuracy. It represents the likelihood that a randomly selected successful patient will be ranked higher than a randomly selected unsuccessful patient by any of the algorithms. The AUC (area under the curve) metric measures the performance of a prediction model, with values ranging from 0 to 1. AUC = 1 indicates a perfect forecast, while AUC = 0.5 suggests that the prediction is no better than chance.

Dataiku's ML diagnostics feature was enabled to conduct comprehensive checks on the dataset, modelling parameters, training speed, overfitting, leakage, model checks, ML assertions, and abnormal predictions. A Bayesian search strategy was employed to optimise the hyperparameters of the machine learning models. The search was guided by a probabilistic model that intelligently selected hyperparameter combinations for evaluation. The goal was to find the best-performing set of hyperparameters for the model's task. The search process was limited to exploring five different combinations of hyperparameters. This approach allowed for an efficient and systematic exploration of the hyperparameter space, leading to improved model performance. A super learning model was constructed by combining the predictions of a Random Forest model and an XGBoost model using the "average" method. Each model was trained independently on the training data to capture distinct patterns and relationships. During prediction, the outputs of both models were averaged for each data point, resulting in a final prediction for the super learning model. This approach leverages the strengths of both Random Forest and XGBoost, providing a potentially more robust and accurate prediction by blending the insights from these two diverse algorithms.

3. Results

Dataiku automatically ranks the best-performing interpretable model based on the set performance metric (AUC in this case). The characteristics of the sample are presented in Table 1. It presents an overview of a cohort and only includes gender as well as the top 10 predictors of PSYPROB that were selected as the most essential based on the Shapley values, to keep it concise. The cohort predominantly resides in states such as New York, Colorado, and Illinois. Notably, around 30% had no prior treatment episodes, reflecting a significant proportion seeking treatment for the first time, while diverse referral sources: individuals, legal systems, and community referrals highlight the multifaceted pathways to treatment. In terms of race, the majority of the individuals classified themselves as Black or African American (73.9%), and a range of substance use patterns emerged, encompassing various substances across primary, secondary, and tertiary categories. The significant unemployment rate of 52.3% among the cohort highlights the possible socioeconomic factors at play. The substances encompass alcohol, cocaine/crack, marijuana/hashish, prescription opiates/synthetics, methamphetamine/speed, and various other substances. The diagnostic data indicated a significant occurrence of opioid dependence, with a prevalence rate of 33.8%. Additionally, around 26.3% of individuals received medication-assisted opioid therapy.

Table 1. Baseline characteristics of the cohort (n = 132,128).

Factor	Value	Number (%)
GENDER	Female	132,128 (100)
State (STFIPS)	New York	35,662 (27)
	Colorado	11,247 (8.5)
	Illinois	9351 (7.1)
	Michigan	9161 (6.9)
	North Carolina	8410 (6.4)
	New Jersey	7520 (5.7)
	Indiana	6806 (5.2)
	Connecticut	5502 (4.2)
	Kentucky	4954 (3.7)
	Tennessee	4052 (3.1)
	Missouri	3593 (2.7)
	Pennsylvania	3236 (2.4)
	Ohio	2771 (2.1)
	Other	19,863 (15)

Table 1. Cont.

Factor	Value	Number (%)
Previous substance use treatment episodes (NOPRIOR)	No prior treatment episodes One prior treatment episode Five or more prior treatment episodes Two prior treatment episodes Three prior treatment episodes Four prior treatment episodes	39,112 (29.6) 28,334 (21.4) 24,478 (18.5) 19,212 (14.5) 13,101 (9.9) 7891 (6)
Type of treatment service/setting (SERVICES)	Ambulatory, non-intensive outpatient Rehab/residential, short-term (30 days or fewer) Ambulatory, intensive outpatient Detox, 24-h, free-standing residential Other	70,284 (53.2) 21,110 (16) 15,802 (12) 13,945 (10.6) 10,983 (8.4)
Referral source (PSOURCE)	Individual (includes self-referral) Court/criminal justice referral/DUI/DWI Other community referral Alcohol/drug use care provider Other	62,232 (47.1) 29,059 (22) 15,135 (11.5) 14,176 (10.7) 11,535 (9.7)
Race (RACE)	Black or African American Asian or Pacific Islander White Other	97,677 (73.9) 20,931 (15.8) 8788 (6.7) 4732 (3.5)
Substance use (secondary) (SUB2)	None Cocaine/crack Marijuana/hashish Methamphetamine/speed Alcohol Other opiates and synthetics Other	48,513 (36.7) 19,126 (14.5) 18,044 (13.7) 11,659 (8.8) 10,974 (8.3) 7012 (5.3) 10,246 (12.7)
Substance use (tertiary) (SUB3)	None Marijuana/hashish Alcohol Cocaine/crack Methamphetamine/speed Other	92,205 (69.8) 10,689 (8.1) 6454 (4.9) 5465 (4.1) 3373 (2.6) 13,942 (10.5)
Employment (EMPLOY)	Unemployed Not in labour force Part-time	69,048 (52.3) 51,075 (38.7) 12,005 (9.1)
Diagnostic and Statistical Manual of Mental Disorders diagnosis (DSMCRIT)	Opioid dependence Alcohol dependence Other substance dependence Other mental health condition Cannabis dependence Cocaine dependence Other	44,699 (33.8) 22,077 (16.7) 17,766 (13.4) 14,540 (11) 6567 (5) 6196 (4.7) 20,283 (15.4)
Medication-assisted opioid therapy (METHUSE)	Yes No	34,807 (26.3) 97,321 (73.7)

Table 2 shows the performance matrices for each algorithm applied for binary classification in the test set (N = 26,368). The primary evaluation criterion in this study was the AUC. All AUC values were between 0.631 and 0.817. This range signifies the probability that any of the algorithms would correctly rank a randomly selected woman with co-occurring mental and substance use disorders higher than one without such disorders. As hypothesised, the super learning model showed the largest AUC of 0.817, demonstrating robust predictive capability. The performance of the super learning model is closely followed by XGBoost with an AUC of 0.809. Several ensemble techniques such as Random Forest (AUC = 0.807) and Extra Trees (AUC = 0.803) showed significant discriminatory ability, closely following the top-performing algorithm. Meanwhile, conventional methods such as Gradient-Boosted Trees (AUC = 0.799) and Single-Layer Perceptron (AUC = 0.776) demonstrated comparable but slightly lower AUC scores. Nevertheless, the utilisation of K Nearest Neighbors (grid) resulted in a relatively reduced prediction accuracy, as indicated by an AUC of 0.670. Interestingly, models employing Deep Neural Network architecture exhibited the least satisfactory performance among the investigated algorithms, achieving an AUC of 0.631. These findings highlight the superiority of the proposed ensemble-based approach in achieving higher AUC values and therefore more successful binary classification in this experimental environment.

Table 2. Performance matrices for each algorithm applied for binary classification in the test set (N = 26,368).

Model	AUC	Accuracy	Precision	Recall	F1 Score
Random Forest	0.807	0.742	0.734	0.923	0.818
Gradient Boosted Trees	0.799	0.733	0.726	0.921	0.812
XGBoost	0.809	0.745	0.739	0.918	0.819
Extra Trees	0.803	0.738	0.733	0.916	0.814
SGD	0.778	0.725	0.728	0.898	0.804
Deep Neural Network	0.631	0.628	0.628	1	0.771
Single Layer Perceptron	0.776	0.721	0.718	0.916	0.805
K Nearest Neighbors (grid)	0.670	0.661	0.655	0.971	0.782
Super Learning	0.817	0.751	0.743	0.926	0.825

Table 3 provides the mean and standard deviation (SD) for each metric across the different models. Based on these findings, the "super learning" model emerged as the better option, as it consistently demonstrated high performance across various parameters with low variability.

Table 3. Mean and standard deviation of key metrics across the evaluated models.

Metric	Mean	Standard Deviation (SD)
AUC	0.772	0.059
Accuracy	0.713	0.037
Precision	0.711	0.037
Recall	0.935	0.032
F1 Score	0.804	0.020

Figure 2 provides a visual representation of the AUC in the test set (n = 26,368) for the super learning model. The super learning model exhibited the highest AUC among all models, boasting an AUC of 0.817, a score that is typically considered a strong performance for prediction models. Other matrices for the super learning model include accuracy (0.751), precision (0.743), recall (0.926), and F1 score (0.825). This outcome underscores the model's strong ability to distinguish women with co-occurring mental and substance use disorders from those without.

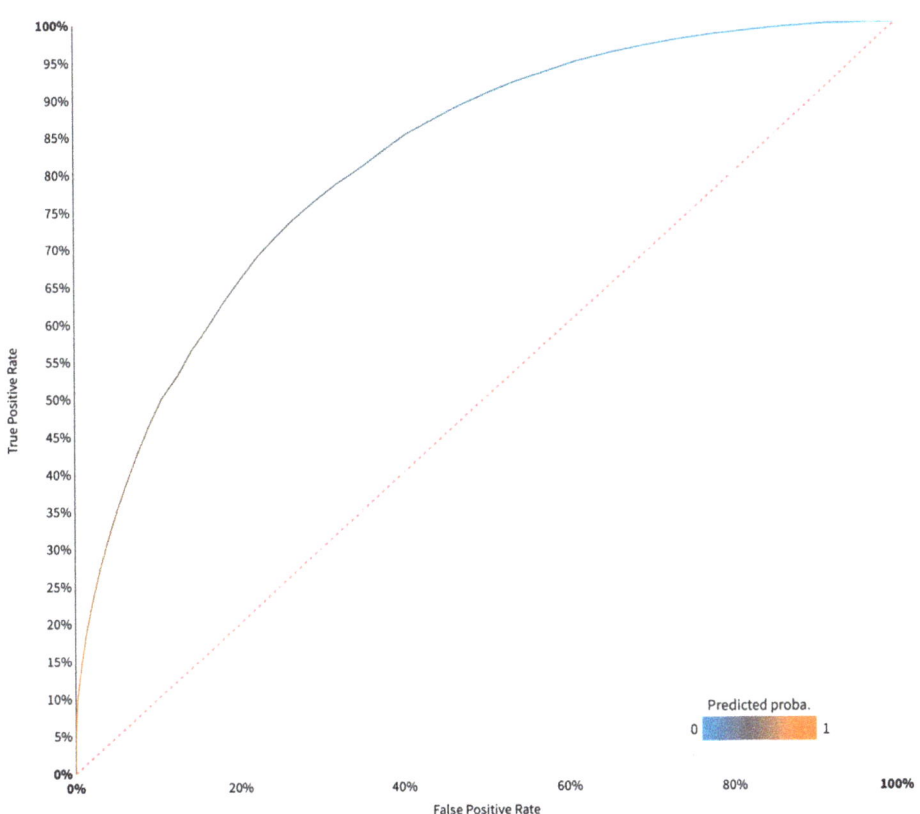

Figure 2. Distribution of the performance metric (AUC) of the super learning model.

4. Discussion

This section offers a discussion on the application, limitations, and future prospects of the research findings. It highlights the practical implications, potential challenges, and opportunities for further progress in the field of co-occurring mental health and substance use disorders among women.

4.1. Application

In ML, classification emerges as a vital task, involving the nuanced prediction of target classes for individual data instances [28]. Achieving optimal performance on diverse datasets necessitates the careful selection of suitable individual classifiers. The challenge lies in pinpointing the most suitable data mining or machine learning model tailored to a specific problem. To tackle this complexity, researchers often deploy an array of models to ascertain the utmost performance for a given scenario. AutoML platforms are appealing pre-packaged tools for constructing predictive models using healthcare data [47]. In this study, the AutoML interface was employed to forecast and differentiate the simultaneous co-occurrence of mental health and substance use disorders in women. Notably, AutoML consistently demonstrates enhanced precision and specificity across various research investigations. By harnessing the capabilities of AutoML, the study automated critical tasks encompassing model selection, hyperparameter optimisation, and feature engineering. This streamlined approach simplifies the analytical pipeline and substantiates an elevation in the accuracy of prediction models, marking a promising stride within computational health research.

A significant novelty of our study represents the statistical analysis using an AutoML interface to predict co-occurring mental and substance use disorders in women. This research serves as a practical demonstration of the presented statistical methods utilising an AutoML interface within a real-world context, offering valuable insights into predictive analytics in health-related domains.

The research finding showcasing the performance of the super learning model in distinguishing co-occurring mental health and substance use disorders among women carries substantial potential for transformative impact. The super learning model comprised two base learners: a Random Forest model and an XGBoost model, and it outperformed the individual base learners. The super learning model's accuracy in identification would enable early identification of women at risk of co-occurring mental health and substance use disorders. Women who receive substance use treatment that is tailored to their gender experience a longer duration of stay in treatment and have a higher probability of maintaining abstinence after completing treatment [1]. The emergence of more accurate and timely diagnosis has significant consequences for the development of improved treatment techniques, aimed at reducing the complications, illness, and death associated with these disorders [26]. Efficient resource allocation would be facilitated as the model's precision allows healthcare providers to focus on those at elevated risk, ensuring that support and treatment resources are channelled where they can yield the most significant benefits.

4.2. Limitations

AutoML platforms expedite the process of developing machine learning pipelines, and the models they produce can be used as initial frameworks for constructing predictive models. It is crucial to approach the integration of such a model with caution when determining the best output levels based on the research topic, considering ethical considerations, data security, and ongoing clinical supervision to ensure that its application aligns with the envisioned positive impact. The study acknowledges the fear of stigma preventing women from seeking substance abuse treatment, leading to a lower likelihood of them pursuing help compared to men [10], highlighting a potential limitation in real-world application. Although the super learning model demonstrated enhanced accuracy in differentiating co-occurring mental health and substance use disorders in women, it is important to acknowledge its limitations, including the possibility of false positives and false negatives. While the potential benefits of early identification and intervention on the health of women are promising, it may require time for these effects to become evident. Further research and validation are necessary to validate and measure these possible long-term benefits.

4.3. Future Prospects

The utilisation of AutoML platforms, as demonstrated by the study's implementation of Dataiku, signifies a progression towards enhancing patient outcomes in the medical domain, particularly in efficiently analysing and examining large collections of patient data. The implementation of streamlined methodologies and enhanced diagnostic procedures enhances the efficiency of healthcare operations, while potentially preserving resources. This could reduce the need for physical infrastructure such as storage rooms, as data administration and utilisation become more optimised. The research results regarding the performance of the super learning model have the potential to bring about significant changes, especially in the early detection of women who are at risk of experiencing both mental health and substance use issues simultaneously. Early diagnosis enables proactive intervention, customised support, and trauma-informed treatments [48], which address the fear of social disapproval and encourage more compassionate approaches to women's mental well-being. The research highlights that the model's accuracy in allocating resources effectively could help overcome the obstacles related to stigma, leading to improved health outcomes for both impacted women and their families and communities. Ultimately, the precise forecasts generated by the model have the potential to accelerate progress in

5. Conclusions

This study investigated the potential of AutoML for predicting co-occurring mental health and substance use disorders among women using TEDS-A data for 2020. Employing advanced statistical and machine learning techniques through Dataiku's AutoML interface, a super learning model achieved a high AUC of 0.817, demonstrating robust predictive capability. These findings highlight the promise of AutoML in healthcare, particularly the super learning model's potential as a diagnostic tool for early identification of co-occurring disorders in women. Future research should focus on disseminating knowledge about AutoML's advantages and ethical considerations in healthcare integration. Collaboration with policymakers, medical associations, and patient advocacy groups is crucial for establishing guidelines on responsible implementation, data privacy, and continuous performance monitoring. This holistic approach ensures maximising the model's benefits while adhering to the highest ethical standards, safeguarding patient well-being and privacy.

Author Contributions: Conceptualisation, N.A. and P.K.; methodology, N.A. and P.K.; software, N.A. and P.K.; validation, N.A., P.K., M.A. and J.S.; formal analysis, N.A. and P.K.; writing—original draft preparation, N.A. and P.K.; writing—review and editing, N.A., P.K., M.A. and J.S.; supervision, M.A. and J.S.; project administration, P.K. All authors have read and agreed to the published version of the manuscript.

Funding: This research received no external funding.

Institutional Review Board Statement: Not applicable.

Informed Consent Statement: Not applicable.

Data Availability Statement: Publicly available datasets were analyzed in this study. The data can be found here: https://www.datafiles.samhsa.gov/dataset/treatment-episode-data-set-admissions-2020-teds-2020-ds0001 (accessed on 2 June 2023).

Conflicts of Interest: Author Padmaja Kar was employed by the company St Vincent's Care Services. The remaining authors declare that the research was conducted in the absence of any commercial or financial relationships that could be construed as a potential conflict of interest.

References

1. Louison, L.; Green, S.L.; Bunch, S.; Scheyett, A. The problems no one wants to see: Mental illness and substance abuse among women of reproductive age in North Carolina. *North Carol. Med. J.* **2009**, *70*, 454–458. [CrossRef]
2. Stewart, D.; Ashraf, I.; Munce, S. Women's mental health: A silent cause of mortality and morbidity. *Int. J. Gynecol. Obstet.* **2006**, *94*, 343–349. [CrossRef] [PubMed]
3. Kokane, S.S.; Perrotti, L.I. Sex Differences and the Role of Estradiol in Mesolimbic Reward Circuits and Vulnerability to Cocaine and Opiate Addiction. *Front. Behav. Neurosci.* **2020**, *14*, 74. [CrossRef] [PubMed]
4. McCaul, M.E.; Roach, D.; Hasin, D.S.; Weisner, C.; Chang, G.; Sinha, R. Alcohol and women: A brief overview. *Alcohol. Clin. Exp. Res.* **2019**, *43*, 774. [CrossRef]
5. Fox, H.C.; Sinha, R. Sex differences in drug-related stress-system changes: Implications for treatment in substance-abusing women. *Harv. Rev. Psychiatry* **2009**, *17*, 103–119. [CrossRef] [PubMed]
6. Prieto-Arenas, L.; Díaz, I.; Arenas, M.C. Gender differences in dual diagnoses associated with cannabis use: A review. *Brain Sci.* **2022**, *12*, 388. [CrossRef]
7. Ruiz, M.A.; Douglas, K.S.; Edens, J.F.; Nikolova, N.L.; Lilienfeld, S.O. Co-occurring mental health and substance use problems in offenders: Implications for risk assessment. *Psychol. Assess.* **2012**, *24*, 77–87. [CrossRef]
8. Forster, M.; Rogers, C.J.; Tinoco, S.; Benjamin, S.; Lust, K.; Grigsby, T.J. Adverse childhood experiences and alcohol related negative consequence among college student drinkers. *Addict. Behav.* **2023**, *136*, 107484. [CrossRef]
9. Larsen, J.L.; Johansen, K.S.; Mehlsen, M.Y. What kind of science for dual diagnosis? A pragmatic examination of the enactive approach to psychiatry. *Front. Psychol.* **2022**, *13*, 825701. [CrossRef]
10. Agterberg, S.; Schubert, N.; Overington, L.; Corace, K. Treatment barriers among individuals with co-occurring substance use and mental health problems: Examining gender differences. *J. Subst. Abus. Treat.* **2020**, *112*, 29–35. [CrossRef]
11. Acion, L.; Kelmansky, D.; van der Laan, M.; Sahker, E.; Jones, D.; Arndt, S. Use of a machine learning framework to predict substance use disorder treatment success. *PLoS ONE* **2017**, *12*, e0175383. [CrossRef]

12. Miranda, O.; Fan, P.; Qi, X.; Wang, H.; Brannock, M.D.; Kosten, T.R.; Ryan, N.D.; Kirisci, L.; Wang, L. DeepBiomarker2: Prediction of Alcohol and Substance Use Disorder Risk in Post-Traumatic Stress Disorder Patients Using Electronic Medical Records and Multiple Social Determinants of Health. *J. Pers. Med.* **2024**, *14*, 94. [CrossRef]
13. Adams, R.S.; Jiang, T.; Rosellini, A.J.; Horváth-Puhó, E.; Street, A.E.; Keyes, K.M.; Cerdá, M.; Lash, T.L.; Sørensen, H.T.; Gradus, J.L. Sex-Specific Risk Profiles for Suicide Among Persons with Substance Use Disorders in Denmark. *Addiction* **2021**, *116*, 2882–2892. [CrossRef]
14. Aishwarya, N.; Yathishan, D.; Alageswaran, R.; Manivannan, D. AutoML Based IoT Application for Heart Attack Risk Prediction. In Proceedings of the Decision Intelligence Solutions, Singapore, 2–3 March 2023; 2023; pp. 19–29.
15. Kundu, A.; Chaiton, M.; Billington, R.; Grace, D.; Fu, R.; Logie, C.; Baskerville, B.; Yager, C.; Mitsakakis, N.; Schwartz, R. Machine Learning Applications in Mental Health and Substance Use Research Among the LGBTQ2S+ Population: Scoping Review. *JMIR Med Inf.* **2021**, *9*, e28962. [CrossRef] [PubMed]
16. Johnstone, S.; Dela Cruz, G.A.; Kalb, N.; Tyagi, S.V.; Potenza, M.N.; George, T.P.; Castle, D.J. A systematic review of gender-responsive and integrated substance use disorder treatment programs for women with co-occurring disorders. *Am. J. Drug Alcohol Abus.* **2023**, *49*, 21–42. [CrossRef] [PubMed]
17. Waring, J.; Lindvall, C.; Umeton, R. Automated machine learning: Review of the state-of-the-art and opportunities for healthcare. *Artif. Intell. Med.* **2020**, *104*, 101822. [CrossRef] [PubMed]
18. Obermeyer, Z.; Powers, B.; Vogeli, C.; Mullainathan, S. Dissecting racial bias in an algorithm used to manage the health of populations. *Science* **2019**, *366*, 447–453. [CrossRef] [PubMed]
19. Mustafa, A.; Rahimi Azghadi, M. Automated Machine Learning for Healthcare and Clinical Notes Analysis. *Computers* **2021**, *10*, 24. [CrossRef]
20. Beam, A.L.; Kohane, I.S. Big Data and Machine Learning in Health Care. *JAMA* **2018**, *319*, 1317–1318. [CrossRef] [PubMed]
21. Rajkomar, A.; Dean, J.; Kohane, I. Machine learning in medicine. *N. Engl. J. Med.* **2019**, *380*, 1347–1358. [CrossRef]
22. Tsamardinos, I.; Charonyktakis, P.; Papoutsoglou, G.; Borboudakis, G.; Lakiotaki, K.; Zenklusen, J.C.; Juhl, H.; Chatzaki, E.; Lagani, V. Just Add Data: Automated predictive modeling for knowledge discovery and feature selection. *NPJ Precis. Oncol.* **2022**, *6*, 38. [CrossRef] [PubMed]
23. Thomaidis, G.V.; Papadimitriou, K.; Michos, S.; Chartampilas, E.; Tsamardinos, I. A characteristic cerebellar biosignature for bipolar disorder, identified with fully automatic machine learning. *IBRO Neurosci. Rep.* **2023**, *15*, 77–89. [CrossRef] [PubMed]
24. Naser, M.Z. Machine learning for all! Benchmarking automated, explainable, and coding-free platforms on civil and environmental engineering problems. *J. Infrastruct. Intell. Resil.* **2023**, *2*, 100028. [CrossRef]
25. Perotte, A.; Pivovarov, R.; Natarajan, K.; Weiskopf, N.; Wood, F.; Elhadad, N. Diagnosis code assignment: Models and evaluation metrics. *J. Am. Med. Inf. Assoc.* **2014**, *21*, 231–237. [CrossRef] [PubMed]
26. Zhuhadar, L.P.; Lytras, M.D. The Application of AutoML Techniques in Diabetes Diagnosis: Current Approaches, Performance, and Future Directions. *Sustainability* **2023**, *15*, 13484. [CrossRef]
27. Barenholtz, E.; Fitzgerald, N.D.; Hahn, W.E. Machine-learning approaches to substance-abuse research: Emerging trends and their implications. *Curr. Opin. Psychiatry* **2020**, *33*, 334–342. [CrossRef]
28. Kabir, M.F.; Ludwig, S.A. Enhancing the Performance of Classification Using Super Learning. *Data-Enabled Discov. Appl.* **2019**, *3*, 5. [CrossRef]
29. Van der Laan, M.J.; Rose, S. *Targeted Learning: Causal Inference for Observational and Experimental Data*; Springer: Berlin/Heidelberg, Germany, 2011; Volume 4.
30. Laan, M.J.V.D.; Polley, E.C.; Hubbard, A.E. Super Learner. *Stat. Appl. Genet. Mol. Biol.* **2007**, *6*. [CrossRef]
31. Comartin, E.B.; Burgess-Proctor, A.; Harrison, J.; Kubiak, S. Gender, Geography, and Justice: Behavioral Health Needs and Mental Health Service Use Among Women in Rural Jails. *Crim. Justice Behav.* **2021**, *48*, 1229–1242. [CrossRef]
32. Zhao, Q.; Kong, Y.; Henderson, D.; Parrish, D. Arrest Histories and Co-Occurring Mental Health and Substance Use Disorders Among Women in the USA. *Int. J. Ment. Health Addict.* **2023**. [CrossRef]
33. SAMHSA. *Treatment Episode Data Set Admissions (TEDS-A) 2020*; SAMHSA: Rockville, MD, USA, 2023.
34. Standeven, L.R.; Scialli, A.; Chisolm, M.S.; Terplan, M. Trends in cannabis treatment admissions in adolescents/young adults: Analysis of TEDS-A 1992 to 2016. *J. Addict. Med.* **2020**, *14*, e29–e36. [CrossRef]
35. Baird, A.; Cheng, Y.; Xia, Y. Use of machine learning to examine disparities in completion of substance use disorder treatment. *PLoS ONE* **2022**, *17*, e0275054. [CrossRef]
36. Yang, J.C.; Roman-Urrestarazu, A.; Brayne, C. Differences in receipt of opioid agonist treatment and time to enter treatment for opioid use disorder among specialty addiction programs in the United States, 2014–2017. *PLoS ONE* **2019**, *14*, e0226349. [CrossRef]
37. Pozo-Luyo, C.A.; Cruz-Duarte, J.M.; Amaya, I.; Ortiz-Bayliss, J.C. Forecasting PM2.5 concentration levels using shallow machine learning models on the Monterrey Metropolitan Area in Mexico. *Atmos. Pollut. Res.* **2023**, *14*, 101898. [CrossRef]
38. Egger, R. *Software and tools. Applied Data Science in Tourism: Interdisciplinary Approaches, Methodologies, and Applications*; Springer: Cham, Switzerland, 2022; pp. 547–588.
39. Tapeh, A.T.G.; Naser, M.Z. Artificial Intelligence, Machine Learning, and Deep Learning in Structural Engineering: A Scientometrics Review of Trends and Best Practices. *Arch. Comput. Methods Eng.* **2023**, *30*, 115–159. [CrossRef]

40. Sahker, E.; Acion, L.; Arndt, S. National analysis of differences among substance abuse treatment outcomes: College student and nonstudent emerging adults. *J. Am. Coll. Health* **2015**, *63*, 118–124. [CrossRef]
41. Glasheen, C.; Pemberton, M.R.; Lipari, R.; Copello, E.A.; Mattson, M.E. Binge drinking and the risk of suicidal thoughts, plans, and attempts. *Addict. Behav.* **2015**, *43*, 42–49. [CrossRef]
42. Alang, S.M. Sociodemographic disparities associated with perceived causes of unmet need for mental health care. *Psychiatr. Rehabil. J.* **2015**, *38*, 293. [CrossRef] [PubMed]
43. Huang, J.-C.; Tsai, Y.-C.; Wu, P.-Y.; Lien, Y.-H.; Chien, C.-Y.; Kuo, C.-F.; Hung, J.-F.; Chen, S.-C.; Kuo, C.-H. Predictive modeling of blood pressure during hemodialysis: A comparison of linear model, random forest, support vector regression, XGBoost, LASSO regression and ensemble method. *Comput. Methods Programs Biomed.* **2020**, *195*, 105536. [CrossRef]
44. Hong, W.; Zhou, X.; Jin, S.; Lu, Y.; Pan, J.; Lin, Q.; Yang, S.; Xu, T.; Basharat, Z.; Zippi, M. A comparison of XGBoost, random forest, and nomograph for the prediction of disease severity in patients with COVID-19 pneumonia: Implications of cytokine and immune cell profile. *Front. Cell. Infect. Microbiol.* **2022**, *12*, 819267. [CrossRef]
45. Meng, D.; Xu, J.; Zhao, J. Analysis and prediction of hand, foot and mouth disease incidence in China using Random Forest and XGBoost. *PLoS ONE* **2021**, *16*, e0261629. [CrossRef] [PubMed]
46. Fawcett, T. An introduction to ROC analysis. *Pattern Recognit. Lett.* **2006**, *27*, 861–874. [CrossRef]
47. Romero, R.A.A.; Deypalan, M.N.Y.; Mehrotra, S.; Jungao, J.T.; Sheils, N.E.; Manduchi, E.; Moore, J.H. Benchmarking AutoML frameworks for disease prediction using medical claims. *BioData Min.* **2022**, *15*, 15. [CrossRef] [PubMed]
48. Apsley, H.B.; Vest, N.; Knapp, K.S.; Santos-Lozada, A.; Gray, J.; Hard, G.; Jones, A.A. Non-engagement in substance use treatment among women with an unmet need for treatment: A latent class analysis on multidimensional barriers. *Drug Alcohol Depend.* **2023**, *242*, 109715. [CrossRef] [PubMed]

Disclaimer/Publisher's Note: The statements, opinions and data contained in all publications are solely those of the individual author(s) and contributor(s) and not of MDPI and/or the editor(s). MDPI and/or the editor(s) disclaim responsibility for any injury to people or property resulting from any ideas, methods, instructions or products referred to in the content.

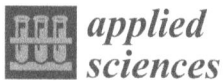

Article

A Novel Criticality Analysis Method for Assessing Obesity Treatment Efficacy

Shadi Eltanani [1,*], Tjeerd V. olde Scheper [1], Mireya Muñoz-Balbontin [1], Arantza Aldea [1], Jo Cossington [2], Sophie Lawrie [2], Salvador Villalpando-Carrion [3], Maria Jose Adame [3], Daniela Felgueres [3], Clare Martin [1] and Helen Dawes [4]

[1] School of Engineering, Computing and Mathematics, Faculty of Technology, Design and Environment, Oxford Brookes University, Wheatley Campus, Wheatley, Oxford OX33 1HX, UK; tvolde-scheper@brookes.ac.uk (T.V.o.S.); aaldea@brookes.ac.uk (A.A.); cemartin@brookes.ac.uk (C.M.)

[2] Centre for Movement and Occupational Rehabilitation Sciences (MOReS), Oxford Brookes University, Oxford OX3 0BP, UK; jcossington@brookes.ac.uk (J.C.); sophielawrie@hotmail.co.uk (S.L.)

[3] Hospital Infantil de Mexico Federico Gomez, Mexico City 06720, Mexico; villalpandoca@himfg.edu.mx (S.V.-C.); mariajose@adame.com.mx (M.J.A.); danielafelgueresn@gmail.com (D.F.)

[4] National Institute for Health and Care Research (NIHR) Exeter Biomedical Research Centre, University of Exeter, St Luke's Campus, Exeter EX1 2LU, UK; h.dawes@exeter.ac.uk

* Correspondence: seltanani@brookes.ac.uk

Citation: Eltanani, S.; olde Scheper, T.V.; Muñoz-Balbontin, M.; Aldea, A.; Cossington, J.; Lawrie, S.; Villalpando-Carrion, S.; Adame, M.J.; Felgueres, D; Martin, C.; et al. A Novel Criticality Analysis Method for Assessing Obesity Treatment Efficacy. *Appl. Sci.* **2023**, *13*, 13225. https://doi.org/10.3390/app132413225

Academic Editors: Arkady Voloshin, Chien-Hung Yeh, Wenbin Shi, Xiaojuan Ban, Men-Tzung Lo and Shenghong He

Received: 18 August 2023
Revised: 2 November 2023
Accepted: 7 December 2023
Published: 13 December 2023

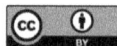

Copyright: © 2023 by the authors. Licensee MDPI, Basel, Switzerland. This article is an open access article distributed under the terms and conditions of the Creative Commons Attribution (CC BY) license (https:// creativecommons.org/licenses/by/ 4.0/).

Abstract: Human gait is a significant indicator of overall health and well-being due to its dependence on metabolic requirements. Abnormalities in gait can indicate the presence of metabolic dysfunction, such as diabetes or obesity. However, detecting these can be challenging using classical methods, which often involve subjective clinical assessments or invasive procedures. In this work, a novel methodology known as Criticality Analysis (CA) was applied to the monitoring of the gait of teenagers with varying amounts of metabolic stress who are taking part in an clinical intervention to increase their activity and reduce overall weight. The CA approach analysed gait using inertial measurement units (IMU) by mapping the dynamic gait pattern into a nonlinear representation space. The resulting dynamic paths were then classified using a Support Vector Machine (SVM) algorithm, which is well-suited for this task due to its ability to handle nonlinear and dynamic data. The combination of the CA approach and the SVM algorithm demonstrated high accuracy and non-invasive detection of metabolic stress. It resulted in an average accuracy within the range of 78.2% to 90%. Additionally, at the group level, it was observed to improve fitness and health during the period of the intervention. Therefore, this methodology showed a great potential to be a valuable tool for healthcare professionals in detecting and monitoring metabolic stress, as well as other associated disorders.

Keywords: human gait; criticality analysis; support vector machine

1. Introduction

Human gait, the intricate orchestration of biomechanical movements during ambulation, stands as a pivotal aspect of human motor function with far-reaching implications for an individual's health and overall wellbeing [1–3]. This intricate phenomenon, however, is not a static entity. It is subject to perturbations stemming from a diverse array of factors, encompassing injuries, diseases, disorders, and external conditions, thereby engendering deviations from established norms and the emergence of irregular or aberrant gait patterns [4–6].

The traditional methodologies employed in gait analysis, predominantly reliant upon observational techniques, possess inherent limitations marked by subjectivity and interobserver variability [7]. These methodologies, furthermore, confront difficulties in adequately encapsulating the nuanced, multifaceted, and quantitative attributes inherent in gait, particularly when confronted with intricate patterns stemming from underlying pathologies [8].

In the contemporary landscape of medical diagnostics, artificial intelligence (AI) has emerged as a promising frontier, bearing the capacity to substantially enhance gait analysis and expedite the detection of gait-related disorders [9,10]. Its proficiency in the processing of extensive datasets, identification of latent patterns, and facilitation of early diagnoses offers substantial promise [11]. Nonetheless, AI grapples with intricate challenges in the realm of gait analysis, stemming from the dynamic nature of gait itself and the intricate interplay of a multitude of contributory factors [11].

In response to these exigencies, this paper introduces Criticality Analysis (CA) as an innovative and robust AI tool primed for precise identification of abnormal or irregular gait patterns, thereby indicating the presence of latent disorders or ailments. Beyond its diagnostic prowess, CA serves as a dynamic tool for the continuous monitoring of disorder progression and the systematic tracking of treatment efficacy over temporal trajectories. This innovative paradigm promises to empower medical practitioners in their clinical decision making in relation to gait-related disorders, ultimately effecting substantial enhancements in patient outcomes and the broader landscape of healthcare.

The paper is structured as follows: Section 2 outlines a methodology employing mathematical models to assess critical aspects of human gait, emphasising the integration of mathematical modeling and criticality analysis in the context of gait study. In Section 3, the methodology applied to the Criticality Analysis of Diabetic Gait in Children (CARDIGAN) dataset is detailed, covering data collection, feature extraction, criticality analysis data representation, and spatiotemporal analysis. Section 4 explores the experimental results of the CARDIGAN dataset, including the analysis of Receiver Operating Characteristic (ROC) Curves, the calculation of Area Under the Curve (AUC), and the determination of the decision boundary of the support vector method. Section 5 provides a concise summary of the overarching results, while Section 6 concludes by highlighting the key findings of the research.

2. Mathematical Model-Driven Criticality Analysis for Human Gait Assessment

The complexities of human locomotion have long intrigued researchers who strive to decode the dynamic, self-organised patterns underlying gait. With each step, the intricately choreographed motions blur the boundary between conscious control and automated processes. Gait is governed by nonlinear phenomena, including emergent oscillations, traveling waves, and spiraling coordination, which evolve across spatiotemporal scales. To decipher the chaotic fluctuations disrupting normal walking, mathematical models become indispensable, capturing nuanced biomechanics within the motor control system [12]. Particularly intriguing is the analysis of disruptions propelling gait into criticality, marked by surges in kinetic energy and resulting in near power-law and exponential dynamics. The human locomotive system, while captivating, lacks comprehensive models characterising its dynamics across both temporal and spatial dimensions. Simplified models often cannot fully capture the complex control mechanisms translating network behavior into stable, coordinated movement patterns across space. Therefore, developing sophisticated models is crucial for decoding the inherent complexities of human gait and locomotion.

In this paper, we employ a nonlinear biochemical enzyme control model to conduct a comprehensive analysis of human gait dynamics, shedding new light on the intricate biomechanical processes underlying locomotion [13]. In this paper, the investigation is centered on elucidating the specific role of biochemical reactions in shaping gait patterns. This meticulous exploration of biochemical intricacies allows for discerning their profound influence on the overall coordination and characteristics of human gait. This modeling approach gains particular relevance when examining scenarios where particular biochemical pathways are suspected to be pivotal factors contributing to gait abnormalities or adaptations, as often observed in various pathological conditions.

The model utilises a control mechanism to stabilise external perturbations to the motor system by precisely calibrating the quantity of enzyme in relation to the concentration of one of the variables, f. The model also represents the control process of two enzymes that govern the formation of the extracellular matrix, m, from soluble filaments, f. The proteinase, p, deconstructs the matrix into filaments, while transglutaminase, g, reassembles the filaments into the matrix. The extracellular matrix, m, is continually generated by adjacent cells, r_{im}, at a constant rate, with each protein undergoing catalytic processes proportional to p. The bifurcation parameter, r_{im}, acts as an external turbulent input to the control model. The dynamics governing the rate of enzyme production, specifically enzymes p and g, are influenced by the Rate Control of Chaos (RCC). This approach employs a series of nonlinear rate equations, as illustrated in Equations (4)–(7), to describe the temporal evolution of system variables. A key control term in these rate equations contains variable f, which has a strong nonlinear influence on the dynamics. The RCC confines this control term using a rate control function, as depicted in Equation (1), that restricts its divergence rate, thereby stabilising the overall system behavior. The adjustable parameters in the rate control function allow tuning the intensity of control applied to the chaotic dynamics. Meanwhile, the criticality analysis involves examining the phase space representation of outputs f and m, which correspond to concentrations of soluble filaments and extracellular matrix, respectively. The phase space plot with f on the x-axis and m on the y-axis illustrates the time-dependent evolution of nonlinear dynamics. As parameters are varied, the system exhibits complex phenomena, including bistability, limit cycles, spiralling trajectories, and chaos, particularly near critical transition points. Analysing the geometric patterns within the phase portrait provides valuable insights into the mechanisms underpinning self-organised criticality. Characteristics such as the number and stability of fixed points, oscillations, excitability, and susceptibility to perturbations can be deduced from phase space topology. Additionally, the fractal-like features within the phase portrait unveil the self-similar, scale-invariant nature of critical fluctuations. Moreover, this representation facilitates the quantification of nonlinear correlations that capture the intricacies of coupled dynamics. Therefore, phase space-based criticality analysis unveils the system's rich nonlinear behavior, phase transitions, and emergent complexity resulting from self-organised criticality.

$$q_f = \frac{f}{f + \mu_f}, \tag{1}$$

$$\sigma_p(q_f) = f_p e^{(x_p q_f)}, \tag{2}$$

$$\sigma_g(q_f) = f_g e^{(x_g q_f)}, \tag{3}$$

$$\frac{dm}{dt} = k_g \frac{fg}{K_G + f} - \frac{mp}{1 + m} + r_{im}, \tag{4}$$

$$\frac{df}{dt} = -k_g \frac{fg}{K_G + f} + \frac{mp}{1 + m} - \frac{fp}{1 + f}, \tag{5}$$

$$\frac{dp}{dt} = \sigma_p(q_f) \gamma \frac{f^n}{K_R^n + f^n} - k_a p^2, \tag{6}$$

$$\frac{dg}{dt} = \sigma_g(q_f) \beta \frac{f^l}{K_S^l + f^l} - k_{deg} \frac{gp}{K_{deg} + g}. \tag{7}$$

Mathematically speaking, the CA model has several parameters, including $\gamma = 0.026$, $\beta = 0.00075$, $K_R = 4.5$, $K_S = 1$, $K_G = 0.1$, $K_{deg} = 1.1$, $k_g = k_{deg} = 0.05$, and $k_a = \frac{k_{deg}}{K_{deg}} = 0.0455$. Hill numbers n and l are also set to four. Bifurcation parameter r_{im} exhibits a wide range of dynamic behaviors, including stable periodic cycles, bistability, and chaos. This parameter remains constant for all oscillators within the chaotic domain. Additionally, an external input is applied as a perturbation to the r_{im} parameter as described in Equation (8). This parameter links different oscillators together by using a relative scale contribution from all other oscillators. RCC control parameters presented in Equations (1)–(3) ($f_p = f_g = 1$, $x_p = x_g = -1$, and $\mu_f = 2$) are kept constant throughout the experiment simulations in this paper, but can have different values that allow the local oscillator possibility to change its oscillatory orbits.

$$r_{im}^i = \sum_{j=1, j \neq i}^{n} w_j m_j + \varepsilon. \tag{8}$$

The connectivity strength between various oscillators, represented by w_j, can range from 0.00011, 0.00012, to 0.00025. External perturbations, represented by ε, are uniformly distributed according to a Gaussian distribution and scaled within the domain of $[-1, 1]$. These perturbations are observed over a range of evolution steps to explore the varying oscillatory cycles they produce. In this paper, a connectivity strength of $w_j = 0.0002$ was selected from the chaotic domain of the underlying oscillators to assess its effect on the dynamics while maintaining overall stability.

The network of nonlinear models in this paper consists of 16 oscillators, each of which can adjust their local dynamics to adapt to external perturbations from their neighboring oscillators. The simulation of the entire model was carried out using EuNeurone software (v2.3, 2013) and the Fehlberg-RK method as a fixed step integration for Ordinary Differential equations (ODEs). The total unweighted dynamics, represented by M and F in Equations (9) and (10), were measured as the net sum of the individual oscillators, allowing for observation by a remote observer who would otherwise be unable to detect the individual oscillators.

$$M = \sum_{i=1}^{n} m_i, \tag{9}$$

$$F = \sum_{i=1}^{n} f_i. \tag{10}$$

The CA method described in this paper has previously been applied in research, leveraging its capabilities to generate dynamic and scale-free nonlinear data representations, which in turn facilitate the precise detection of disturbances associated with human gait [14]. Subsequently, CA combined these encoded representations with the SVM algorithm, enhancing superior detection accuracy. This synergy surpasses traditional methods that lack the CA approach in terms of performance and robustness. Hence, this innovative CA approach allows for the generation of nonlinear data representations that are well suited for training conventional classifiers [15].

3. Methodology

The proposed CA method for classifying human gait disorders includes a framework consisting of several key components, including data collection, data processing, feature extraction, and the use of the SVM technique. This methodology is illustrated in Figure 1.

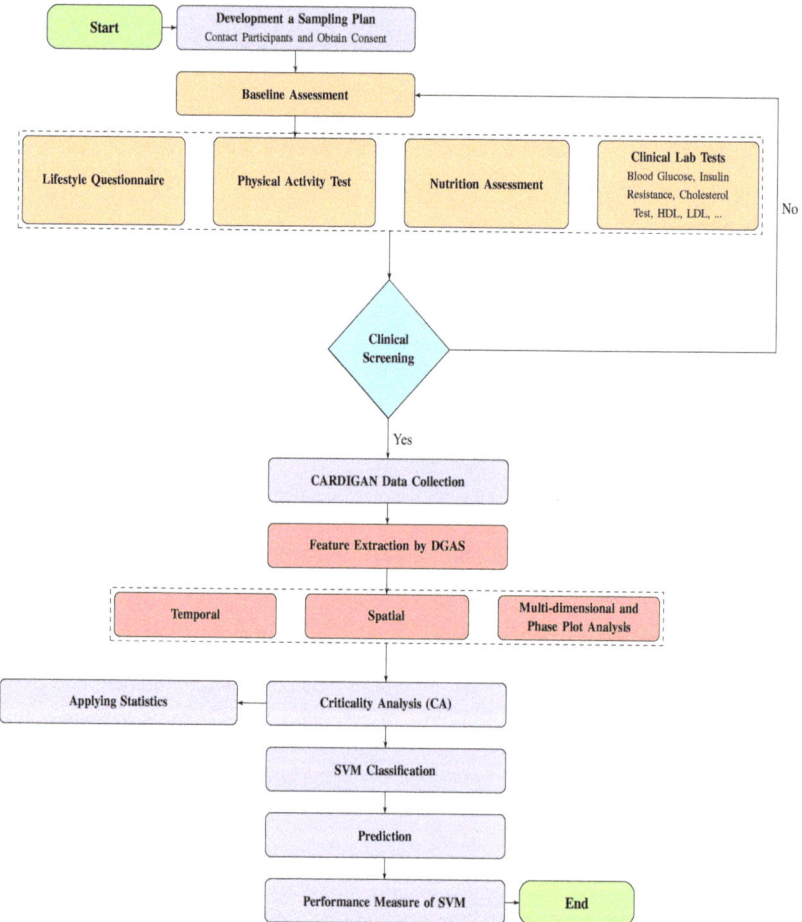

Figure 1. The flowchart of the proposed CARDIGAN methodology is presented.

3.1. Data Collection

The study assembled a heterogeneous cohort of 50 adolescent subjects, comprising individuals diagnosed with obesity, those with diabetes, and a cohort of healthy controls, all of whom were thoroughly recruited from Mexico Children's Hospital. Among the healthy control group, 19 were males, and there was one female participant, with ages ranging from 10 to 15 years, weights spanning from 40 to 83 kg, heights from 133 to 172.9 cm, and BMIs from 21.16 to 34. The participants with obesity included 16 males and 4 females, aged between 10 and 17 years, with weights ranging from 36 to 106.4 kg, heights spanning from 129 to 179 cm, and BMIs from 17.64 to 35.5. Meanwhile, diabetic participants consisted of 10 females aged 12 to 13 years, with weights ranging from 74.5 to 76.2 kg, heights from 159 to 159.7 cm, and BMIs from 29.5 to 30.4. It is crucial to underscore that due to an inadequate volume of available diabetic data points, the analysis was restricted to data from 20 healthy controls and 20 participants diagnosed with obesity, ensuring the robustness of the findings while acknowledging data limitations. The participants underwent a 6-week intervention program aimed at improving fitness and reducing weight. Gait analysis was conducted at baseline, immediately after the intervention, and at 3- and 6-month follow-ups. Gait analysis involved participants walking back and forth over a 30 m track for 6 min while wearing an inertial measurement unit sensor on their lower back. The gait data were anonymised, and approval was obtained before analysis.

Assessment was based on the use of an inertial measurement movement sensor (IMU), placed on the fourth lumbar vertebra located on the top left of the anatomical position of the lumber spine, known as the body Centre of Mass (CoM). The sensor was designed to be incredibly flexible, providing for mobility in many different planes including flexion, extension, side bending, and rotation. Gait analysis was conducted for participants using a standardised 6 m test, wherein an IMU was attached to the lower back to capture triaxial accelerometer and gyroscope data at a frequency of 100 Hz. For individuals with DPN (Diabetic Peripheral Neuropathy), the assessment took place at OCDEM (Oxford Centre for Diabetes, Endocrinology, and Metabolism) in a dedicated obstacle-free corridor. The methodology employed for deriving gait parameters has been comprehensively described in previous studies. The spatiotemporal parameters obtained from the 6 min walking test encompassed step time (measured in milliseconds), cadence (expressed in steps per minute), stride length (in meters), and walking speed (in meters per second). Furthermore, gait control parameters, which encompass measures of dynamic stability and gait variability, were evaluated utilising various instruments such as accelerometers, force plates, or motion capture technology. These assessments aimed to quantify fluctuations in temporal aspects (e.g., stride time), spatial aspects (e.g., step length), and comprehensive whole-body kinematics (e.g., segment angles). The parameters assessed included Beta (expressed in degrees), SDa (measured in arbitrary units), SDb (also in arbitrary units), ratio (in a dimensionless unit), and walk ratio (in millimeters per steps per minute). These parameters have been identified as indicators of neuro motor control [16,17]. The dynamics of their walking activity were monitored using the Polar Team tracking system [18].

3.2. Feature Extraction Method for Analysing Gait Data

The CARDIGAN dataset, which was collected utilising a 3-dimensional accelerometer, gyroscope, and magnetometer IMU sensor, was analysed utilising DataGait Analysis Software (DGAS) (v11.1, 2019). Developed as a standalone software analysis package by the Movement Science Group at Oxford Brookes University using LabVIEW2011 (National Instruments, Ireland), DGAS employs quaternion rotation matrices and double integration to transpose the accelerations frame of the z-axis from the object to the global system, thereby allowing for the measurement of translatory vertical CoM accelerations during walking and the achievement of a relative change in position. As referenced in [18], upward CoM measurements determine the global quality of human gait parameters. DGAS extracts critical features of individuals' gait for the purpose of classification. In this context, it becomes feasible to differentiate between biologically distinct masculine and feminine gait patterns, taking into account not only the spatiotemporal parameters that capture gait dynamics at specific time points but also the potential impact of their respective body shapes or dimensions on these distinctions. In gait analysis, a multitude of parameters are employed to comprehensively understand the complexities of human locomotion. Temporal parameters encompass fundamental measurements such as Step Time, which quantifies the duration from the initial contact of one foot to the subsequent contact of the opposite foot, and Stride Time, which denotes the time interval between successive initial contacts of the same foot. Cadence adds another layer of insight, representing the number of steps taken per unit of time. Meanwhile, spatial parameters offer dimensions to gait assessment; Step Length measures the distance between successive initial contacts of the same foot, and Stride Length extends this to cover the span from one foot's initial contact to the following foot's contact. The rate of position change during gait, known as Velocity, is calculated by the ratio of stride length to stride time. In addition, multi-dimensional parameters introduce complexity: Duty Factor gauges the percentage of the gait cycle during which each foot remains on the ground, while the Froude Number serves as a dimensionless speed parameter reflecting the interplay of centripetal and gravitational forces during walking. Finally, the Walk Ratio denotes the relationship between cadence and mean step length, offering insights into the neuromotor control of gait. Within the realm of Phase Plot Analysis, distinctive parameters emerge: Beta Angle, a measure of stability, is the angle of the primary gait phase plot axis relative to the vertical axis; SDa and SDb represent standard deviations describing the distribution of phase plot points, with SDa reflecting stability and SDb pertaining to rhythm; and Ratio (SDa/SDb) serves as a relative rhythm stability indicator. The raw data from the accelerometer are processed using DGAS software, which is founded on the inverted pendulum approach. This conversion results in 17 parameters that are used to assess the physical characteristics of each individual. These 17 gait features serve as inputs for perturbing the criticality analysis model, as represented by Equations (4) and (7), respectively. Table 1 displays the list of the 17 gait parameters.

Table 1. Extracted Gait Features.

Gait Parameter	Measurement	Unit
Temporal	Step Time	(ms)
	Step Time (Left)	(ms)
	Step Time (Right)	(ms)
	Stride Time	(ms)
	Cadence	(steps/min)
Spatial	Step Length (Left)	(m)
	Step Length (Right)	(m)
	Stride Length	(m)
	Velocity	(m/s)
Multi-dimensional	Duty Factor Double Stance	(%)
	Duty Factor Single Stance	(%)
	Froude Number	(au)
	Walk Ratio	(mm/steps/min)
Phase Plot Analysis	Beta Angle	(Degree (°))
	SDa	(au)
	SDb	(au)
	Ratio = SDa/SDb	(Dimensionless)

3.3. Gait Data Representation and Spatiotemporal Analysis Using Criticality Analysis

Criticality Analysis is a method used to represent complex multivariate data patterns in a simplified form, typically in the form of a phase plot portrait or manifold. This method involves analysing the data in multiple dimensions and identifying patterns or structures that are most critical to understanding the underlying dynamics of the system. The extracted features by DGAS were used as perturbation inputs to the CA model represented by Equations (4) and (7), respectively. This aided in gaining a deeper understanding of the underlying mechanisms and dynamics of the system under study. The visual representations of gait regulation and coordination between spatial and temporal domains are depicted in Figures 2–7 through phase plot orbits. Well-regulated gait was characterised by smooth and narrow orbits, whereas dysfunctional gait control was evident in irregular and variable orbits. These phase plots served as a means to distinguish between healthy and pathological gaits by evaluating the dynamics of spatiotemporal coordination. These phase plots demonstrated clear differences between the gait patterns of the healthy control and obesity groups over the 6-week period. Specifically, in the healthy control group, the phase plots exhibited a consistent pattern characterised by smooth and regular oscillations with steady amplitudes and frequencies. These findings were indicative of a well-maintained, rhythmic gait pattern that demonstrated excellent coordination and balance. Notably, the orbits in this group remained relatively narrow, which underscored the efficiency of their biomechanics and the minimal occurrence of side-to-side body motion. In contrast, the obesity group displayed phase plots that deviated from the healthy control group's pattern. These plots appeared more irregular and distorted, with variable amplitudes and wider orbits, suggesting a compromised sense of balance and increased lateral swaying during gait. Furthermore, these phase plots exhibited more abrupt changes in direction, indicating the need for sudden adjustments to maintain stability. These observations were reflective of a slower and more effortful gait, likely resulting from the additional weight burdening the joints and muscles in individuals with obesity. Moreover, both groups exhibited a common trend of declining gait consistency over the 6-week observation period, potentially attributable to the onset of fatigue effects. The healthy control group, despite its initial robust gait pattern, displayed a gradual decrease in consistency, reflecting the possibility of accumulating fatigue from repeated gait assessments. The obesity group, already experiencing challenges in maintaining gait regularity, showed a similar decline in consistency, accentuating the toll that prolonged observation sessions might take on their gait patterns. This convergence in declining gait consistency underscores the importance of considering potential fatigue factors in the interpretation of gait analysis results across different population groups.

Examining the gait patterns across the 6-week period, in Figure 2 (Week 1), the healthy group displayed a tight circular cluster, indicating consistent gait cycles. In contrast, the obesity group showed more elongated, scattered orbits, reflecting a higher degree of variability in gait. As we progressed to data depicted in Figure 3 (Week 2), the healthy group continued to maintain a tight cluster, while the obesity group's orbits, though still dispersed, appeared somewhat more rounded, suggesting some improvement in gait coordination compared to that of Week 1. Figure 4 (Week 3) portrayed the healthy group with a very tight cluster, indicative of highly consistent gait, while the obesity group exhibited more elongated orbits with flatter tops, indicating instability in their gait pattern. In Figure 5 (Week 4), the healthy control cluster became somewhat looser, possibly due to accumulating fatigue. The obesity group's orbits remained uneven but showed a slightly improved level of coordination compared to Week 3. Figure 6 (Week 5) demonstrates the healthy control group's cluster becoming more dispersed, reflecting increasing gait variability. On the other hand, the obesity group's plots were highly scattered with jagged trajectories, suggesting a worsening of gait control. Finally, in Figure 7 (Week 6), both groups display more dispersed orbits than in previous weeks, indicating the potential impact of fatigue on gait consistency in both groups. The obesity group's orbits appeared slightly more rounded than in Week 5, hinting at some recovery in coordination, although the overall trend indicated challenges in maintaining consistent gait patterns.

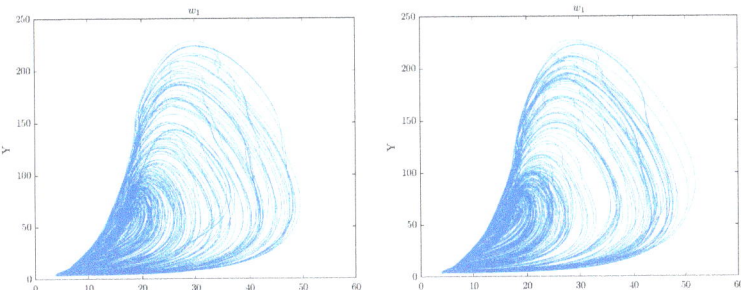

Figure 2. Comparison of phase space plots of walk patterns for healthy control and obesity groups in the clinical gait experiment conducted in w_1 is presented. Healthy control walk patterns are shown on the left while obesity walk patterns are shown on the right.

In this paper, we utilised a kernel SVM classifier to distinguish between the obesity and healthy groups based on phase plot data. The choice of kernel SVM is particularly well suited for this analysis due to the inherently nonlinear and complex nature of the data. Phase plot data, representing dynamic patterns of physiological processes, often exhibit intricate and nonlinear relationships. Traditional linear classifiers may struggle to capture the patterns present in such data. However, the kernel SVM is designed to address this challenge by mapping the data into a higher-dimensional space, where complex patterns become more separable. It leverages a diverse set of kernel functions, including radial basis function (RBF), to effectively transform the data into a format where it can distinguish between the obese and healthy groups. This approach enables the identification of hidden patterns, making it an ideal choice for this study, and ensures that the classification approach is capable of handling the inherent nonlinearity in the phase plot data, facilitating the reliable and accurate differentiation of the two groups. Figures 16–18 demonstrate the decision boundary generated by kernel SVM, highlighting its effectiveness in distinguishing between obese and healthy control groups using phase plot data.

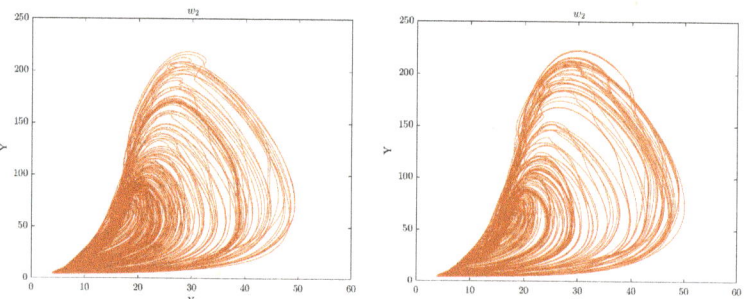

Figure 3. Comparison of phase space plots of walk patterns for healthy control and obesity groups in the clinical gait experiment conducted in w_2 is presented. Healthy control walk patterns are shown on the left while obesity walk patterns are shown on the right.

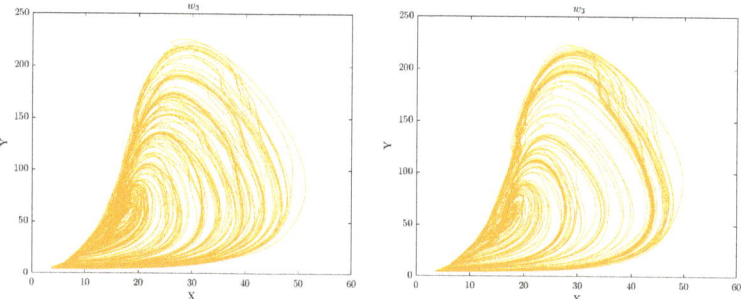

Figure 4. Comparison of phase space plots of walk patterns for healthy control and obesity groups in the clinical gait experiment conducted in w_3 is presented. Healthy control walk patterns are shown on the left while obesity walk patterns are shown on the right.

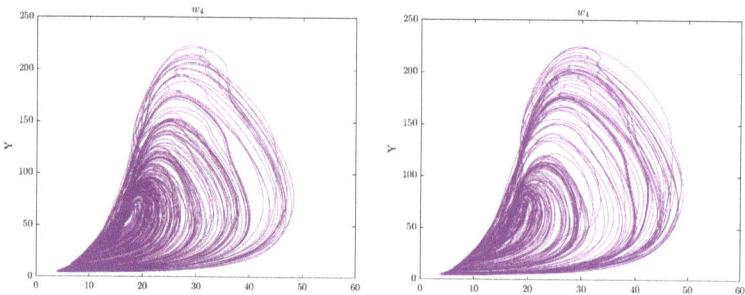

Figure 5. Comparison of phase space plots of walk patterns for healthy control and obesity groups in the clinical gait experiment conducted in w_4 is presented. Healthy control walk patterns are shown on the left while obesity walk patterns are shown on the right.

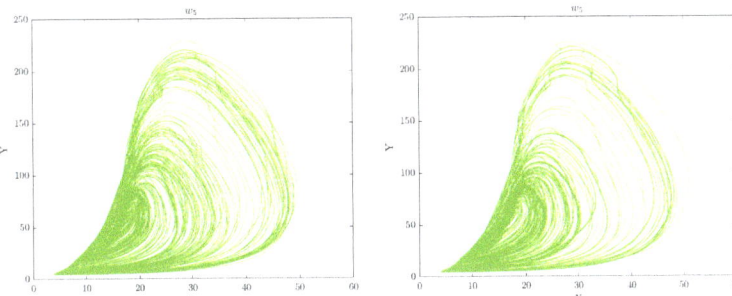

Figure 6. Comparison of phase space plots of walk patterns for healthy control and obesity groups in the clinical gait experiment conducted in w_5 is presented. Healthy control walk patterns are shown on the left while obesity walk patterns are shown on the right.

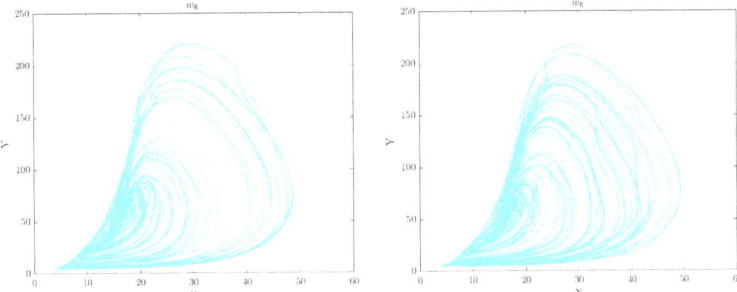

Figure 7. Comparison of phase space plots of walk patterns for healthy control and obesity groups in the clinical gait experiment conducted in w_6 is presented. Healthy control walk patterns are shown on the left while obesity walk patterns are shown on the right.

Figures 8 and 9 serve as invaluable tools for assessing the dynamic nature of gait progression throughout the 6-week study period. These graphical representations offered a comprehensive view of the data by plotting the peak values extracted from each phase plot orbit as discrete data points for every week. Consequently, these visualisations effectively generated trajectories that unveiled nuanced alterations in gait patterns over time. Fundamentally, each data point within these trajectories captured the maximum step length achieved during a specific gait cycle, encapsulating the essence of gait performance. By plotting these peak values across the 6-week observation window, an intuitive visual perspective emerged on how maximal step length evolved across multiple visits. Furthermore, these peak values functioned as numerical metrics that concisely represented the range of variability, which is an informative measure quantifying the degree of variation in maximal step length from one week to the next. To provide a rigorous statistical summary of this variation over time, standard deviation (SD) of the peak values for each participant was calculated. This SD became a pivotal indicator, with a higher value signifying a greater degree of inconsistency in the maximal step length achieved across different weeks. Consequently, comparing SD values before and after the intervention yielded a quantitative assessment of whether gait improved (resulting in a lower SD) or deteriorated (resulting in a higher SD). This analytical approach enabled the precise quantification of the impact of the intervention on gait stability and consistency, offering valuable insights into the effectiveness of the intervention. In Figure 8, which pertains to healthy controls, the majority of trajectories exhibited minimal fluctuation, remaining relatively level throughout the study duration. This observation signified consistent gait patterns from week to week, characterised by limited variation in peak values. Conversely, in Figure 9, representing the obesity group, the trajectories displayed greater irregularity, featuring discernible peaks and troughs across the weeks. This pattern indicated increased instability in gait parameters, with significant variations in the peak values across the different visits. As an illustrative example, participant P14 was considered. In Figure 8, P14's trajectory remained consistently around 0.55, demonstrating a steady gait with little variation over time. However, in Figure 9, P14's trajectory exhibited a drop from approximately 0.7 to 0.4 by Week 3 before subsequently rebounding. This trajectory pattern suggested that P14's gait became more irregular during the course of the study but later exhibited improvement. Complementing these trajectories, the standard deviation bars visually represented the extent of variability across the 6 weeks. In Figure 8, P14's standard deviation bars were notably small, confirming minimal fluctuation and consistent gait during the pre-intervention period. In contrast, Figure 9 portrayed larger standard deviation bars, indicating increased inconsistency in gait patterns when P14 was in an obese state. Overall, these quantitative comparisons between Figures 8 and 9 provided valuable insights into the differences in gait stability and variability between individuals with obesity and healthy controls. These trajectories, coupled with the standard deviation bars, facilitated the rigorous tracking and assessment of gait changes for each participant throughout the 6-week study period.

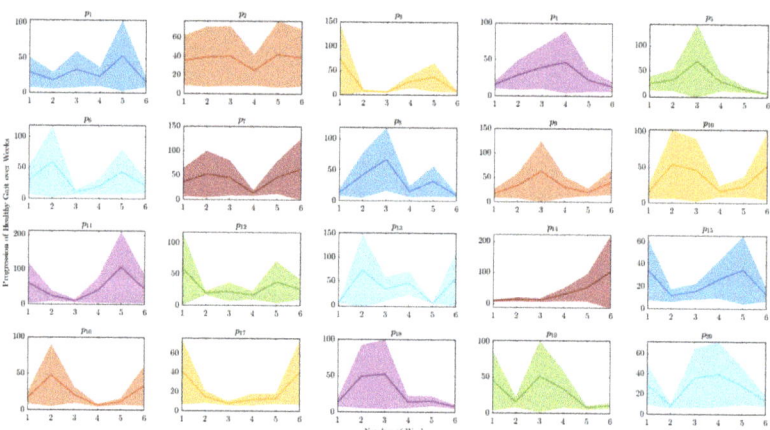

Figure 8. The advancement of normal walking patterns for each person over a 6-week period is shown.

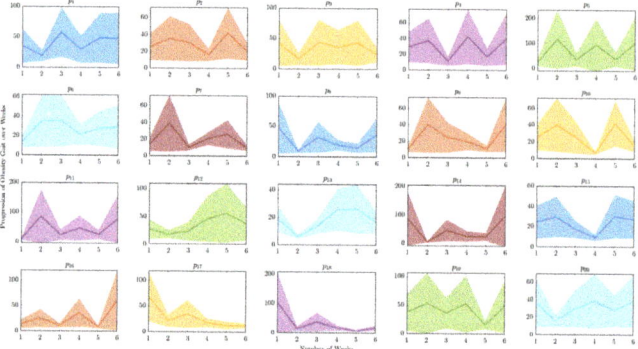

Figure 9. Tracking the improvement in gait for managing obesity for each person over a 6-week period is shown.

4. Experiment Results

In this section, we present the findings of our experimental investigation, which encompasses the performance of the SVM classifier in identifying gait patterns for both healthy control and obese groups. Additionally, we examine the impact of various Kernel SVM model parameters on classification performance. A comprehensive analysis of the generalisation performance of the SVM classifier is also presented, including the Receiver Operating Characteristic (ROC) curve, the area under the ROC curve, and the SVM decision classification boundary. The results demonstrate the potential of using SVM in combination with a controlled CA model for accurate detection of gait patterns associated with healthy controls and individuals with obesity.

4.1. Receiver Operating Characteristic (ROC) Curve

The Receiver Operating Characteristic (ROC) curve is a graphical representation of the performance of a binary classifier system as the discrimination threshold is varied [19]. In the context of SVM, the ROC curve is used to evaluate the performance of the SVM classifier in classifying data samples into two different classes. The ROC curve plots the true positive rate (TPR) (sensitivity) against the false positive rate (FPR) ($\approx 1 - $ TNR) at various threshold settings. Figures 10–12 illustrate the ROC curves for the best pair of σ and C values that satisfy the highest accuracy during the entire trial period.

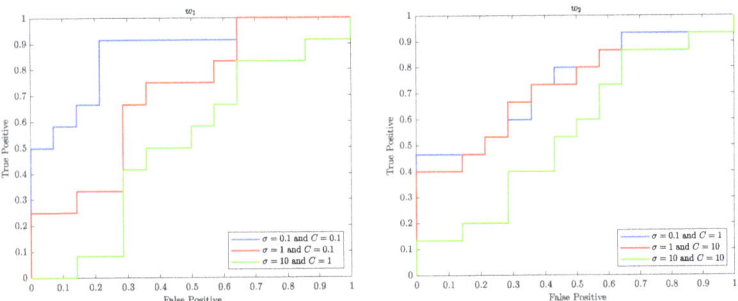

Figure 10. The relationship between True Positive Rate (Sensitivity) and False Positive Rate (1-Specificity) at various threshold levels, as determined by the kernel function of the SVM, is displayed through the ROC curves of w_1 and w_2.

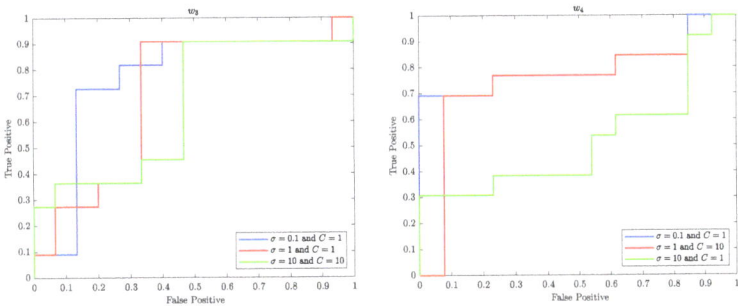

Figure 11. The relationship between True Positive Rate (Sensitivity) and False Positive Rate (1-Specificity) at various threshold levels, as determined by the kernel function of the SVM, is displayed through the ROC curves of w_3 and w_4.

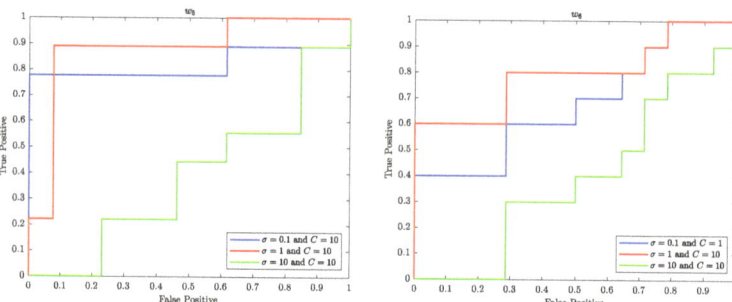

Figure 12. The relationship between True Positive Rate (Sensitivity) and False Positive Rate (1-Specificity) at various threshold levels, as determined by the kernel function of the SVM, is displayed through the ROC curves of w_5 and w_6.

The ROC plots (Figures 10–12) show that, in the context of SVM, parameter C controls the trade-off between maximising the margin and minimising the misclassification error. When the value of C is smaller, such as $C = 0.1$, the margin becomes wider, but there are more instances of misclassifications. Conversely, a larger value of C, such as $C = 10$, leads to a narrower margin, but with a reduced number of misclassifications. Parameter σ is used to control the width of the Kernel Gaussian function that is used to map the input data into a higher-dimensional space, where a linear boundary can be found. A larger value of σ results in a wider Gaussian function, which leads to a softer decision boundary and a higher bias, while a smaller value of σ results in a narrower Gaussian function, which leads to a harder decision boundary and a higher variance.

When σ is small, the decision boundary is more sensitive to input data, which can lead to overfitting. On the other hand, when σ is large, the decision boundary is less sensitive to input data, which can lead to underfitting. Therefore, the value of σ has an impact on generalisation performance of the SVM.

A good value for C and σ is the one that balances the trade-off of bias and variance, that is, a good balance between overfitting and underfitting.

The ROC curves shown in Figures 10–12 perform well with $\sigma = 0.1$ and 1 for various values of C of the SVM, which is likely because the classifier is able to find a good balance between overfitting and underfitting by adjusting the value of C and σ which in turn results in good performance.

4.2. The Area under the Curve (AUC)

The area under the ROC curve is a measure of the performance of a binary classifier [20]. In the context of SVM, the AUC represents the ability of the classifier to distinguish between positive and negative classes. A higher AUC value indicates that the classifier is able to correctly classify more instances of the positive class as positive, while also correctly classifying more instances of the negative class as negative. An AUC of 1.0 represents a perfect classifier, while an AUC of 0.5 represents a classifier that performs no better than random guessing.

Figures 13–15 show how the performance of the SVM model changes as the regularisation parameter strength C is varied. Regularisation parameter C controls the trade-off between maximising the margin (the distance between the decision boundary and the closest training instances) and minimising the classification error. When C is small, the model focuses more on maximising the margin, which can lead to a simpler decision boundary but also a higher classification error. As C is increased, the model focuses more on minimising the classification error, which can lead to a more complex decision boundary but also lower classification error. From Figures 13–15, if the AUC increases as C increases, it means that the model's performance is improving as regularisation strength C increases. This may suggest that the model is underfitting the data when C is small and that increasing the regularisation strength helps to improve the model's performance. On the other hand, if the AUC decreases as C increases, it means that the model's performance worsens as the regularisation strength increases. This may suggest that the model is overfitting the data when C is small and that increasing regularisation strength C causes the model to become too simplistic and lose important information from the data.

The optimal value of C is where the AUC is the highest; this is the sweet spot where the model is able to balance the trade-off between maximising the margin and minimising the classification error in a way that leads to the best classification performance.

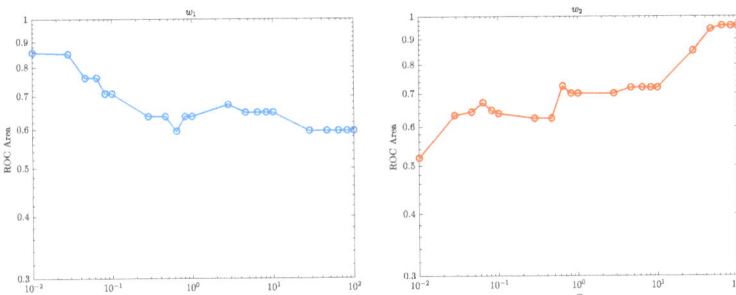

Figure 13. The relationship between the AROC and regularisation parameter C for w_1 and w_2 is presented.

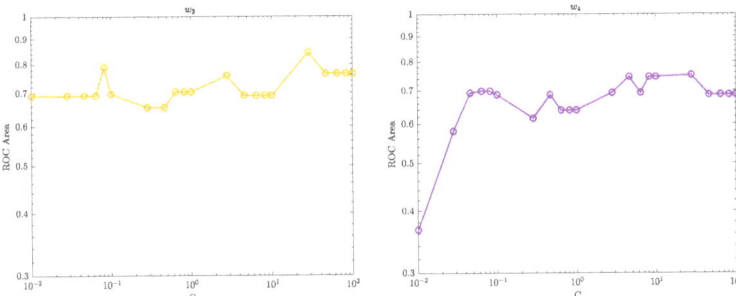

Figure 14. The relationship between the AROC and regularisation parameter C for w_3 and w_4 is presented.

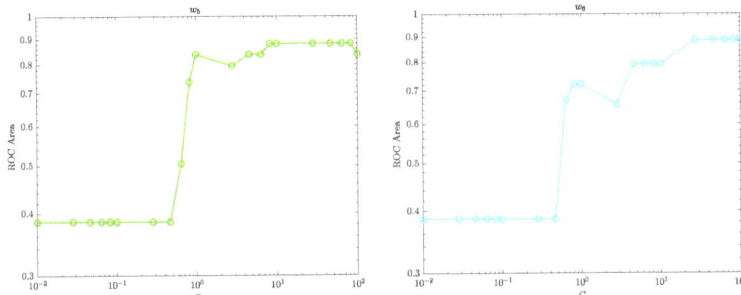

Figure 15. The relationship between the AROC and regularisation parameter C for w_5 and w_6 is presented.

4.3. The Classification Decision Boundary of SVM

The decision boundary of an SVM classifier is determined by the support vectors, which are the data points closest to the boundary. Parameters C and σ, also known as regularisation and kernel parameters, respectively, control the width of the margin and the shape of the decision boundary. For instance, when σ is set to 0.1 and C is set to 1, the decision boundary becomes complex and more influenced by the individual data points. The width of the margin becomes relatively small and the classifier more sensitive to the presence of outliers, as the algorithm tries to minimise misclassification errors. Moreover, when σ is set to 0.1 and C is set to 10, the decision boundary is even more complex as C has a greater influence on the decision boundary. The width of the margin is even smaller and the classifier is even more sensitive to outliers. Furthermore, when σ is set to 0.1 and C is set to 0.1, the decision boundary is relatively simple as C has a much smaller influence on the decision boundary. The width of the margin is relatively large and the classifier is less sensitive to outliers.

The classification boundaries of the SVM model are depicted in Figures 16–18 using the best classification parameters, enabling the model to accurately categorise participants into the appropriate group.

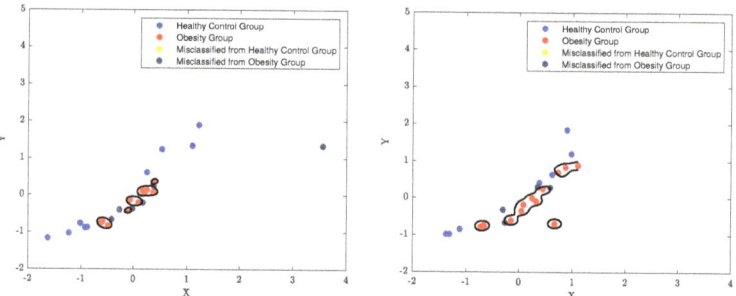

Figure 16. The boundary that separates the healthy control walk patterns from the obesity patterns in an SVM model, with RCC control parameters $f_p = 1$, $f_g = 1$, $x_p = -1$, $x_g = -1$, $\mu_f = 2$, and $\sigma = 0.1$ and $C = 0.1$ for w_1 and $\sigma = 0.1$ and $C = 1$ for w_2, is shown.

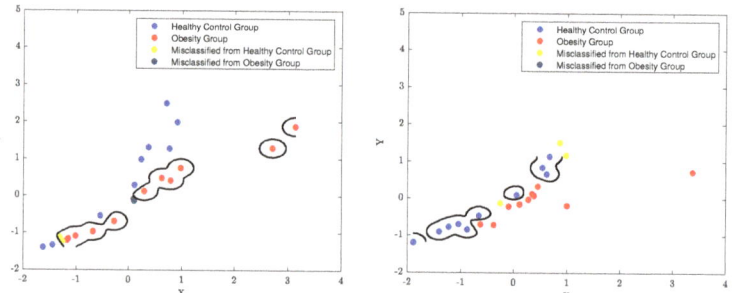

Figure 17. The boundary that separates the healthy control walk patterns from the obesity patterns in an SVM model, with RCC control parameters $f_p = 1$, $f_g = 1$, $x_p = -1$, $x_g = -1$, $\mu_f = 2$, and $\sigma = 0.1$ and $C = 1$ for w_3 and w_4, is shown.

The overall performance of the proposed SVM model is evaluated in Figure 19, where the best classification parameters ($\sigma = 0.1$ and $C = 0.1$) result in the optimal generalisation performance. The 6-week evaluation of the SVM shows fluctuating accuracy in classifying participants into the healthy control and obesity groups. A high accuracy reflects consistent participant characteristics, facilitating accurate classification by the SVM, whereas a low accuracy indicates high variability in participant characteristics, making classification challenging. In individuals with obesity, the influence of various factors, including walk speed, affects the results depicted in Figure 19. The figure demonstrates that the highest accuracy is observed during the initial week, but experiences a significant decline in the third week. Subsequently, there is a slight improvement in the fourth week, followed by further declines in the fifth and sixth weeks. The fluctuation in the accuracy of the SVM model during the 6-week period, despite the uniform diet and exercise regimen followed by the participants, could be attributed to various reasons such as variations in compliance levels, where some participants may have been more diligent in adhering to the regimen than others, leading to different classifications into healthy control or obesity groups. Other factors include individual differences such as genetics, medical history, and personal habits, measurement inaccuracies, and changes in any of the systems (metabolic, neuromuscular, cardiovascular) altering participant characteristics over time, even when following the prescribed diet and exercise regimen. Participants' stress levels or health status could impact their classification as it could alter variables affecting their gait and hence classification into healthy control or obesity groups.

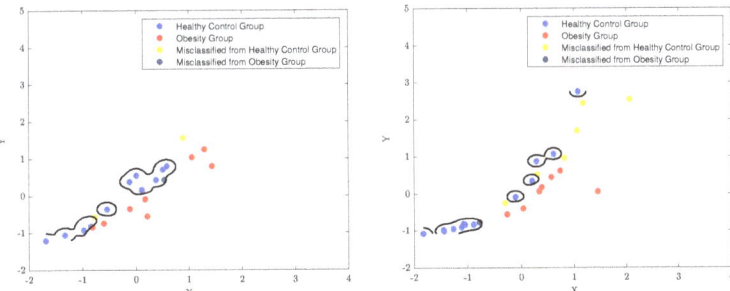

Figure 18. The SVM decision boundary that separates the healthy control walk patterns from the obesity patterns in an SVM model, with RCC control parameters $f_p = 1$, $f_g = 1$, $x_p = -1$, $x_g = -1$, $\mu_f = 2$, and $\sigma = 0.1$ and $C = 10$ for w_5 and $\sigma = 0.1$ and $C = 1$ for w_6, is shown.

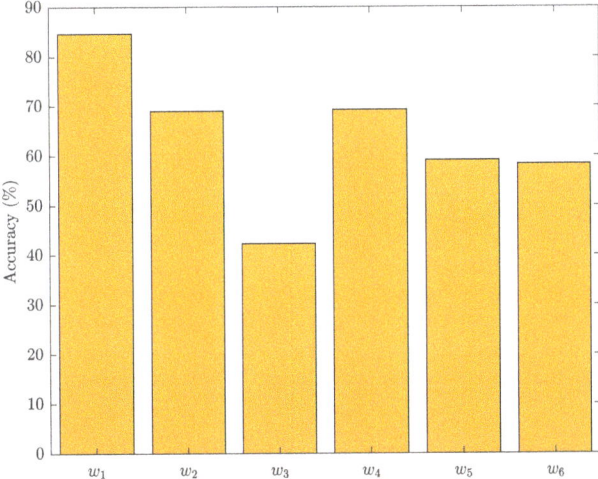

Figure 19. The classification performance of SVM over a 6-week (w_1–w_6) period is presented.

5. Discussion

The primary aim of the comprehensive study was to assess the effectiveness of obesity treatment interventions through the application of a unique CA approach. Simultaneously, the investigation delved into the intricate dynamics of gait patterns, particularly within the context of obesity. This multifaceted exploration sought to provide a deeper understanding of gait patterns and evaluate the potential of the CA methodology combined with SVM classification in gait analysis within the context of obesity treatment assessment. This multidimensional exploration sought to not only quantify gait variability, but also ascertain the robustness of our CA-SVM methodology for gait classification. Throughout the 6-week study period, SVM classification accuracy exhibited significant fluctuations, with the highest accuracy recorded in the initial week, followed by substantial declines in Weeks 3 through 6. These fluctuations highlight the dynamic nature of SVM model's ability to categorise gait patterns over time. Notably, these variations are not arbitrary but reflect shifts in participant characteristics that significantly impact classification outcomes.

All participants adhered to a uniform diet and exercise regimen during the study, making it evident that individual factors beyond the protocol influenced gait patterns and SVM classifications each week. Factors such as compliance, genetics, medical history, stress levels, or changes in metabolic/neuromuscular systems likely played a role. The SVM accuracy metric robustly quantifies the influence of these individual characteristics on classification performance. ROC curves and AUC values provide insights into the model's proficiency in distinguishing between healthy and obese gait patterns. Optimal model performance occurred under specific parameter settings, $\sigma = 0.1$ and $C = 1$ or 10, where AUC values were maximised. These results confirm the exceptional generalisation capabilities of the SVM model when applied to unseen data and underscore the effectiveness of our CA-SVM methodology in extracting relevant features from gait data.

Visual representations, in the form of phase plots, vividly illustrate the distinctions between healthy and obese gait patterns achieved through the CA method. The phase plots reveal that obese gait patterns are characterised by slower and more labored movements, while healthy gait patterns are smoother and more fluid. These differences align with expectations, given the increased joint stress and stiffness associated with obesity. Phase plots affirm that CA effectively distinguishes between the two groups by revealing interpretable spatio-temporal gait characteristics.

The spatio-temporal analysis quantifying variability in gait progression over a 6-week period offers valuable insights. Notably, wider variability is observed among obese participants compared to their healthy counterparts. This underscores CA's capacity to elucidate subtle yet evolving patterns through phase plot analysis and its competence in quantifying gait variability. Lastly, classification accuracy results, ranging from 78.2% to 90%, strongly validate the efficacy of the CA method in dimensionality reduction and data representation, enhancing classification performance. CA successfully transforms complex gait patterns into lower-dimensional trajectories discernible by the SVM algorithm, leading to high accuracy. This demonstrates CA's proficiency in extracting essential features and capturing nonlinear relationships, enabling precise classification and establishing it as an effective data representation strategy.

6. Conclusions

The Criticality Analysis method for nonlinear data representation can be effectively used to represent gait data and highlight medical conditions. The variability and detection of changes over time highlight the ability of the method to determine changes in gait in response to clinical intervention. The potential to assess clinical disorders using only gait is an exciting development especially for long-term or complex disorders associated with metabolic stress. The combination of nonlinear data representation with supervised machine learning methods can significantly improve the assessment of a patient's status and improve the likelihood of positive outcomes by enabling objective assessment during treatment.

Author Contributions: Conceptualisation, S.E.; methodology, S.E. and T.V.o.S.; validation, S.E.; formal analysis, S.E.; investigation, S.E.; data curation, H.D., J.C., A.A., C.M., M.M.-B., S.L., S.V.-C., M.J.A. and D.F.; writing—original draft preparation, S.E.; writing—review and editing, S.E. and T.V.o.S.; visualisation, S.E.; supervision, T.V.o.S. All authors have read and agreed to the published version of the manuscript.

Funding: This work was supported by a Newton Fund Institutional Links grant (grant ID: 432368181) under the Newton–Mosharafa Fund partnership between the United Kingdom and Mexico. The grant was funded by the UK Department for Business, Energy and Industrial Strategy (BEIS) and delivered by the British Council. The funding supported collaboration activities between Oxford Brookes University and Hospital Infantil de Mexico Federico Gomez under the Newton Institutional Links program administered by the British Council.

Institutional Review Board Statement: Not applicable.

Informed Consent Statement: Not applicable.

Data Availability Statement: In accordance with the General Data Protection Regulation (GDPR) guidelines, the database utilised in this study is maintained in a confidential and secure manner within the purview of the Faculty of Health and Life Sciences at Oxford Brookes University. Owing to privacy considerations, access to the dataset is restricted to authorised personnel only.

Acknowledgments: The authors gratefully acknowledge the support provided by the British Council under the Newton Fund Institutional Links program for making this collaboration possible. We also acknowledge our institutional partners Oxford Brookes University and Hospital Infantil de Mexico Federico Gomez for their support and contribution.

Conflicts of Interest: The authors declare no conflict of interest.

References

1. Kuo, A.D.; Donelan, J.M. Dynamic principles of gait and their clinical implications. *Phys Ther.* **2010**, *90*, 157–174. [CrossRef] [PubMed]
2. Clark, J.E.; Phillips, S.J. A longitudinal study of intralimb coordination in the first year of independent walking: A dynamical systems analysis. *Child Dev.* **1993**, *64*, 1143–1157. [CrossRef] [PubMed]
3. Dingwell, J.B.; Cusumano, J.P. Nonlinear time series analysis of normal and pathological human walking. *Chaos* **2000**, *10*, 848–863. [CrossRef] [PubMed]
4. Glazier, D.S. Metabolic Scaling in Complex Living Systems. *Systems* **2014**, *2*, 451–540. [CrossRef]
5. Hausdorff, J.M.; Mitchell, S.L.; Firtion, R.; Peng, C.K.; Cudkowicz, M.E.; Wei, J.Y.; Goldberger, A.L. Altered fractal dynamics of gait: Reduced stride-interval correlations with aging and Huntington's disease. *J. Appl. Physiol.* **1997**, *82*, 262–269. [CrossRef] [PubMed]
6. Alam, U.; Riley, D.R.; Jugdey, R.S.; Azmi, S.; Rajbhandari, S.; D'Août, K.; Malik, R.A. Diabetic Neuropathy and Gait: A Review. *Diabetes Ther.* **2017**, *8*, 1253–1264. [CrossRef] [PubMed]
7. Toro, B.; Nester, C.; Farren, P. A review of observational gait assessment in clinical practice. *Physiother. Theory Pract.* **2003**, *19*, 137–149. [CrossRef]
8. Pirker, W.; Katzenschlager, R. Gait disorders in adults and the elderly: A clinical guide. *Wien. Klin. Wochenschr.* **2017**, *129*, 81–95. [CrossRef]
9. Sipari, D.; Chaparro-Rico, B.D.M.; Cafolla, D. SANE (Easy Gait Analysis System): Towards an AI-Assisted Automatic Gait-Analysis. *Int. J. Environ. Res. Public Health* **2022**, *19*, 10032. [CrossRef]
10. Guo, Q.; Jiang, D. Method for Walking Gait Identification in a Lower Extremity Exoskeleton Based on C4.5 Decision Tree Algorithm. *Int. J. Adv. Robot. Syst.* **2015**, *12*, 30.
11. Harris, E.J.; Khoo, I.-H.; Demircan, E. A Survey of Human Gait-Based Artificial Intelligence Applications. *Front. Robot. AI* **2022**, *8*, 749274. [CrossRef] [PubMed]
12. McGrath, M.; Howard, D.; Baker, R. The strengths and weaknesses of inverted pendulum models of human walking. *Gait Posture* **2015**, *41*, 389–394. [CrossRef] [PubMed]
13. Berry, H. Chaos in a Bienzymatic Cyclic Model with Two Autocatalytic Loops. *Chaos Solitons Fractals* **2003**, *18*, 1001–1014. [CrossRef]
14. Eltanani, S.; olde Scheper, T.V.; Dawes, H. A Novel Criticality Analysis Technique for Detecting Dynamic Disturbances in Human Gait. *Computers* **2022**, *11*, 120. [CrossRef]
15. olde Scheper, T.V. Criticality Analysis: Bio-inspired Nonlinear Data Representation. *arXiv* **2023**, arXiv:2305.14361.
16. Rota, V.; Perucca, L.; Simone, A.; Tesio, L. Walk ratio (step length/cadence) as a summary index of neuromotor control of gait: Application to multiple sclerosis. *Int. J. Rehabil. Res.* **2011**, *34*, 265–269. [CrossRef] [PubMed]

17. Mobbs, R.J.; Perring, J.; Raj, S.M.; Maharaj, M.; Yoong, N.K.M.; Sy, L.W.; Fonseka, R.D.; Natarajan, P.; Choy, W.J. Gait metrics analysis utilizing single-point inertial measurement units: A systematic review. *Mhealth* **2022**, *8*, 9. [CrossRef] [PubMed]
18. Esser, P.; Dawes, H.; Collett, J.; Howells, K. Insights into Gait Disorders: Walking Variability Using Phase Plot Analysis, Parkinson's Disease. *Gait Posture* **2013**, *38*, 648–652. [CrossRef]
19. Nahm, F.S. Receiver operating characteristic curve: Overview and practical use for clinicians. *Korean J. Anesthesiol.* **2022**, *75*, 25–36. [CrossRef]
20. Bradley, A.P. The use of the area under the ROC curve in the evaluation of machine learning algorithms. *Pattern Recognit.* **1997**, *30*, 1145–1159. [CrossRef]

Disclaimer/Publisher's Note: The statements, opinions and data contained in all publications are solely those of the individual author(s) and contributor(s) and not of MDPI and/or the editor(s). MDPI and/or the editor(s) disclaim responsibility for any injury to people or property resulting from any ideas, methods, instructions or products referred to in the content.

Article

A Modified and Effective Blockchain Model for E-Healthcare Systems

Basem Assiri

Computer Science Department, Jazan University, Jazan 82917, Saudi Arabia; bas0911@hotmail.com or babumussmar@jazanu.edu.sa

Abstract: The development of e-healthcare systems requires the application of advanced technologies, such as blockchain technology. The main challenge of applying blockchain technology to e-healthcare is to handle the impact of the delay that results from blockchain procedures during the communication and voting phases. The impacts of latency in blockchains negatively influence systems' efficiency, performance, real-time processing, and quality of service. Therefore, this work proposes a modified model of a blockchain that allows delays to be avoided in critical situations in healthcare. Firstly, this work analyzes the specifications of healthcare data and processes to study and classify healthcare transactions according to their nature and sensitivity. Secondly, it introduces the concept of a fair-proof-of-stake consensus protocol for block creation and correctness procedures rather than famous ones such as proof-of-work or proof-of-stake. Thirdly, the work presents a simplified procedure for block verification, where it classifies transactions into three categories according to the time period limit and trustworthiness level. Consequently, there are three kinds of blocks, since every category is stored in a specific kind of block. The ideas of time period limits and trustworthiness fit with critical healthcare situations and the authority levels in healthcare systems. Therefore, we reduce the validation process of the trusted blocks and transactions. All proposed modifications help to reduce computational costs, speed up processing times, and enhance security and privacy. The experimental results show that the total execution time using a modified blockchain is reduced by about 49% compared to traditional blockchain models. Additionally, the number of messages using modified blockchain is reduced by about 53% compared to the traditional blockchain model.

Keywords: parallelism; distributed systems; modified blockchain technology; personal health records; e-healthcare

Citation: Assiri, B. A Modified and Effective Blockchain Model for E-Healthcare Systems. *Appl. Sci.* **2023**, *13*, 12630. https://doi.org/10.3390/app132312630

Academic Editor: Gianluca Lax

Received: 25 October 2023
Revised: 21 November 2023
Accepted: 22 November 2023
Published: 23 November 2023

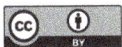

Copyright: © 2023 by the author. Licensee MDPI, Basel, Switzerland. This article is an open access article distributed under the terms and conditions of the Creative Commons Attribution (CC BY) license (https://creativecommons.org/licenses/by/4.0/).

1. Introduction

Technological development plays vital roles in areas of life such as healthcare, education, tourism, national security, and others. In the field of healthcare, healthcare agencies compete through applying advanced technologies to improve their throughput, management, control, and services with reduced costs. One important step toward this direction is to use electronic personal health records (EPHRs), which supports the use of other technologies [1]. The use of EPHRs involves cloud storage, which allows for more control, availability, and accessibility [2,3]. However, having EPHRs in cloud storage is called a centralized parallel and distributed system, which has a single point of failure.

Blockchain technology is one kind of distributed system that runs in a decentralized manner [4], in which multiple transactions are processed and grouped into one block. The blocks are listed in one ledger. Copies of the ledger are distributed among all nodes, such that every node has an updated copy of the ledger. The nodes are devices that belong to the blockchain network, and they are authorized to store and validate transactions and blocks. Actually, transactions are executed by users, but they cannot confirm (commit) those transactions. The blockchain nodes (miners) perform processing of transactions to confirm them. During this process, the miners compete in transaction processing to create a block of transactions using some consensus mechanisms, such as proof-of-work (PoW) or proof-of-stake (PoS) [5]. Then, the miner who succeeds in creating a new block proposes that block to other miners in order to verify it. If this block is verified, then it is added to the ledger; otherwise, it is ignored [6,7]. The blockchain processes are executed as follows:

- Proposal: A miner verifies transactions and proposes a new block to other miners (they will act as validators);
- Verification: The validators validate the proposed block and send their votes to the others to either confirm or decline (commit or abort) the proposed block;
- Consensus: After receiving the votes of all validators, every validator checks the votes of the majority. Accordingly, the block is committed and either added to the ledger or not.

On the other hand, healthcare utilizes various data sources, such as healthcare professionals and the Internet of Things (IoT). Firstly, healthcare professionals have different levels of authority and trustworthiness, and this is also connected with the criticality of healthcare situations. For example, in emergency cases, doctors and nurses should access EPHRs to read or update them directly without any delay; for these purposes, blockchain procedures such as permission or voting cannot be applied. Secondly, IoT, including sensors, smartphones, and wearable mobile devices, provides real-time data as these devices sense and reflect data directly [8]. These devices are able to facilitate or perform some actions [9–11]. Actually, wearable mobile devices can be embedded in clothes or accessories such as watches, bracelets, glasses, jewelry, etc. [12]. There are also other, complicated kinds of wearable devices that can be embedded into the human body. This allows for the improvement of healthcare follow-up and services. It helps in tracking life signs and monitoring patients' situations [13]. However, such real-time technology is challenged by delays caused by blockchain procedures [14]. Moreover, these tools usually have limited storing, processing, and energy capabilities, which would also be challenged by blockchain procedures such as mining, validating, voting and storing processes [15].

Applying blockchain technology to e-healthcare has many advantages, such as decentralization, security, privacy, anonymity, transparency, reliability, and fault tolerance. However, the main challenge is to handle the impact of the latency that results from blockchain procedures during the communication and voting phases. The impacts of latency in blockchains negatively influence systems' efficiency, performance, real-time processing, and quality of services. To the best of our knowledge, this is the first work that modifies the blockchain model to cope with e-healthcare authority levels and real-time specifications.

This work proposes a modified model of a blockchain that is used to store, process, and manage data in the field of e-healthcare. Firstly, this work studies and classifies healthcare data according to their nature and sensitivity. It investigates and analyzes the roles and authorities that are interwoven with data access and processing. Secondly, understanding the nature of transaction is an important step at the beginning of this work. Unfortunately, many works apply blockchain technology without studying the implications of using transactions, which obviously shows a lack of understanding of transaction specifications. Therefore, the proposed model modifies the shape of data within the blocks, since the regular form of transaction is not required for all data, operations, and processes. Thirdly, it also introduces a modified form of PoS that implies the fairness of the proof-of-queue protocol (PoQ). The proposed protocol is called fair-proof-of-stake (FPoS). Actually, in PoS, the chance of creating and validating blocks is given according to the amount of stake the miner puts in, which causes difficulty for new miners. The PoQ, on the other hand, queues miners and gives a fair chance to every miner. The proposed FPoS uses the block creation and correctness procedure of PoS for a specific number of cycles; then, it gives chances to the miners waiting in the queue (but they cannot compete in the PoS manner). Fourthly, it presents a modified procedure for block verification that relaxes the verification for some trusted transactions and blocks. Obviously, all proposed modifications help to reduce costs, support processing speed-up, and enhance security and privacy. The experimental results show that the total execution time using the modified blockchain was reduced by about 49% comparing to traditional blockchain model. Additionally, the number of messages using modified blockchain was reduced by about 53% compared to the traditional blockchain model.

The rest of this paper is organized as follows: Related work is described in Section 2. Section 3 shows the analysis of healthcare specifications. Section 4 introduces the modified blockchain model that suits e-healthcare specifications. Section 5 illustrates the numerical analysis and the experimental results. Section 6 discusses the advantages of the proposed model, while Section 7 concludes the paper.

2. Related Work

Blockchain technology was used firstly in Bitcoin cryptocurrency [16], and then in other cryptocurrencies such as Ripple, Litecoin, Ethereum, and Zcash [17]. It was introduced to avoid the centralization and control of third parties [18]. Since then, researchers have applied blockchain technology in many other fields, such as healthcare, education, judiciary, etc. [19,20].

Blockchain-distributed architecture is supported by consensus protocols to ensure the correctness of the processes. Different consensus protocols are used, such as PoW, which applies the solutions of some mathematical puzzles with some specifications. The results of such mathematical puzzles are used to hash the proposed block, and the miners use them to verify the correctness of the block [5]. Another consensus protocol is PoS, by which miners use their own coins as guarantees and according to which they have the chance to propose or validate the blocks, which also gives them a chance to win more coins [5]. Proof-of-space allows users to propose their own hard disks and hardware to process and secure the blockchain. According to the given space, the miner has a higher chance. Another protocol is the practical Byzantine fault tolerance (PBFT) consensus protocol, where the number of fault votes should not exceed one-third of the votes [21].

In addition, wearable devices help to sense, collect, and send data and to receive alerts, as well as to share updates and information. This improves healthcare processes and services for all stockholders [11]. Many research has investigated the use of wearable devices in healthcare for patient monitoring [22], recognition, and assistance, as well as for research purposes [23].

Many researchers have linked blockchains with wearable devices to support users, healthcare providers, and insurance companies [24–26]. In such research, the advantages of using blockchain with wearable devices, such as decentralization, distribution, transparency, robustness, availability, automation, traceability, reliability, ownership protection, privacy, and security are investigated, and some of these advantages intersect with each other. In contrast, some work has highlighted the blockchain's disadvantages, such as energy consumption, computational cost, traffic flow latency, and scalability [27]. In response, many works have provided modified blockchain models [28] and modified transactions [29]. Blockchains have been used in healthcare systems for storage security [30], EPHR sharing [31], insurance processes [32], pharmaceutical supply chains [33], patient monitoring [34], organ transplant management [35], clinical trial support [36], and IoT data management [37]. However, to the best of our knowledge, this is the first work that has targeted e-healthcare authority levels, in addition to reducing latency and processing time, using a relaxed blockchain model.

3. Healthcare System's Specifications

Before we move on to integrating blockchain technology with a healthcare system, this paper illustrates some important points related to the healthcare system. Such an analysis allows us to frame the specifications of healthcare data and processes. Accordingly, the blockchain model will be adjusted. The analysis of healthcare specifications is presented as follows:

- *Healthcare system's stockholders*: The main healthcare system's stockholders are patients, doctors, nurses, dentists, health technicians, and administration staff [38].
- *EPHR general privacy*: Patients' information in EPHRs can be revealed for specific purposes, but only if the personal identities are hidden [39]. Such information can be revealed for specific purposes, like research or awareness-raising campaigns. Dealing with EPHRs is very sensitive, even with hidden identities, as they could be negatively exploited by politicians, marketplaces, or businesses.
- *EPHR with healthcare stakeholders*: No patients' information and EPHRs should be hidden form doctors, nurses, dentists, or health technicians [39]. The data can be accessed under a non-disclosure agreement. However, some EPHR information, such as identities or mental and psychological issues, should be hidden from co-members such as volunteers and students who join healthcare teams.
- *EPHR privacy levels*: Different privacy levels are assigned to EPHRs. For example, EPHRs would require specific privacy levels [39,40] for politicians, military leaders, and famous people compared to the public.
- *Updating EPHR*: Different parts of EPHRs can be updated by doctors, nurses, dentists, or health technicians. Indeed, everyone who is part of the healthcare staff can update specific related parts without restriction. However, we should restrict updates that are irrelevant to the roles within the healthcare team [41].
- *Direct update of EPHR*: Most EPHR updates require the approval of the primary or main doctor. Primary doctors do not need any approval, and they can authorize others to directly update the relevant parts or sections without any approval [42].
- *Financial Transactions*: Financial transactions can be accessed or updated by the authorized people, although the approval of any operation is required [32].
- *Latency*: Latency or delays that result from approval are critical in some emergency cases and scenarios.
- *System considerations*: The development of any healthcare system should consider the general regulations, ethical obligations, and cultural influence. For example, cases of abortion, transgender status, and violence should be treated according to the laws and culture perspectives, which differ from one place to another.

4. Modified Blockchain Model

Blockchain technology introduces decentralized and distributed architecture that is combined with supported algorithms and procedures. The blockchain has nodes that are fully connected to each other and share copies of the same ledger. The algorithm starts by confirming the correctness of transactions and groups them in blocks. Only one of the miners can propose a new block. This miner is decided based on different consensus mechanisms, such as PoW, PoS, PoQ, or PBFT. Then, the other miners validate and vote on the approval of the proposed block. According to the votes of the majority (consensus), the block is approved and added to ledger; otherwise, it is ignored and another block is proposed. In fact, every miner has to update their copy the ledger based on the consensus.

In this paper, the blockchain procedure is modified according to the guidance of the results of the healthcare specifications in Section 3. The details of the modifications are explained in the following subsections.

4.1. Transaction Process

Understanding the nature of transactions is important. Unfortunately, many works apply blockchain technology without studying the implication of using transactions, which obviously indicates a lack of understanding of transaction specifications.

A regular operation reads data or updates it directly in the main memory. However, a transaction consists of one or more operations. These operations involve either reading a piece of data or writing a piece of data. The operations within a transaction are executed one by one in a temporary memory (buffer). In the end, the transaction is committed or aborted. Committing a transaction means that the results of all operations are reflected from the temporary memory to the main memory, while aborting a transaction means that the results of all operations are neglected and the temporary memory is freed. In addition, by using a transactional system, many operations and transaction are executed in parallel, which increases the throughput (number of executed transactions per time). It also speeds up the processing system with minimal costs. Another advantage is the ability to roll back and retrieve the correct data. The transactional system is supported by software and hardware resources.

4.2. Mining

The mining process has two basic steps. Firstly, the correctness of the transactions is confirmed, and they are placed into a new block. Secondly, a consensus protocol such as PoW or PoS is followed to obtain a chance of proposing the new block to others for validation and votes, which is explained in the following section. Now, let us focus on the correctness of transactions; indeed, there are two kinds of transactions: read and update. The read transaction only includes read operations, while the update transaction includes at least one write operation, as shown in Figure 1. Actually, Figure 1 shows examples of different kinds of transactions. T1 is a read transaction that includes only one read operation, which returns the value of the variable *a*. At the end, the transaction tries to commit (TryC). T2 is a read transaction that includes multiple read operations for the variables *a*, *b*, and *c*. T3 is an update transaction that includes only one write operation, which updates the value of the variable *a* with the value 5. T4 is a update transaction that includes multiple write operations to update the variables *a*, *b*, and *c*, consequently with the values 1, 2, and 3. T5 is an update transaction that includes multiple read and write operations, which read variable *a*, write to *a*, then read variable *c*.

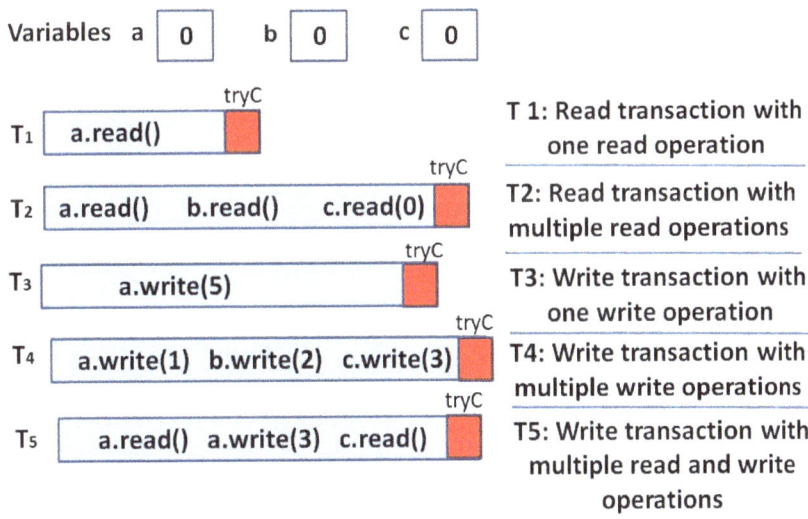

Figure 1. Kinds of transactions.

Furthermore, since transactions run in parallel and in isolation, the effects of the operations appear after transaction is committed. This means that the changes that result from transaction operations are not visible to the system until it commits. This may allow for inaccurate data to be read (not up to data), and may cause conflict among transactions, as illustrated in Figure 2. In fact, running a read transaction in parallel does not have any negative impact, since the values of the memory data are stable. However, update transactions change the value of the memory content. Figure 2 gives an example of four transactions running in parallel and shows how the conflicts caused the abortion of some transactions. T1, T2, and T3 are read transactions, while T4 is an update transaction. The operations of those transactions accessed some memory variables, namely, a = 0, b = 0, c = 0, and d = 0. Actually, T1 read variable *a* (returning a = 0), *c* (returning c = 0), and *d* (returning d = 0). T2 read variables *a* (returning a = 0) and *b* (returning b = 1), which means that T4 changed the value of *b* and had already committed. T3 read variable *b* (returning b = 0) and *d* (returning d = 1). This means that T3 read *b* before the commitment of T4, and *d* afterward. T4 read variable *a* (returning a = 0) and updated the values of *b* (returning b = 1) and *d* (returning d = 1).

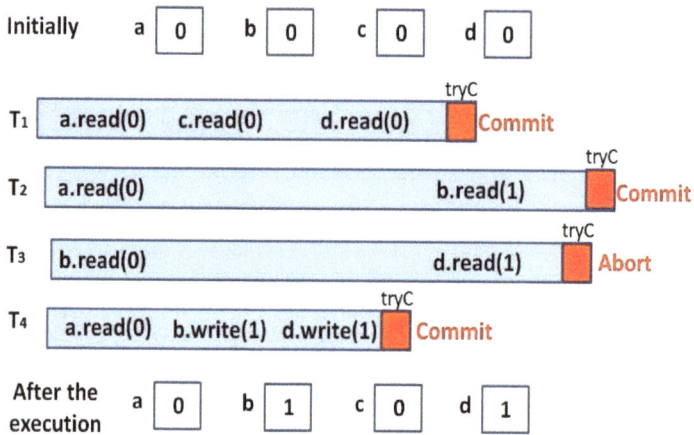

Figure 2. An Example of parallel execution of four transactions to illustrate the conflicts that caused the abortion of T4.

In fact, the correctness of the execution of parallel transaction is confirmed when the results of parallel execution match any correct serialized execution. In other words, the transactions in parallel execution must be ordered in a logical way. Considering our example in Figure 2, T1 can be considered as the first executed transaction, since it returned all original values of *a*, *c*, and *d*. T4 can be considered as the second executed transaction, since it read the original values of *a* and updated the value of *b* (b = 1) and *d* (d = 1). T2 can be considered as the third executed transaction, since it read the original values of *a* (no concurrent transaction has updated *a*) and *b* (returning b = 1), where the *b* value had been updated by T4. However, T3 must be aborted and ignored in the process of ordering; it could not be ordered before T4 as it read d = 1, which could only be seen after the commitment of T4, and it could not be ordered after T4 as it read b = 0, clearly ignoring the change in variable *b* that took place after T4 was committed.

One last example is shown in Figure 3 to explain the conflicts between two update transactions. Let us have one bank account, called the hospital bank account (*h*), and let h = 10,000, which means that the hospital bank account contains USD 10,000. Now, let there be two transactions, T1 and T2, that belong to different patients and are executed in parallel. The first patient pays USD 100 as the cost of some blood tests (T1), while the other pays USD 500 for medical examination (T2). In this way, T1 should read the value of *h* and add a value of 100, while T2 should read the value of *h* and add a value of 500. Since both T1 and T2 are executed in parallel, both of them will read the original value of *h*. This means that T1 will add 100 to 10,000, and at the end, it will write h = 10,100, while T2 will add 500 to 10,000, and at the end it writes h = 10,500. The last results of both transactions are incorrect, since the value of *h* after the commitment of T1 and T2 should be 10,600. Consequently, one of the transactions must be aborted and rolled back, then executed again after the commitment of the other. Let us say that T2 is aborted, then executed again after the commitment of T1: it sees h = 10,100, and by adding 500, the result becomes h = 10,600.

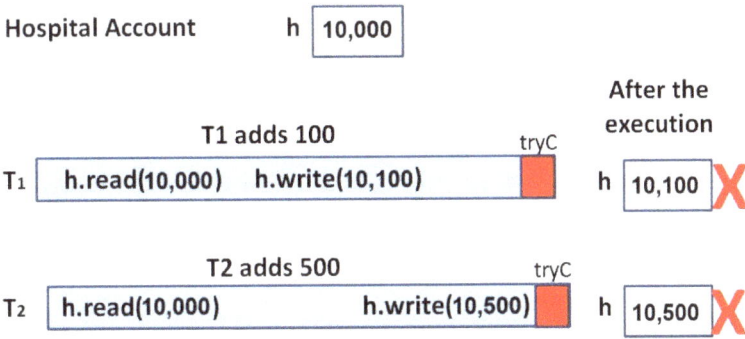

Figure 3. The conflict between two update transactions.

Aborting some transactions to guarantee correctness is one of the disadvantages of transactional processing systems, because it costs time, energy, effort to maintain and it does not suit healthcare systems. To cope with such an issue, some works relax the correctness property as they allow us to read some stale data (not up to date) [43], but such strategies might be harmful in cases of sensitive data, such as in the healthcare system.

4.3. Fair-Proof-of-Stake

In addition, we introduce the concept of fair-proof-of-stake (FPoS). Actually, the traditional PoS is a consensus mechanism that allows a miner to create a new block and validate the proposed block according to the number of coins a miner stakes. A miner who stakes a large amount has more to lose it in case the block has not been verified. This enhances the confidentiality of miners and the security of the system. However, new miners who have just joined the blockchain usually do not have enough to stake or to compete with old miners. On the other hand, PoQ queues miners in a fair manner, for example, using timestamps. However, all miners have the same chance regardless of their trustworthiness or confidentiality. For such issues, FPoS is proposed to balance the ideas of PoS and PoQ. The system assigns a ratio—say, $x{:}y$—such that the system applies PoS for x cycles, then applies PoQ for y cycles. For example, if the ratio is 10:1, then the one with higher stakes takes a chance, and this is repeated 10 times. Then, at cycle number 11, the first miner in the queue (it might be a newly joined miner or a miner with few stakes) is given a chance to create or validate a block. Obviously, the ratio can be changed over time according to the need of the system. In short, FPoS helps to motivate nodes with low processing capabilities or low credit to participate in mining processes; gives more of a chance to the trustworthy miners; and provides flexibility, as the ratio is decided according to the system's nature and data sensitivity.

Algorithm 1 shows FPoS, setting the FPoS ratio $x{:}y$ (Line 2). At the beginning, if any node N_i wants to be selected as a miner, it has to stake some coins to join the stake list (*flag* = 1), or it joins the queue (*flag* = 2). Any other value of the *flag* will lead to an error (Lines 7–15). Then, FPoS selects a miner from the stake list x times. Every time, it selects the node of the maximum stake (Lines 17–19). After that, y times, it selects a miner from the queue (Lines 20–22). Finally, it starts over and sets the counters to zero (Lines 23–24).

Algorithm 1: FPoS

1.	**// Initialization:**
2.	**Input:** x, y; // Insert x:y ratio for FPoS
3.	counter1 = 0;
4.	counter2 = 0;
5.	flag; // Flage to join miner lists
6.	// Node N_i joins miner lists by inserting 1 to stake coins or 2 to joins Queue;
7.	**Switch** (flag):
8.	**Case** flag = 1;
9.	$N_i \to$ Stake(); // Node stakes some coins
10.	**break;**
11.	**Case** flag = 2;
12.	$N_i \to$ Queue; // Node is enqueued
13.	**break;**
14.	**default:**
15.	*error()*; // flag $\neq$ 1 or 2
16.	// Now the FPoS selects miners
17.	**While** counter1 < x;
18.	miner$\leftarrow$maxStake();
19.	counter1++;
20.	**While** counter2 < x;
21.	miner$\leftarrow$Queue();
22.	counter2++;
23.	goto(line 3);

4.4. Trusted Transactions

In healthcare systems, there are different kinds of operations and privileges. Firstly, some members of medical team are authorized to read and update specific parts of EPHR. Therefore, they can access their parts directly, without permission (before the access) or approval (after the execution of operations). This means that they can execute and update memory directly in a non-transactional manner. Our model keeps them in a transactional manner, but it relaxes the validation process for such transactions. This is called a level-one trusted transaction, denoted as *TrustedT1*. Secondly, some healthcare practitioners can access data for reading, but any updates require approval by a primary doctor, for example. This form can be called a level-two trusted transaction, denoted as *TrustedT2*. The third kind of process requires approval for both reading and updating, which can be executed in a regular transaction manner denoted as *T*. In fact, the data that come from IoT or wearable devices is processed using regular *T*. Moreover, coordinating parallel transactions can be solved through some efficient leader election algorithms [44], where the primary doctor acts as the leader of the medical team and organizes the access to the EPHR.

Another important issue is focusing on the content of the transaction. One example is the transaction of Bitcoin, which includes information about the sender, receiver, and amount. There are different patterns of transactions in e-health systems, such as read transactions and update transactions for EPHR, as well as financial transactions for insurance and other related process. Unlike Bitcoin's transactions, where the sender and receiver identities appear to the public, in healthcare transactions, patients' identities should be hidden for privacy purposes using smart contracts and encryption, as explained later on in Section 6.2.

4.5. Blocks and Trusted Blocks

Having different kinds of transactions allows us to have different kinds of blocks. There are three kinds of blocks: *Block1* includes *TrustedT1*, *Block2* includes *TrustedT2*, and regular *Block* includes *T*. Since *TrustedT1* transactions do not need approval, miners do not need to spend time or effort to verify them. They just checks the authorization of the performer of the transactions, and so they receive the minimum reward (which can be some amount of coins of any cryptocurrency). Moreover, *Block2* includes *TrustedT2*. For *TrustedT2*, read transactions do not need approval and are treated as *TrustedT1*. This only requires verification that the transaction has already been approved by the primary doctor, so miners receive an average amount in reward. Update transactions in *TrustedT2*, however, require the correctness of the transactions to be validated and the approval to be verified, and the miner receives a higher reward. However, miners receive the maximum reward for verifying *T* and, consequently, *Block*. Figure 4 shows a copy of a ledger that has a chain composed of different kinds of blocks. It also shows that each type of block has the hash of the previous block, the hash of the current block, and specific kinds of transactions. Indeed, *Block1* includes *TrustedT1*, *Block2* includes *TrustedT2*, and regular *Block* includes regular transactions (*T*).

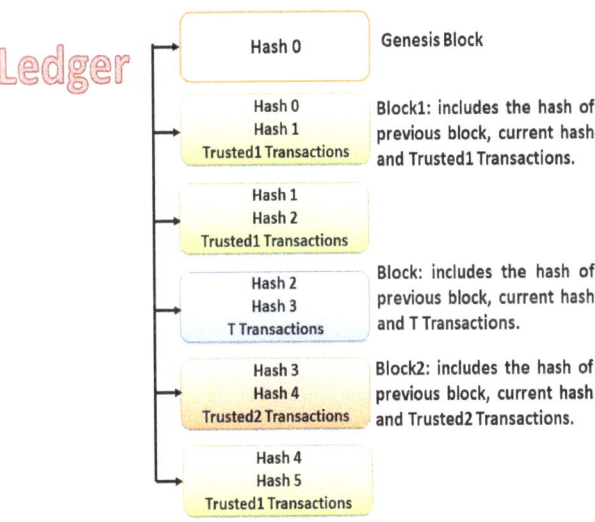

Figure 4. The ledger in the proposed blockchain model, containing three kinds of blocks, namely, Block, Block1 and Block2. Every kind of block includes a specific kind of transaction.

4.6. The Proposed Algorithm

The blockchain algorithm consists of three stages: proposing, voting, and consensus. The proposing stage includes transactional correctness, block creations, hash calculation, and casting a new block through FPoS to the others. All proposing steps have already been explained in the previous sections. The current section shows the validation and consensus processes, as well as the preliminaries and the algorithm.

4.6.1. Proposal Sending and Validating

At this level, the validator group is prepared. The validator group includes the number of miners who are going to validate the proposed block. The process includes sending the proposed block to every member of the validator group. Clearly, having a large number of validators enhances the accuracy and correctness of the validation process, but it also uses a large number of communication messages and increased processing. In our model, *Block1* requires the minimum number of validators—say, three validators. The odd number of validators helps to satisfy consensuses. *Block2* requires an average number of validators, while a regular *Block* require more validators. As mentioned earlier, the validators are selected according to the FPoS procedure. After nominating the members of the validator group, the proposed block is sent to all members.

Upon receiving the proposed block, every member validates the block and casts the result to all nodes. The result is either 1, for a valid block, or 0, for an invalid one. Actually, in a regular validation process, the validator checks the proposer's identity (to confirm the authorization), as well as whether the block has been modified after the proposing step, which can be assessed through the block's hash validation. However, validating the content of the block (transactions) is an important step to cope with the sensitivity of healthcare data. In fact, to validate *Block1*, the validators do not validate the transactions, but instead just check that all transactions have been executed by primary doctors. To validate *Block2*, the validator should check that all read transactions have been executed by authorized members and that all update transactions are correct, updated by authorized members, and approved by primary doctors. For regular *Block*, the validator should check that all transactions are correct, executed by authorized members, and approved by primary doctors. Finally, every validator casts the validation results (vote).

4.6.2. Consensus

Upon receiving the validation results from all validators, every node counts the valid and invalid votes to calculate the votes of the majority. According to the majority, if the block is valid, it is linked to the ledger; otherwise, the block is rejected and ignored. Indeed, the consensus is a procedure that can vary from one system to another. For example, a consensus of the majority can be reached by confirming a mathematical puzzle or by reaching a majority of 51% of the votes, while in other systems, it requires at least 2/3 of votes, which suits our model. The sensitivity of healthcare data and the nature of technology require higher percent for the consensus procedure.

4.6.3. Preliminaries and Notations

As shown in Algorithm 2, the blockchain process starts with node N_i, which mines T_i transactions to validate them, and then fills a new block B_i with the validated transactions considering the block size *Bsize*. Indeed, there are three kinds of transactions and, consequently, three kinds of blocks (Lines 9–29). Then, nodes compete to find hash and propose a new block using FPoS (Lines 31–33). Next, the blockchain algorithm assigns the validator group *voters* according to the kind of block using *validateor_size()*, then casts the block (Lines 34–35).

As mentioned earlier, according to the block type, validators have different levels of validation processes (Lines 37–44). They cast their votes (Line 45), which are either 1 for correct or *0* for not correct, as shown in Algorithm 3.

In Algorithm 4, upon receiving the votes, the consensus decision is made according to the votes of the majority to commit the new block and either add it to L_i or abort it.

Algorithm 2: Modified Blockchain Algorithm (Proposing)

1.   // Initialization:
2.   L; // The current ledger
3.   T; // Transaction
4.   B; // The current block
5.   Bsize← x; // x is an integer representing the block size
6.   **Proposing stage:**
7.   // Create B_i
8.   // For any node N_i: decides what kinds of transactions to validate;
9.   **Switch** (T_i):
10.   Case *TrustedT1*:
11.   For j = 0 to j < Bsize
12.   if (valid *TrustedT1* == True)
13.   *TrustedT1*→*Block1*;
14. B_i→*Block1*;

Algorithm 2 *Cont.*

15.   break;
16.   Case *TrustedT2*:
17.   For j = 0 to j < Bsize
18.   if (valid *TrustedT2* == True)
19.   *TrustedT2*→*Block2*;
20. B_i→*Block2*;
21.   break;
22.   Case *T*:
23.   For j = 0 to j < Bsize
24.   if (valid *T* == True)
25.   *T*→*Block*;
26. B_i→*Block*;
27.   break;
28.   default:
29.   exit(0);
30.   // After B_i is created, hash B_i, use FPoS, decide validators group and cast B_i
31. B_i→*hash()*;
32.   While ((B_i→*FPoS()*) == false)
33.   Wait();
34.   *validateor_size(B_i)*;
35.   *Cast(B_i)*;

Algorithm 3: Modified Blockchain Algorithm (Voting)

36.   // According B_i Kind determines the level of validation, then vote
37.   Case B_i →*TrustedT1*:
38.   *Low_validation()*;
39.   break;
40.   Case B_i →*TrustedT2*:
41.   *Normal_validation()*;
42.   break;
43.   default: // When B_i →*T*
44.   *high_validation()*;
45.   *Vote()*;

Algorithm 4: Modified Blockchain Algorithm (Consensus)

46.   // According to the vote of majority B_i is added to L_i or is aborted
47.   if (*majority()* == True)
48.   *message(Commit)*;
49. B_i →L_i
50.   else
51.   *message(Abort)*;

5. Experimental Results

In this paper, the blockchain procedures are modified according to the guidance of the results of the healthcare specifications. The experiment focuses on a modified blockchain for healthcare, which relaxes blockchain procedures for some blocks. As mentioned earlier, the modified blockchain has three kinds of blocks depending on what kind of transactions are in the block. The experiment simulates traditional blockchain procedures and modified blockchain procedures. It compared the performances of both, focusing on total execution time. The experiment was run on OS-Window 10 using Java as the programming language and an Intel Core (TM) i7 CPU, with 2.90 GHz and 4 GB (RAM). Every test was run for five times, and the average is shown.

5.1. Execution Time

In fact, the experiment created 12,000 transactions, including 6000 read transactions and 6000 update transactions. The read transactions were divided into three categories: *TrustedT1* (2000 transactions), *TrustedT2* (2000 transactions), and *T* (2000 transactions); the same categories are applicable to the update transactions. After the execution of the transactions, the blockchain procedure was executed to verify the transactions and store the verified ones in a blockchain ledger.

For simplicity, in this experiment, we built a blockchain of ten nodes. The block creation was fairly distributed among the ten nodes, as every cycle-one node proposed a new block of size 50 transactions (every block contained 50 transactions). The block also had a hash number which represented the content of the block, including the identity of the creator node, for authentication. After the block creation step, it was sent to the other nodes for verification.

Actually, a traditional blockchain treats all transactions with the same procedures, while a modified blockchain relaxes the validation of all *TrustedT1* and the read transactions from *TrustedT2*. The update transactions from *TrustedT2* and all *T* were treated as in a traditional blockchain. Consequently, the execution time of *Block1* was the minimum, the execution time of *Block2* was average, and the execution time of *Block* was the maximum. Figure 5 shows the total execution time for the traditional blockchain and modified blockchain, where the modified blockchain reduced the execution time by about 49% since about 33% of blocks were the *Block1* type, about 33% of blocks were the *Block2* type, and about 33% of blocks were the *Block* type, while all blocks of the traditional blockchain were the *Block* type.

In addition, Figure 6 illustrates the detailed execution time for the validation process of the read and update transactions for *Block1*, *Block2*, and *block*. It shows how relaxation reduced the execution time. Actually, for *Block1*, it only checked the hash for the block, since the transactions came from trusted executers. The same thing applied to read transactions in *Block2*, but for update transactions, it validated each transaction, then checked the hash for the block. For *block*, it validated each transaction (both the read and update ones) and the hash for the block.

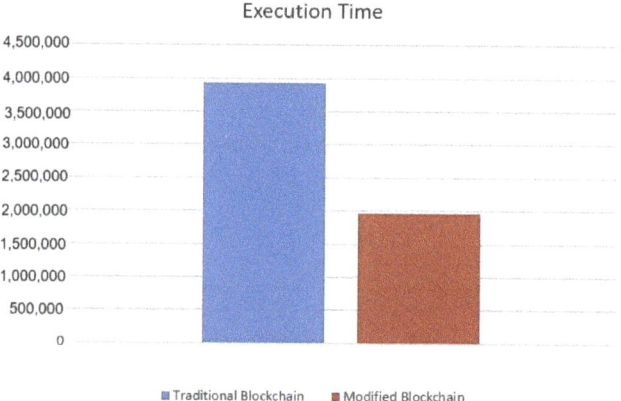

Figure 5. Total execution time for the traditional blockchain and modified blockchain.

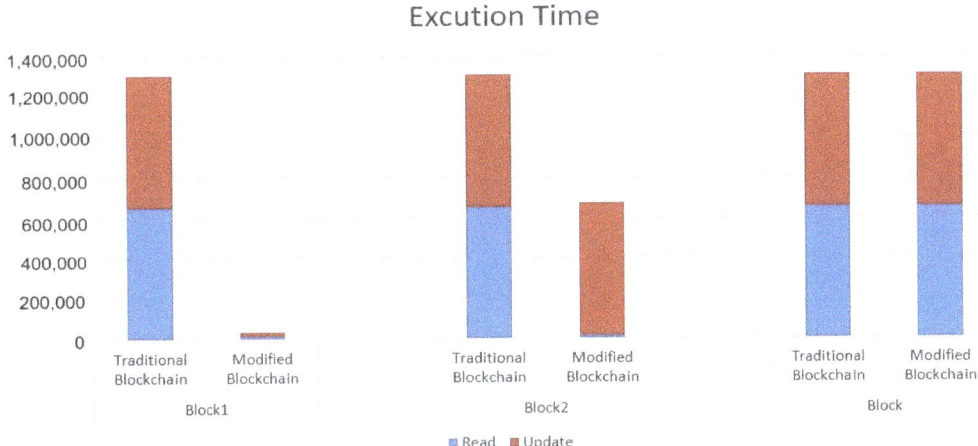

Figure 6. The detailed execution time for the validation process of read and write transactions within Block1, Block2, and Block using a traditional blockchain and a modified blockchain.

5.2. Numrical Analysis for the Number of Messages

The decentralization characteristic of a blockchain requires a large number of messages. In fact, the miner node sends the proposed block to all other nodes for validation; say n nodes require n messages. Then, every node validates the proposed block and sends the vote to all others (excluding itself), which costs $n(n-1)$ messages. After that, every node calculates the majority of votes and send the consensus decision to all others (excluding itself), which costs another $n(n-1)$ messages. The number of messages for this blockchain process is presented below:

$$b(n + (2(n(n-1)))) \tag{1}$$

where b is the total number of blocks and n is the number of nodes.

The modified blockchain reduces the validation process as well as the number of validators for *Block1* to the minimum—say, only three nodes (in our proposal).

It also reduces the number of validators for *Block2* to the average—say only six nodes (in our proposal)—while the number of validators for *Block* will be ten for both the traditional and the modified blockchain. Using our experiment's specifications, there were 4000 *TrustedT1* (both reads and updates), 4000 *TrustedT2* (both reads and updates) and 4000 *T* (both reads and updates). Since the block size was 50 transactions, there were 80 *Block1*, 80 *Block2*, and 80 *Block*. Figure 7a shows the relationship between the number of messages and the number of nodes where the number of blocks was constant (50 blocks). It highlights the total number of messages for *Block1*, which was 1200 messages; 5280 messages for *block2*; and 15,200 messages for *Block*. By increasing the number of nodes, the number of messages increased exponentially. Figure 7b demonstrates the relationship between the number of messages and number of blocks where the number of nodes was constant (10 nodes). By increasing the number of blocks, the number of messages increased linearly.

Figure 8, illustrates the total number of messages the modified blockchain which includes 80 *Block1*, 80 *Block2* and 80 *Block*, 240 total. It also shows the total number of messages for the traditional blockchain that includes 240 blocks of type *Block*. Obviously, the total number of messages using modified blockchain is reduced by about 53% compared to the traditional blockchain model.

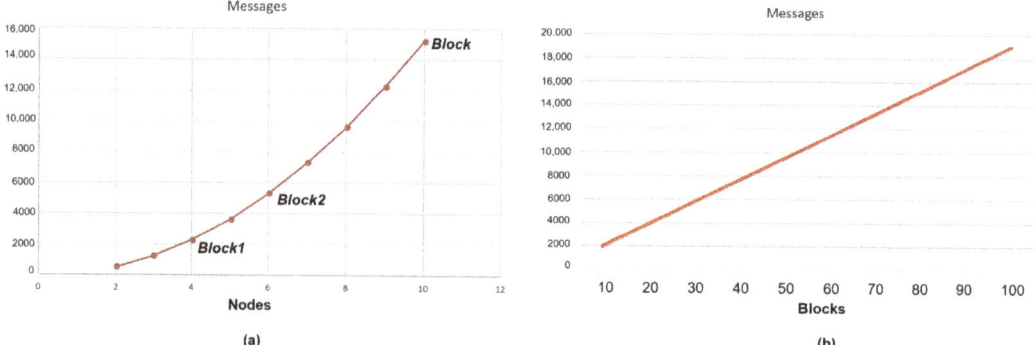

Figure 7. (a) Shows the Relationship between Number of Messages and Number of Nodes where the Number of Blocks is Constant, Highlighting the Number of Messages for Block1, Block2 and Block; (b) Shows the Relationship between Number of Messages and Number of Blocks where the Number of Nodes is Constant.

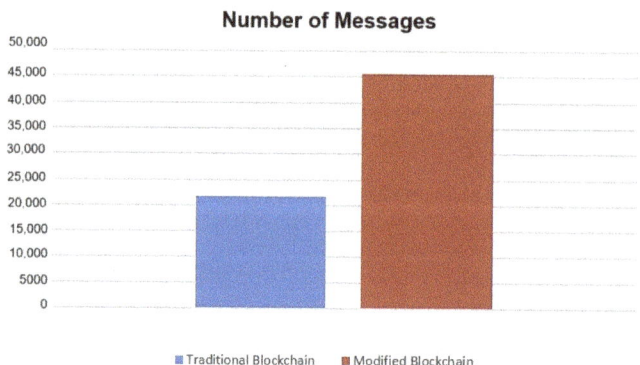

Figure 8. The number of messages using traditional blockchain and modified blockchain.

6. Discussion

This section discusses blockchain technology in general, as well as the proposed modified blockchain that is illustrated in this work. It also discusses the IoT and wearable device specifications which may enhance our model.

6.1. Decentralization

One of the main characteristics of using blockchain technology is decentralization, where the blockchain eliminates the central authority, since every node and device in the blockchain network can generate data and all decisions are made according to the consensus. This allows for fault tolerance, as it does not have a single point of failure. This means the system keeps running even if there are some faulty or failed components. In addition, every node in the blockchain has an up-to-date copy of the data, which helps to avoid centralized data storage. Actually, this supports data availability, accessibility, and recovery if needed [20]. However, it costs more space, time, computation, communication, and energy to manage the data's consistency.

6.2. Security

Another important feature of blockchain technology is security, which also includes authentication, authorization, and privacy. The structure of a blockchain allows us to have multiple copies of data ledgers, which facilitates discovery and recovery in case of data misusing or corruption issues. Every block in the ledger is secured through a hash number that considers the content of the current block and the hash of the previous block in the ledger. This prevents any change in the ledger or the blocks as the chain of the hash numbers is changed, which can be directly discovered, and the approval of such a change is reached through consensus, which makes it impossible.

Moreover, a blockchain allows direct communication between any two nodes, which helps to authenticate every communication. The authentication is performed using smart contracts and encryption. Smart contracts include some conditions, and if those conditions are satisfied, specific actions are taken. It is an automatic code that is immutable (cannot be changed) and distributed (so every node knows the actions it takes) [26]. In our model, every node and device in the blockchain has a unique ID, authority, privilege, and role, which are listed in a smart contract. Upon any communication, the nodes or devices authenticate each other through smart contract. This also helps to validate whether the communication or the requested action is authorized. This is implemented using a private or public key, which allows for validated authorization of access or updates to any data. This guarantees privacy and control. Furthermore, the transferred data and patient identities are encrypted for privacy purposes. In fact, according to the healthcare specifications, there are different levels of data sensitivity, and there are specific considerations for some patients, such as some governmental or military officials. Thus, different levels of security protocols, encryption techniques, and privacy procedures can be applied.

6.3. Performance

It is important to discuss the performance in cases of applying blockchains in healthcare systems. As mentioned earlier, applying blockchain technology has a negative impact on the space, as a copy of the data is attached to every node. It also costs a large number of messages exchanges to perform blockchain tasks such as proposing, voting, and consensus. In addition, the cost of computation increases as a result of decentralization, in which every validator runs validation processes and processes for consensus calculations [1].

On the other hand, the use of blockchain technology results in many advantages that enhance its performance. In fact, having direct communication among nodes and devices speeds up communication. In addition, having smart contracts within a blockchain enables the automation of processes and actions. In fact, smart contracts and consensus decisions both give more reliability to blockchain technology. Another vital advantage of blockchain technology is scalability, where large numbers of IoT sensors, wearable devices, users' devices, and others can be adapted. Blockchains also facilitate the management, coordination, and cooperation of heterogeneous components within systems. One of the main advantages is the ability to manage the components and identities of users, processes, services and ownerships. Those elements interweave many processes and are subject to change over time, which is a challenging task.

Moreover, the procedures of validation in blockchains clearly challenge attempts at manipulation. Such features reduce the chances of aborting transactions and blocks, which improves the performance, since these abortions waste execution time. Indeed, all aborted transactions should be rolled back and re-executed again. Some studies have shown that the abortion of read transactions costs about 80% of the total execution time [43].

6.4. Sensors and Wearable Devices

The development of sensors and wearable devices has enhanced their uses in many fields of technology. There are various categories of wearable devices, i.e., clothes like smart shirts, accessories such as watches and earbuds, and embedded wearable devices such as biosensors and smart tattoos. The use of wearable devices has many advantages, such as providing real-time data and responses. It supports data accessibility, availability, automation, and control. On the other hand, wearable devices cause some weaknesses to the systems from the point of view of security, energy, and computation abilities. Actually, most wearable devices use Bluetooth technology for communication, which is considered a vulnerable communication technology from a security perspective. Therefore, it should be supported with advanced security protocols and techniques for key generation, key characteristics, key exchange, and data encryption, as well as to detect malicious and infected devices.

However, having advanced security protocols and techniques is challenged by computation and energy capabilities that are limited as a result of the sizes of wearable devices [15]. In this case, the system should balance the computation and energy capabilities on one side, and security on another side. It also should balance the computation and energy capabilities with the quality of data. Actually, to overcome the challenge of computation, it is recommended to exploit the computation power of other system components or faraway servers [45,46]. It could also outsource the computation and processing tasks in case the data are not sensitive. Moreover, for energy consumption, there are different kinds of energy technology that can be involved in enhancing wearable devices, such as renewable energy that comes from nature (e.g., sun, wind, and body temperature).

6.5. Risk Management

At the end this discussion, it is important to highlight risk management for the modified blockchain model. Firstly, blockchain technology promises to change centralized management by enforcing democratic decision-making techniques through data sharing and voting. However, the modified blockchain model satisfies healthcare specifications by reducing data sharing and voting in response to the authority level and case sensitivity. Such a reduction risks the reliability of the decision-making. Secondly, people's identities are another critical issue, as hiding the identities of doctors would hide their authority levels, which would risk the relaxation of the validation process. Thirdly, using security techniques such as hashing and encryption risks delays data accessibility, which is critical in some healthcare cases. Fourthly, the cultural resistance to the new methods of processing and management that restrict privileges is another challenge. Finally, the automation of data access, processing, communication, and voting is very difficult to adopt in some areas of healthcare system because it may risk lives.

7. Conclusions

Blockchains are a promising type of technology to be applied in healthcare systems. This work introduces a modified model of a blockchain to enhance e-healthcare with blockchain advantages. This work investigates healthcare and transaction specifications to modify the blockchain model. Indeed, it proposes different kinds of transactions and blocks which enable different levels of processing, validation, and security. This allows us to improve the performance, to increase efficiency, and to reduce costs. For future work, it is still challenging to compromise blockchain reliability to reduce time and communication costs. Moreover, it is important to develop a blockchain model that reduces space complexity and energy consumption. It also should enhance wearable device security and computation abilities. These fields will need to discover specific techniques for such improvements.

Funding: This research received no external funding.

Acknowledgments: We would like to acknowledge the assistance of Medical College members at Jazan University for the fruitful sessions of discussions that helped us in understanding and analyzing the roles, authority, data, and processing of healthcare systems.

Conflicts of Interest: The author declares no conflict of interest.

References

1. Assiri, B. October. Leader Election and Blockchain Algorithm in Cloud Environment for E-Health. In Proceedings of the 2019 2nd International Conference on new Trends in Computing Sciences (ICTCS), Amman, Jordan, 9–11 October 2019; pp. 1–6.
2. Kuo, M.H. Opportunities and challenges of cloud computing to improve health care services. *J. Med. Internet Res.* **2011**, *13*, e1867. [CrossRef] [PubMed]

3. Dinh, H.T.; Lee, C.; Niyato, D.; Wang, P. A survey of mobile cloud computing: Architecture, applications, and approaches. *Wirel. Commun. Mob. Comput.* **2013**, *13*, 1587–1611. [CrossRef]
4. Ghosh, P.K.; Chakraborty, A.; Hasan, M.; Rashid, K.; Siddique, A.H. Blockchain application in healthcare systems: A review. *Systems* **2023**, *11*, 38. [CrossRef]
5. Xu, J.; Wang, C.; Jia, X. A survey of blockchain consensus protocols. *ACM Comput. Surv.* **2023**, *55*, 278. [CrossRef]
6. Guo, H.; Yu, X. A survey on blockchain technology and its security. *Blockchain Res. Appl.* **2022**, *3*, 100067. [CrossRef]
7. Assiri, B.; Khan, W.Z. Fair and trustworthy: Lock-free enhanced tendermint blockchain algorithm. *TELKOMNIKA (Telecommun. Comput. Electron. Control)* **2020**, *18*, 2224–2234. [CrossRef]
8. Subhan, F.; Mirza, A.; Su'ud, M.B.M.; Alam, M.M.; Nisar, S.; Habib, U.; Iqbal, M.Z. AI-enabled wearable medical internet of things in healthcare system: A survey. *Appl. Sci.* **2023**, *13*, 1394. [CrossRef]
9. Lee, Y.H.; Medioni, G. RGB-D camera based wearable navigation system for the visually impaired. *Comput. Vis. Image Underst.* **2016**, *149*, 3–20. [CrossRef]
10. Jawale, A.S.; Park, J.S. A security analysis on apple pay. In Proceedings of the 2016 European Intelligence and Security Informatics Conference (EISIC), Uppsala, Sweden, 17–19 August 2016; pp. 160–163.
11. Borowski-Beszta, M.; Polasik, M. Wearable devices: New quality in sports and finance. *J. Phys. Educ. Sport* **2017**, *20*, 1077–1084.
12. Vidal, M.; Turner, J.; Bulling, A.; Gellersen, H. Wearable eye tracking for mental health monitoring. *Comput. Commun.* **2012**, *35*, 1306–1311. [CrossRef]
13. Wijsman, J.; Grundlehner, B.; Liu, H.; Hermens, H.; Penders, J. Towards mental stress detection using wearable physiological sensors. In Proceedings of the 2011 Annual International Conference of the IEEE Engineering in Medicine and Biology Society, Boston, MA, USA, 30 August–3 September 2011; pp. 1798–1801.
14. Tyagi, A.K.; Dananjayan, S.; Agarwal, D.; Thariq Ahmed, H.F. Blockchain—Internet of Things Applications: Opportunities and Challenges for Industry 4.0 and Society 5.0. *Sensors* **2023**, *23*, 947. [CrossRef] [PubMed]
15. Yugank, H.K.; Sharma, R.; Gupta, S.H. An approach to analyse energy consumption of an IoT system. *Int. J. Inf. Technol.* **2022**, *14*, 2549–2558. [CrossRef]
16. Nakamoto, S. *Bitcoin: A Peer-to-Peer Electronic Cash System*. Decentralized Business Review. 2008. p. 21260. Available online: https://bitcoin.org/bitcoin.pdf (accessed on 1 October 2023).
17. Andrianto, Y.; Diputra, Y. The effect of cryptocurrency on investment portfolio effectiveness. *J. Financ. Account.* **2017**, *5*, 229–238. [CrossRef]
18. Akcora, C.G.; Gel, Y.R.; Kantarcioglu, M. Blockchain networks: Data structures of Bitcoin, Monero, Zcash, Ethereum, Ripple, and Iota. *Wiley Interdiscip. Rev. Data Min. Knowl. Discov.* **2022**, *12*, e1436. [CrossRef] [PubMed]
19. Crosby, M.; Pattanayak, P.; Verma, S.; Kalyanaraman, V. Blockchain technology: Beyond bitcoin. *Appl. Innov.* **2016**, *2*, 71.
20. Kuo, T.T.; Kim, H.E.; Ohno-Machado, L. Blockchain distributed ledger technologies for biomedical and health care applications. *J. Am. Med. Inform. Assoc.* **2017**, *24*, 1211–1220. [CrossRef] [PubMed]
21. Chen, Y.; Li, M.; Zhu, X.; Fang, K.; Ren, Q.; Guo, T.; Chen, X.; Li, C.; Zou, Z.; Deng, Y. An improved algorithm for practical byzantine fault tolerance to large-scale consortium chain. *Inf. Process. Manag.* **2022**, *59*, 102884. [CrossRef]
22. Pantelopoulos, A.; Bourbakis, N.G. A survey on wearable sensor-based systems for health monitoring and prognosis. *IEEE Trans. Syst. Man Cybern. Part C* **2009**, *40*, 1–12. [CrossRef]
23. Baig, M.M.; Gholamhosseini, H.; Connolly, M.J. A comprehensive survey of wearable and wireless ECG monitoring systems for older adults. *Med. Biol. Eng. Comput.* **2013**, *51*, 485–495. [CrossRef]
24. Lara, O.D.; Labrador, M.A. A survey on human activity recognition using wearable sensors. *IEEE Commun. Surv. Tutor.* **2012**, *15*, 1192–1209. [CrossRef]
25. Al Sadawi, A.; Hassan, M.S.; Ndiaye, M. A survey on the integration of blockchain with IoT to enhance performance and eliminate challenges. *IEEE Access* **2021**, *9*, 54478–54497. [CrossRef]
26. Liang, X.; Zhao, J.; Shetty, S.; Liu, J.; Li, D. Integrating blockchain for data sharing and collaboration in mobile healthcare applications. In Proceedings of the 2017 IEEE 28th Annual International Symposium on Personal, Indoor, and Mobile Radio Communications (PIMRC), Montreal, QC, Canada, 8–13 October 2017; pp. 1–5.
27. Ometov, A.; Bardinova, Y.; Afanasyeva, A.; Masek, P.; Zhidanov, K.; Vanurin, S.; Sayfullin, M.; Shubin, V.; Komarov, M.; Bezzateev, S. An overview on blockchain for smartphones: State-of-the-art, consensus, implementation, challenges and future trends. *IEEE Access* **2020**, *8*, 103994–104015. [CrossRef]
28. Esposito, C.; De Santis, A.; Tortora, G.; Chang, H.; Choo, K.K.R. Blockchain: A panacea for healthcare cloud-based data security and privacy? *IEEE Cloud Comput.* **2018**, *5*, 31–37. [CrossRef]
29. Assiri, B.; Busch, C. Approximately opaque multi-version permissive transactional memory. In Proceedings of the 2016 45th International Conference on Parallel Processing Workshops (ICPPW), Philadelphia, PA, USA, 16–19 August 2016; pp. 393–402.
30. Arbabi, M.S.; Lal, C.; Veeraragavan, N.R.; Marijan, D.; Nygård, J.F.; Vitenberg, R. A survey on blockchain for healthcare: Challenges, benefits, and future directions. *IEEE Commun. Surv. Tutor.* **2022**, *25*, 386–424. [CrossRef]
31. Shashi, M. Leveraging Blockchain-based electronic health record systems in healthcare 4.0. *Int. J. Innov. Technol. Explor. Eng.* **2022**, *12*, 102407. [CrossRef]
32. Rahimi, N.; Gudapati, S.S.V. Emergence of blockchain technology in the healthcare and insurance industries. In *Blockchain Technology Solutions for the Security of Iot-Based Healthcare Systems*; Academic Press: Cambridge, MA, USA, 2023; pp. 167–182.

33. Ghadge, A.; Bourlakis, M.; Kamble, S.; Seuring, S. Blockchain implementation in pharmaceutical supply chains: A review and conceptual framework. *Int. J. Prod. Res.* **2023**, *61*, 6633–6651. [CrossRef]
34. Shukla, M.; Sethi, D.; Bindal, L.; Mani, K.; Upadhyay, K.; Sharma, M. Patient Monitoring System using Blockchain and IoT Technology. *Recent Adv. Electr. Electron. Eng.* **2023**, *16*, 449–459. [CrossRef]
35. Hawashin, D.; Jayaraman, R.; Salah, K.; Yaqoob, I.; Simsekler, M.C.E.; Ellahham, S. Blockchain-based management for organ donation and transplantation. *IEEE Access* **2022**, *10*, 59013–59025. [CrossRef]
36. Abdu, N.A.A.; Wang, Z. Blockchain Framework for Collaborative Clinical Trials Auditing. *Wirel. Pers. Commun.* **2023**, *132*, 39–65. [CrossRef]
37. Sharma, P.; Namasudra, S.; Chilamkurti, N.; Kim, B.G.; Gonzalez Crespo, R. Blockchain-based privacy preservation for IoT-enabled healthcare system. *ACM Trans. Sens. Netw.* **2023**, *19*, 1–17. [CrossRef]
38. Combi, C.; Pozzi, G.; Veltri, P. (Eds.) *Process Modeling and Management for Healthcare*; CRC Press: Boca Raton, FL, USA, 2017.
39. Bosanac, D.; Stevanovic, A. Trust in E-Health System and Willingness to Share Personal Health Data. In *Informatics and Technology in Clinical Care and Public Health*; IOS Press: Amsterdam, The Netherlands, 2022; pp. 256–259.
40. Calnan, M.; Ferlie, E. Analysing process in healthcare: The methodological and theoretical challenges. *Policy Politics* **2003**, *31*, 185–193. [CrossRef]
41. Samost-Williams, A.; Nanji, K.C. A systems theoretic process analysis of the medication use process in the operating room. *Anesthesiology* **2020**, *133*, 332–341. [CrossRef]
42. Lv, Z.; Qiao, L. Analysis of healthcare big data. *Future Gener. Comput. Syst.* **2020**, *109*, 103–110. [CrossRef]
43. Assiri, B.; Busch, C. Approximate count and queue objects in transactional memory. In Proceedings of the 2017 IEEE International Parallel and Distributed Processing Symposium Workshops (IPDPSW), Lake Buena Vista, FL, USA, 29 May–2 June 2017; pp. 894–903.
44. Numan, M.; Subhan, F.; Khan, W.Z.; Assiri, B.; Armi, N. Well-organized bully leader election algorithm for distributed system. In Proceedings of the 2018 International Conference on Radar, Antenna, Microwave, Electronics, and Telecommunications (ICRAMET), Serpong, Indonesia, 1–2 November 2018; pp. 5–10.
45. Chong, Y.W.; Ismail, W.; Ko, K.; Lee, C.Y. Energy harvesting for wearable devices: A review. *IEEE Sens. J.* **2019**, *19*, 9047–9062. [CrossRef]
46. Rashid, N.; Al Faruque, M.A. Energy-efficient real-time myocardial infarction detection on wearable devices. In Proceedings of the 2020 42nd Annual International Conference of the IEEE Engineering in Medicine & Biology Society (EMBC), Montreal, QC, Canada, 20–24 July 2020; pp. 4648–4651.

Disclaimer/Publisher's Note: The statements, opinions and data contained in all publications are solely those of the individual author(s) and contributor(s) and not of MDPI and/or the editor(s). MDPI and/or the editor(s) disclaim responsibility for any injury to people or property resulting from any ideas, methods, instructions or products referred to in the content.

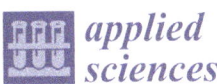

Article

The Centralization and Sharing of Information for Improving a Resilient Approach Based on Decision-Making at a Local Home Health Care Center

Guillaume Dessevre [1,*], Cléa Martinez [1], Liwen Zhang [1,2], Christophe Bortolaso [2] and Franck Fontanili [1]

1. Industrial Engineering Center, IMT Mines Albi, 81000 Albi, France; clea.martinez@mines-albi.fr (C.M.); liwen.zhang@berger-levrault.com (L.Z.); franck.fontanili@mines-albi.fr (F.F.)
2. Berger-Levrault, 31670 Labège, France; christophe.bortolaso@berger-levrault.com
* Correspondence: guillaume.dessevre@mines-albi.fr

Featured Application: In this article, we propose a resilient approach toward the centralization and sharing of information for improving the decision-making of caregivers in local healthcare centers in addition to reducing the number of late arrivals, the total time of late arrivals, and the number of routes ending after the work end time. Coupled with a connected IT tool, such as a smartphone application, this approach would improve the working lives of caregivers.

Abstract: Home care centers face both an increase in demand and many variations during the execution of routes, compromising the routes initially planned; robust solutions are not effective enough, and it is necessary to move on to resilient approaches. We create a close-to-reality use case supported by interviews of staff at home health care centers, where caregivers are faced with unexpected events that compromise their initial route. We model, analyze, and compare two resilient approaches to deal with these disruptions: a distributed collaborative approach and a centralized collaborative approach, where we propose a centralization and sharing of information to improve local decision-making. The latter reduces the number of late arrivals by 11%, the total time of late arrival by 21%, and halves the number of routes exceeding the end of work time (contrary to the distributed collaborative approach due to the time wasted reaching colleagues). The use of a device, such as a smartphone application, to centralize and share information thus, allows better mutual assistance between caregivers. Moreover, we highlight several possible openings, like the coupling of simulation and optimization, to propose a more resilient approach.

Keywords: home health care routing and scheduling problem; resilience; information sharing; discrete event simulation; optimization

Citation: Dessevre, G.; Martinez, C.; Zhang, L.; Bortolaso, C.; Fontanili, F. The Centralization and Sharing of Information for Improving a Resilient Approach Based on Decision-Making at a Local Home Health Care Center. *Appl. Sci.* **2023**, *13*, 8576. https://doi.org/10.3390/app13158576

Academic Editor: Roger Narayan

Received: 16 May 2023
Revised: 13 July 2023
Accepted: 18 July 2023
Published: 25 July 2023

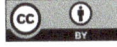

Copyright: © 2023 by the authors. Licensee MDPI, Basel, Switzerland. This article is an open access article distributed under the terms and conditions of the Creative Commons Attribution (CC BY) license (https:// creativecommons.org/licenses/by/ 4.0/).

1. Introduction

Thanks to scientific developments and concurrent improvements in healthcare, hygiene, nutrition, and social conditions, the life expectancy of humans has consistently increased in the developed world over the last century, coupled with a steadily declining birth rate over the course of recent decades, has resulted in an increasingly aging population. In 2020, 20% of the French population was over 60 years old in France, and according to the *Institut National de la Statistique et des Etudes Economiques*, this will rise to 30% by 2070 [1]. In addition, there is a desire to reduce the demand for medical structures (e.g., hospitals), exerting pressure on people to return home as quickly as possible. As a result, the demand for home health care services has increased sharply in recent years, as well as the number of studies on this topic.

In the scientific literature, the management of home care routes is known as the Home Health Care Routing and Scheduling Problem (HHCRSP) and has been studied for fifty years [2]. The goal is to find the best possible routes according to the characteristics of the problem, e.g., strategies to minimize travel times, maximize the stakeholders' satisfaction, take time windows and difficulty of care visit provisions into consideration, etc. Although the variability of HHCRSP systems is increasingly under scrutiny, most studies are carried out in a deterministic environment. For the past five years, an ever-growing number of publications have considered uncertainties, especially for travel times and visit times. Robust approaches build efficient solutions as long as the uncertainties are bound within a defined interval [3], whereas resilient approaches propose policies to recover after a disruption. In the vehicle routing literature, stochastic routing problems are often tackled with robust approaches, such as chance-constrained programming (CCP), or resilient approaches, such as stochastic programming with recourse (SPR). Gendreau et al. [4] argue that the objective functions in SPRs are more relevant than CCPs in solving a stochastic VRP. Moreover, a typical concern with robust approaches is that they can be too conservative and thus too far from optimality for the nominal problem [5]. That is why robust solutions are effective against small variations but become useless against strong disruptions; it is then necessary to turn to resilient approaches. The study of resilient approaches to counter high-impact disruptions remains one of the gaps to be filled in the spectrum of HHCRSP publications. In addition, it is difficult to find a clear, realistic, and readily available use case in the scientific literature.

The aim of this paper is to analyze and compare the performance of resilient approaches applied to a use case close to reality, open to the scientific community, and inspired by home health care centers in the department of Tarn (France) in an environment subject to both variations and high-impact disruptions. Two different approaches are analyzed and compared to a baseline approach using discrete event simulations, including an empirical approach modeling what is done today in the home health care centers interviewed and a new approach based on the centralization and sharing of information between caregivers to improve local decision-making. The two main contributions of the article are (1) creating a realistic case study based on home health care center interviews and making it available to the scientific community and (2) proposing a resilient approach based on the centralization and sharing of information for improving local decision-making when routes are disrupted.

This paper is organized as follows: Section 2 is dedicated to the review of literature on publications related to the topic. Then, Section 3 describes the use case and the design of experiments (resilient approaches and disruptions). Section 4 presents the results and analysis. Finally, Section 5 concludes and proposes avenues for further research.

2. Literature Review

The HHCRSP is a highly pertinent issue and is widely studied in the literature, as evidenced by the numerous state-of-the-art published recently [6,7]. In this section, we present an overview of the existing work to contextualize our contribution.

HHCRSP problems cover a wide range of constraints and objectives. They may include typical features of Vehicle Routing Problems (VRPs), such as time windows (hard or soft) [8] and temporal dependencies (precedence, synchronization, or disjunction) [9], but also more specific features related to the field such as continuity of care [10], skill requirements [11], or incompatibilities [12]. The objective is often cost-related, whether it comes to minimizing travel costs or staffing costs [13,14] or is stakeholder-oriented [8].

As a variant of VRP, approaches seeking to address the issues around HHCRSP are manifold. In small instances, exact methods are developed, e.g., mathematical programming [15], logic-based Benders decomposition [16], branch-and-price-and-cut [17], etc. Larger instances are generally solved with classic metaheuristics or approximation algorithms from the operations research field, such as population-based algorithms [18], neighborhood searches [19], and decomposition methods [20].

In practice, caregivers encounter various problems during their route that can impact the remainder of their working day. Hence, deterministic approaches do not enable us to capture the whole complexity of the HHCRSP, at least not at the operational decision-making level. There are an increasing number of articles currently assessing the HHCRSP in view of various types of uncertainties (e.g., stochastic travel times or visit times, patient cancellations, emergencies, vehicle breakdown, etc.) and propose robust or resilient solutions: visits have an expected duration but can last longer [21] or they are normally distributed [11], and travel times are estimated with a kernel regression, for example [22].

In this paper, we focus on two forms of uncertainties regarding visit and travel times: small *variations* due to the stochasticity of the data and more punctual but also more impactful *disruptions*, such as traffic jams. The robustness of a system is defined as the ability "to maintain its function despite internal or external disruption" [23], whereas resilience is "the ability of a system to return to its original state, within an acceptable period of time, after being disturbed" [24]. A *robust* solution is, therefore, used to absorb a *variation*, and a *resilient* approach is used to counter *disruption*. As represented in Figure 1, a robust solution in blue on the left absorbs the variations (represented by σ in orange) around the mean value μ, so these variations do not affect the performance indicators on the bottom, which are protected by this solution. On the right, the disruption has an impact on these indicators, and that is why a resilient approach is necessary to return to a "normal" operating state.

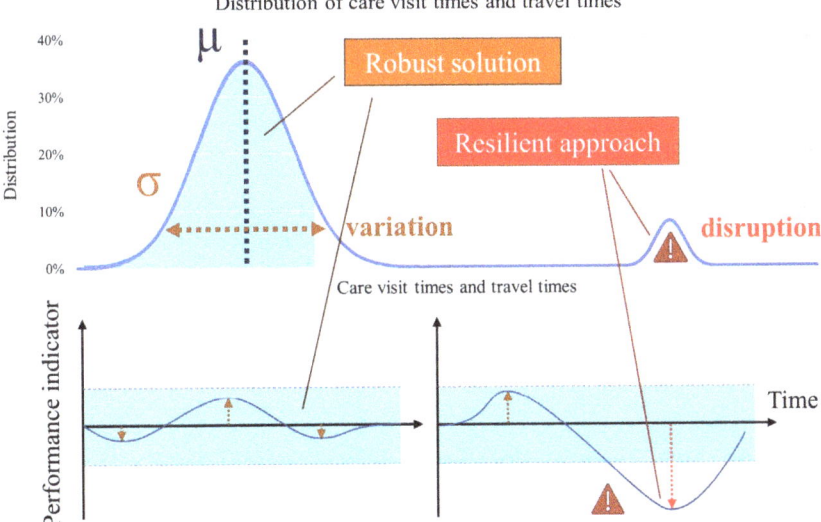

Figure 1. Difference between variation and disruption and between robust solution and resilient approach.

These uncertainties can be addressed at different decision-making levels. Nikzad et al. propose a two-stage stochastic programming model to tackle both uncertain visit and travel times [25], and Zhan et al. propose a mixed-integer linear program and adapt the L-shaped method to solve the HHCRSP with stochastic visit times [26]. Another option to deal with uncertainties is to anticipate different disrupted scenarios and build robust solutions; in the study by Shi et al., each visit and travel time belongs to an uncertainty set based on the theory of budget uncertainty [27]. Since their solutions to the deterministic problem are not robust, they adapt several classic heuristics to build a solution that always remains feasible, despite visit and travel time uncertainties. Cappanera et al. also choose a robust method to study uncertain demands from the patients and illustrate the need for a trade-off between a deterministic optimal solution that is particularly susceptible to any small disruption and an extremely robust solution that is very expensive and often "underused" [28].

Resilient approaches must then be deployed at the operational level to repair the routes in the case of high-impact disruption. Among the classic recourse strategies for stochastic VRP, most of them imply a return to the depot [29], which is not helpful for HHCRSP. Similarly, rescheduling strategies for routing problems may not be suited to HHC applications; Errico et al. study two alternative strategies to solve a VRP with time windows and stochastic service times, which both imply skipping customers [30]. To the best of our knowledge, only three articles propose reactive and resilient solutions to counter high-impact disruptions in the field of HHC. Alves et al. use a multi-agent system to deal with unexpected events, such as vehicle breakdown, where visits are dynamically reassigned to another vehicle [31]. Marcon et al. use a similar two-level architecture with an offline module that assigns caregivers to patients and an online multi-agent module that takes local decisions to optimize the routes [32]. No change in the caregiver–patient assignment is allowed, which prevents any collaboration in case of disruption, and none of these two articles take into account time windows. Yet, we consider temporal constraints as a key element to HHCRSP because delays in care delivery may not only have an impact on the quality of care but also on the satisfaction of the patient. In the study by Yuan et al., patients can cancel their appointments or require new visits during the execution of the routes, so they are re-optimized in real-time with a tabu-search, with the objective of minimizing deviations from the original plan [33]. The possibility of calling in additional workers and the cancellations of requests guarantee a stable workload. In our article, the perturbations on care durations have a major impact on the workload of the caregivers and, thus, on the feasibility of the routes and the quality of care.

In summary, the HHCRSP has been studied for a long time and increasingly in a stochastic environment, where many robust solutions have been proposed in the literature, but few resilient approaches have been published. Moreover, it is difficult to find a use case that is clear, realistic, and available to the scientific community. For this reason, in this article, we propose to examine a realistic use case, the result of numerous interviews, and we analyze and compare two resilient approaches to a baseline one to counter the disruptions of home care routes.

3. Methods

3.1. Use Case Creation

In order to create a realistic use case to share with the HHCRSP scientific community, the staff at seven home health care or service structures were interviewed in the department of Tarn in France during the months of September and October 2022. The aim was to collect information on the working environment, e.g., operating methods, problems encountered, existing and envisaged solutions, tools used, needs, etc. Having identified the challenges of the home care centers, we decided to create a use case inspired by two of these nursing care structures, which have the following characteristics:

1. There are five caregivers performing five routes;
2. Routes start at 7 a.m. from the health care center and end between 12 p.m. and 1 p.m. at the same location;
3. There are 140 care visits to perform, which are requested by 140 patients (one visit per patient);
4. When the caregivers have finished their routes, they can help their colleagues, if needed, or do administrative tasks at the health care center until 1 p.m.;
5. Travel times are often short (usually less than five minutes) and are triangularly distributed more or less 30% around the average value;
6. Care visit times are generally five minutes but can sometimes last 10 min. They are both subject to variations (such as travel times, with the same distribution) and to disruptions (whose distribution is detailed in the design of experiments);
7. Time windows (i.e., time slot during which the caregiver must begin the care visit) last one hour for each visit;
8. There is an early and late tolerance of five minutes, and if the caregiver arrives more than five minutes early, then they must wait before starting the care visit;

9. The website "https://geodatamine.fr/ (accessed on 7 February 2023)" was used to generate random and unidentifiable addresses for patients (e.g., businesses, churches, parking spaces, etc.) around the city of Carmaux (France); the map is presented in Figure 2 on the left (1) where the library *folium* in Python was used to place the patients on a Leaflet map. The health care center was indicated in the city, and the 140 other addresses were randomly distributed to the patients. The website "https://openrouteservice.org/ (accessed on 7 February 2023)" was used by a query in a Python script to create a matrix of real travel times between patients.

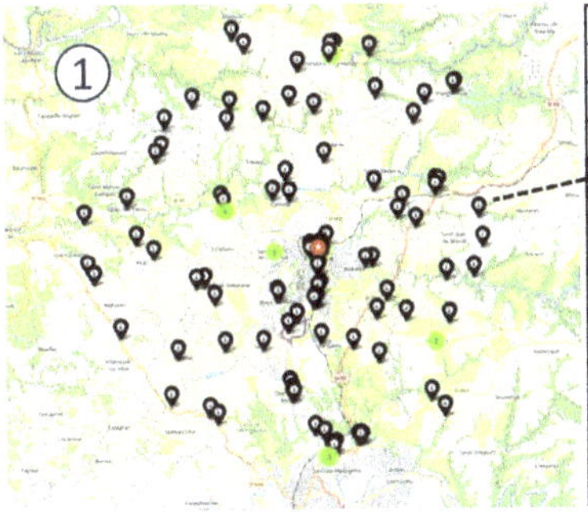

# CareVisit	# Patient	Duration	Time Window	
1	1	5	420	480
2	2	5	600	660
3	3	5	540	600
4	4	10	690	750
5	5	5	600	660
6	6	5	630	690
7	7	5	420	480
8	8	5	420	480
9	9	10	630	690
10	10	10	660	720
11	11	5	630	690
...	...	...	...	...

Figure 2. Map of the surroundings of Carmaux with the patients (in black) and the health care center (in red) on the **left** and examples of care visits with durations and time windows on the **right**.

There are two types of visits: the short visits of 5 min, which represent 75% of the visits, and the long visits lasting 10 min (Figure 2, (2)). Thus, 106 care visits last 5 min, distributed randomly among the patients, and the other 34 last 10 min.

Finally, the time windows must be determined for each visit (Figure 2, (3)). There are 11 possible time windows between 7 a.m. and 1 p.m. (7 a.m.–8 a.m., 7:30 a.m.–8:30 a.m., 11:30 a.m.–12:30 p.m., and 12 p.m.–1 p.m.), evenly distributed among the visits in order to find feasible and realistic solutions.

The map, the coordinates of the addresses, and the care visits file are available in the data archive available at "http://dx.doi.org/10.13140/RG.2.2.28201.98402 (accessed on 15 May 2023)" (Supplementary Material).

3.2. Home Health Care

The discrete-event simulation was chosen as the tool-based method, as it allows complex environments with several sources of variability to be easily modeled and analyzed [34].

The simulation model, represented in Figure 3, is built as follows: (1) the five caregivers are created, and their attributes are assigned to them, then they retrieve the information for their next visit; (2) if they have finished their route, they go back to the center, or they help their colleagues (not represented here, more details in the next subsection); if not (3), the travel time to the next patient is calculated; (4) if the caregiver arrives more than 5 min early at the patient's address, the total number of early arrivals is incremented, and the caregivers wait. If they arrive more than 5 min late, the total number of late arrivals is incremented; and (5) the care visit is carried out before they move on to the next patient.

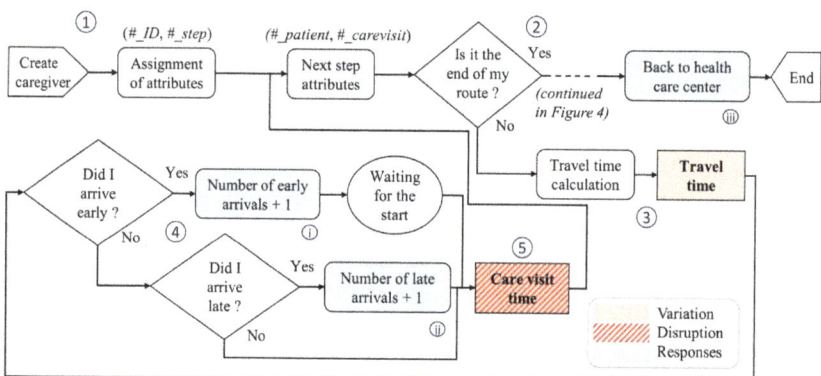

Figure 3. Representation of the main simulation model.

The performance measures of the model are (i) the total number of early arrivals and the cumulative early arrival time; (ii) the total number of late arrivals and the cumulative late arrival time; and (iii) the end time of each route (knowing that a caregiver must normally finish before 1 p.m.).

3.3. Design of Experiments

The Design of Experiments (DoEs) consists of three dimensions detailed below: the three approaches, the different disruptions, and the schedule solutions.

3.3.1. The Resilient Approaches

Two different resilient approaches, as represented in Figure 4 as a complement to the previous figure, are compared to a baseline approach without any collaboration: a distributed collaborative approach (the one used today by the interviewed nursing care structures) and a centralized collaborative approach.

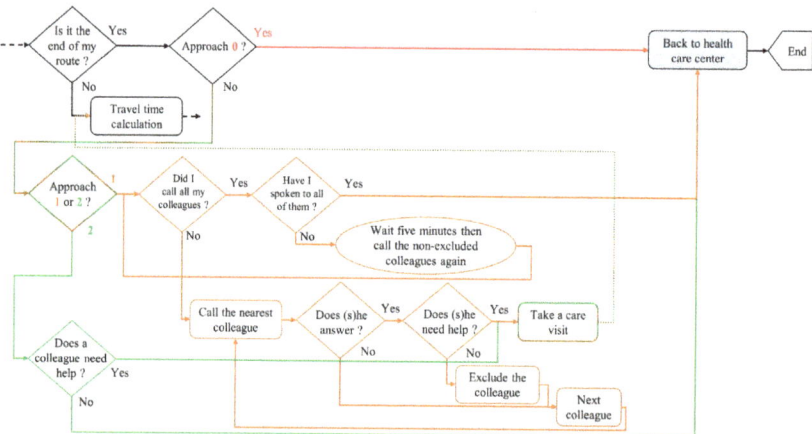

Figure 4. Decision-making algorithm modeling the two resilient approaches and the baseline.

In the baseline approach (named "approach 0" because it is not a resilient approach and is represented in red), there is no cooperation between the caregivers; when a caregiver finishes their route, they return to the health care center to carry out administrative tasks.

In the distributed collaborative approach (named "approach 1" and represented in orange), when a caregiver finishes their route, they try to reach their colleagues to help them. The caregiver knows each colleague's work areas and, therefore, starts by calling those closest to them. A colleague does not answer the call if they are out on a care visit unless the latter is disrupted, whereas a colleague who is driving will always respond using a hands-free kit. If the colleague does not answer the call, the caregiver moves on to the next closest individual. Otherwise, they ask them if they need help (i.e., if they are late because they experienced a disruption during their route). If this is the case, they will take a care visit from them; otherwise, they will remove this colleague from the list and move on to the next one. If they have called and spoken to all their colleagues, they go back to the health care center to carry out administrative tasks. Otherwise, they wait five minutes and call their colleagues who are still on the list again.

In the centralized collaborative approach (named "approach 2" and represented in green), the information is centralized and easily available to everyone. Using a device (e.g., a smartphone application), a caregiver knows directly if their colleagues need help and where they are. If this is the case, they will take a care visit; otherwise, they go back to the health care center to carry out administrative tasks.

Finally, for the two approaches, 1 and 2, there are three possible sub-approaches. These sub-approaches are subsequently named X-1, X-2, and X-3, where X = approach 1 or 2. For X-1 approaches, when a colleague needs help, the available caregiver will take the next care visit closest to them. For X-2, they will take the next care visit indicated on the route, regardless of their distance from the patient. And for X-3, they will take the last care visit on the route.

The three approaches (baseline and the two resilient ones) and the three sub-approaches are summarized in Table 1.

Table 1. Approaches and sub-approaches with their name.

Approaches	
0	Baseline (not a resilient approach)
1-X	Distributed collaborative approach (existing)
2-X	Centralized collaborative approach (innovative)
Sub-approaches	*When I help a colleague, which care visit should I take?*
X-1	The closest to me
X-2	Next on the schedule
X-3	The last of the schedule

3.3.2. The Disruptions

According to the interviews, the disruptions encountered generally last one hour; if a patient dies, for example, a doctor, the family, and the funeral directors must be advised, and the caregivers have to wait until the patient is taken care of, or if a patient is drunk, the caregiver must wait until the patient is sober again to prevent injury.

To first analyze the impact of the variation, a first scenario without variation or disruption was modeled, as well as a second scenario by adding only the variations (modeled by a triangular distribution at ±30% around the mean value).

Then, four disruption scenarios were created: a case with a single one-hour disruption, a case with two 30-min disruptions, a case with two one-hour disruptions, and a case with one two-hour disruption. The disruptions are uniformly distributed among the patients for each replication.

3.3.3. The Schedule Solution

Two schedule solutions were compared: (1) a handmade schedule, as is the case in the health care centers interviewed and (2) an optimized schedule based on the simplified OptaPlanner-oriented model presented by Zhang et al. [35], with the utilization of one embedded "Late Acceptance" metaheuristic for solution generation. The considered constraint is the respect for time windows (to limit the number of late or early arrivals), and the objective function was to minimize travel times.

For the two solutions, represented in Figure 5, the average occupation rates of the caregivers without disruption are 90% and 87%, respectively. The occupation rate includes travel times and care visit times, with the latter representing 55% of the occupation rate on average.

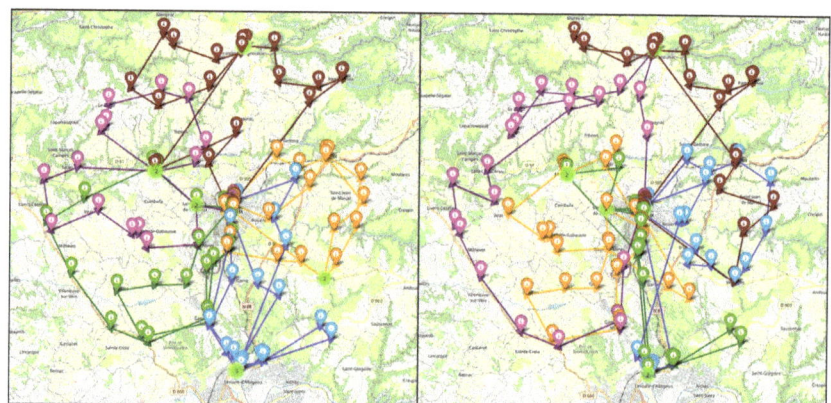

Figure 5. The five routes of the handmade schedule solution on the **left** and the optimized schedule solution on the **right**.

Thus, the DoE is made of 2 × (2 + 7 × 4) = 60 scenarios: two schedule solutions times two scenarios without disruption, plus seven resilient approaches times four scenarios with disruptions.

To ensure that we had significant results, we sought the number of replications necessary for each disruption (i.e., each disturbed patient by an unforeseen event) using the confidence interval method from [36]. Initially, 1000 replications for the same disturbed patient are carried out, where the output data were the total time of late arrival, and the percentage deviation of the confidence interval about the mean time of late arrival is calculated using Equation (1):

$$d = t_{n-1,\alpha/2} \frac{S}{X \times \sqrt{n}} \quad (1)$$

where:

X = average total time of late arrival;
S = standard deviation of the output data from the replications;
n = number of replications;
$t_{n-1,\alpha/2}$ = value from Student's t-distribution, with $n-1$ degree of freedom and a significance level of $\alpha/2$.

We chose a significance level α of 2.5% (i.e., there is a 97.5% probability that the value of the true mean lies within the confidence interval), and we sought a percentage deviation of a maximum of 2.5%. The percentage deviation depending on the number of replications for the first 150 replications is presented in Figure 6.

According to the calculation of the percentage deviation, it takes at least 85 replications per scenario. Therefore, in order to obtain significant and homogeneous results, we performed 100 replications for each scenario (i.e., disturbed patient), which is a total of 14,000 replications since there are 140 patients.

The model and the simulations were made using Python scripts to facilitate the exchange between the different files and applications.

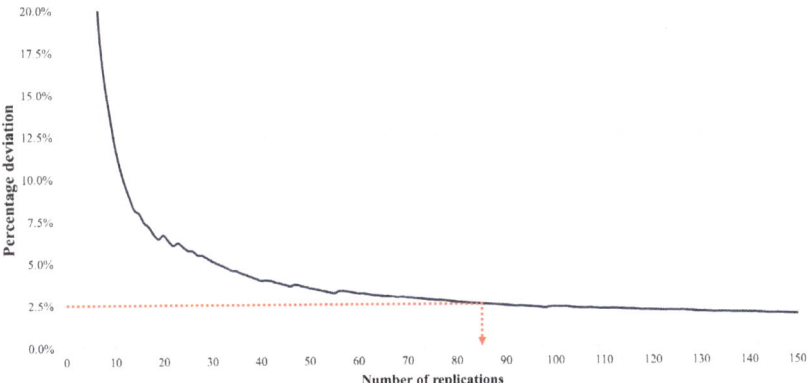

Figure 6. Percentage deviation of the confidence interval about the mean time of late arrival depending on the number of replications where the red arrow shows the number of replications needed.

4. Results

All the results are available in the data archive. For reasons of space, and as it is the most likely outcome, only results on late arrivals for a scenario with a single one-hour disruption are presented in Figure 7. The baseline and the resilient approaches are on the abscissa, the mean total numbers of late arrivals are on the left, the mean total times of late arrival are on the right, and the results for the handmade schedule are hatched, unlike those for the optimized schedule.

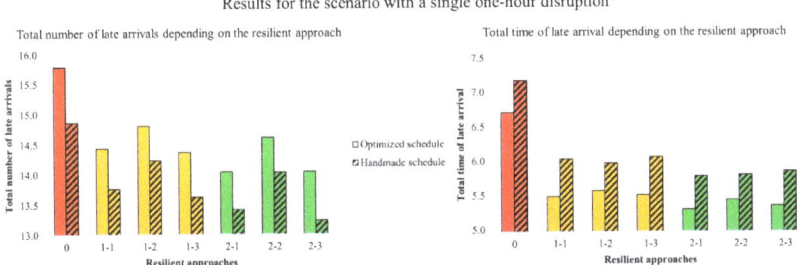

Figure 7. Number of late arrivals (on the **left**) and total time of late arrival (on the **right**) depending on the resilient approach—Scenario with a single one-hour disruption.

The approach 0 in red presents the worst performances: 15.8 late arrivals on average (i.e., 11.3% of care visits are late), with a total of 6.7 h of late arrival in the optimized schedule as well as 14.9 late arrivals and 7.2 h in the handmade schedule. Overall, the two other approaches (in yellow and green) are better, with the X-1 sub-approaches yielding the best results. With approach 1-1, the number of late arrivals is reduced by 9% in the optimized schedule (7% in the handmade one), with the total time of late arrival reduced by 18% (16% in the case of the handmade one). With approach 2-1, the number of late arrivals is reduced by 11% in the optimized schedule (10% in the handmade one), with the total time of late arrival reduced by 21% (19% in the case of the handmade one). The 2-1 approach, therefore, improves performance. The X-2 approaches are the worst performing sub-approaches, while the X-3 performs better than the X-1, with regard to the number of late arrivals but not in terms of the total time of late arrival. Finally, there is a slight difference between the two schedule solutions, but the previous remarks are valid for both.

To better understand the effect of the resilient approaches on the route end times, their distribution and cumulative distribution are presented in Figure 8. Since caregivers must finish before 1 p.m., a dashed blue line has been added to the center of each graph.

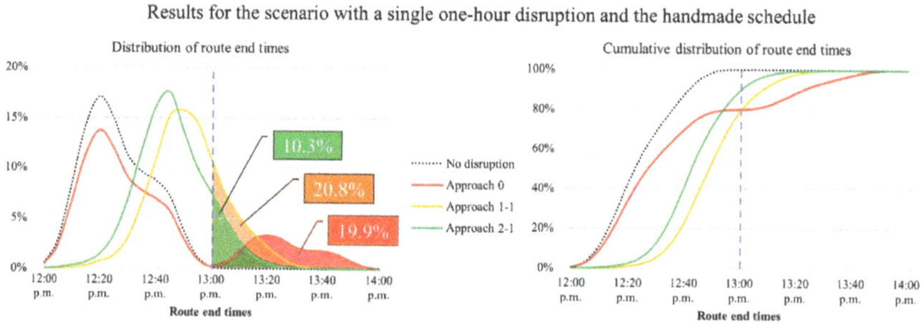

Results for the scenario with a single one-hour disruption and the handmade schedule

Figure 8. Distribution of route end times (on the **left**) and cumulative distribution (on the **right**) for the handmade schedule—Scenario with a single one-hour disruption.

The dotted black curve represents the distribution when there is no disruption: in this case, all routes end before 1 p.m. with an average of 12:24 p.m. With approach 0 in red, the distribution splits into two parts, and 20% of the routes finish after 1 p.m. (this corresponds to the disrupted route out of the five) with an average of 12:36 p.m. With approach 1-1 in yellow, the average rises to 12:50 p.m., with almost 21% of the routes ending after 1 p.m. because of time wasted reaching colleagues. Finally, thanks to approach 2-1 in green, only 10% of the routes go beyond 1 p.m. (i.e., twice less), with the average end time dropping to 12:44 p.m.

Approach 2-1, thus, enables a reduction in the number of late arrivals, the total time of late arrival, and the number of routes ending after 1 p.m.

5. Conclusions and Openings

In this paper, we first created a use case close to reality, which was available to the scientific community working on the HHCRSP. This use case was the result of several interviews with staff at different home health care centers in France. Then, we modeled two different resilient approaches to counter the high-impact disruptions encountered by caregivers on their routes. Hence, we analyzed and compared the existing solution to a baseline approach and a proposal for the centralization and sharing of information to improve local decision-making.

By using discrete event simulation, we showed that the centralized collaborative approach enabled both a reduction in the number of late arrivals and the total time of late arrival, but above, it led to all the number of routes ending before the work end time to be halved (contrary to the distributed collaborative approach). These results hold true, regardless of the number and duration of disruptions we tested, as well as the initial schedule solution (handmade or optimized).

With regard to managerial insights, we recommend that home health care centers:

- Promote the centralization and sharing of information between caregivers to improve mutual aid. The three resilient "2-X" sub-approaches outperform the "1-X" ones according to both the total number of late arrivals, the total time of late arrival, and especially the number of routes finishing before the target end time;
- In cases of mutual assistance between two caregivers, the helper must take the care visit closest to them. Among the three resilient sub-approaches studied, those whose rule is to take the next care visit closest to the helper (the "X-1" sub-approaches) are those that reduce the number of delays and the total time of delay.

To take this line of research further, other resilient approaches are considered, in particular, to improve the response times to disruptions and, thus, reduce recovery time (which we do not discuss in this paper). The coupling of optimization and simulation seems to be a powerful and appropriate tool. Moreover, the simulation plays a double role: firstly, to compare resilient approaches with each other, as is the case here, and secondly, to find a better initial or intermediate schedule solution. Finally, it is also possible to no longer plan the routes but to monitor them in real-time by assigning the care visits on an ongoing basis and taking variations and disruptions in the environment into consideration. However, online scheduling would raise the question of the reliability of real-time communication between the HHC center and the caregivers, which today remains an obstacle to the use of these digital tools in practice.

Supplementary Materials: The following supporting information can be downloaded at: http://dx.doi.org/10.13140/RG.2.2.28201.98402, (Use_Case.zip).

Author Contributions: Literature research, G.D., C.M. and L.Z.; study design, G.D.; data collection, G.D.; data analysis, G.D.; data interpretation, G.D.; writing, G.D., C.M. and L.Z.; supervision, C.B. and F.F.; validation, F.F. All authors have read and agreed to the published version of the manuscript.

Funding: This research was funded by Plan France Relance and Berger-Levrault.

Informed Consent Statement: Informed consent was obtained from all subjects involved in the study.

Conflicts of Interest: The authors declare no conflict of interest.

References

1. INSEE. D'ici 2070, Un Tiers des Régions Perdraient des Habitants—Projections de Population 2018–2070. Available online: https://www.insee.fr/fr/statistiques/6658362 (accessed on 22 March 2023).
2. Fernandez, A.; Gregory, G.; Hindle, A.; Lee, A.C. A Model for Community Nursing in a Rural County. *J. Oper. Res. Soc.* **1974**, *25*, 231–239. [CrossRef]
3. Gabrel, V.; Murat, C.; Thiele, A. Recent advances in robust optimization: An overview. *Eur. J. Oper. Res.* **2014**, *235*, 471–483. [CrossRef]
4. Gendreau, M.; Laporte, G.; Séguin, R. Stochastic vehicle routing. *Eur. J. Oper. Res.* **1996**, *88*, 3–12. [CrossRef]
5. Bertsimas, D.; Sim, M. The Price of Robustness. *Oper. Res.* **2004**, *52*, 35–53. [CrossRef]
6. Cissé, M.; Yalçındağ, S.; Kergosien, Y.; Şahin, E.; Lenté, C.; Matta, A. OR problems related to Home Health Care: A review of relevant routing and scheduling problems. *Oper. Res. Health Care* **2017**, *13–14*, 1–22. [CrossRef]
7. Di Mascolo, M.; Martinez, C.; Espinouse, M.-L. Routing and scheduling in Home Health Care: A literature survey and bibliometric analysis. *Comput. Ind. Eng.* **2021**, *158*, 107255. [CrossRef]
8. Trautsamwieser, A.; Hirsch, P. Optimization of daily scheduling for home health care services. *J. Appl. Oper. Res.* **2011**, *3*, 124–136.
9. Frifita, S.; Masmoudi, M. VNS methods for home care routing and scheduling problem with temporal dependencies, and multiple structures and specialties. *Int. Trans. Oper. Res.* **2020**, *27*, 291–313. [CrossRef]
10. Lahrichi, N.; Lanzarone, E.; Yalçındağ, S. A First Route Second Assign decomposition to enforce continuity of care in home health care. *Expert Syst. Appl.* **2022**, *193*, 116442. [CrossRef]
11. Yuan, B.; Liu, R.; Jiang, Z. A branch-and-price algorithm for the home health care scheduling and routing problem with stochastic service times and skill requirements. *Int. J. Prod. Res.* **2015**, *53*, 7450–7464. [CrossRef]
12. Chaieb, M.; Jemai, J.; Mellouli, K. A decomposition—Construction approach for solving the home health care scheduling problem. *Health Care Manag. Sci.* **2019**, *23*, 264–286. [CrossRef] [PubMed]
13. Bard, J.F.; Shao, Y.; Wang, H. Weekly scheduling models for traveling therapists. *Socioecon. Plann. Sci.* **2013**, *47*, 191–204. [CrossRef]
14. Luna, F.; Cervantes, A.; Isasi, P.; Valenzuela-Valdés, J.F. Grid-enabled evolution strategies for large-scale home care crew scheduling. *Clust. Comput.* **2017**, *21*, 1261–1273. [CrossRef]
15. Liu, R.; Yuan, B.; Jiang, Z. Mathematical model and exact algorithm for the home care worker scheduling and routing problem with lunch break requirements. *Int. J. Prod. Res.* **2017**, *55*, 558–575. [CrossRef]
16. Heching, A.; Hooker, J.N.; Kimura, R. A Logic-Based Benders Approach to Home Healthcare Delivery. *Transp. Sci.* **2019**, *53*, 510–522. [CrossRef]
17. Bard, J.F.; Shao, Y.; Qi, X.; Jarrah, A.I. The traveling therapist scheduling problem. *IIE Trans.* **2014**, *46*, 683–706. [CrossRef]
18. Akjiratikarl, C.; Yenradee, P.; Drake, P.R. PSO-based algorithm for home care worker scheduling in the UK. *Comput. Ind. Eng.* **2007**, *53*, 559–583. [CrossRef]
19. Frifita, S.; Masmoudi, M.; Euchi, J. General variable neighborhood search for home healthcare routing and scheduling problem with time windows and synchronized visits. *Electron. Notes Discrete Math.* **2017**, *58*, 63–70. [CrossRef]
20. Fikar, C.; Hirsch, P. A matheuristic for routing real-world home service transport systems facilitating walking. *J. Clean. Prod.* **2015**, *105*, 300–310. [CrossRef]

21. Carello, G.; Lanzarone, E. A cardinality-constrained robust model for the assignment problem in home care services. *Eur. J. Oper. Res.* **2014**, *236*, 748–762. [CrossRef]
22. Yalçındag, S.; Matta, A.; Sahin, E.; Shanthikumar, J.G. The patient assignment problem in home health care: Using a data-driven method to estimate the travel times of care givers. *Flex. Serv. Manuf. J.* **2016**, *28*, 304–335. [CrossRef]
23. Kitano, H. Biological robustness. *Nat. Rev. Genet.* **2004**, *5*, 826–837. [CrossRef] [PubMed]
24. Christopher, M.; Peck, H. Building the Resilient Supply Chain. 2004. Available online: https://dspace.lib.cranfield.ac.uk/handle/1826/2666 (accessed on 6 March 2023).
25. Nikzad, E.; Bashiri, M.; Abbasi, B. A matheuristic algorithm for stochastic home health care planning. *Eur. J. Oper. Res.* **2021**, *288*, 753–774. [CrossRef]
26. Zhan, Y.; Wang, Z.; Wan, G. Home service routing and appointment scheduling with stochastic service times. *Eur. J. Oper. Res.* **2021**, *288*, 98–110. [CrossRef]
27. Shi, Y.; Boudouh, T.; Grunder, O. A robust optimization for a home health care routing and scheduling problem with consideration of uncertain travel and service times. *Transp. Res. Part E Logist. Transp. Rev.* **2019**, *128*, 52–95. [CrossRef]
28. Cappanera, P.; Scutellà, M.G.; Nervi, F.; Galli, L. Demand Uncertainty in Robust Home Care Optimization. 2017. Available online: http://www.sciencedirect.com/science/article/pii/S0305048316309008 (accessed on 17 April 2018).
29. Oyola, J.; Arntzen, H.; Woodruff, D.L. The stochastic vehicle routing problem, a literature review, part I: Models. *EURO J. Transp. Logist.* **2018**, *7*, 193–221. [CrossRef]
30. Errico, F.; Desaulniers, G.; Gendreau, M.; Rei, W.; Rousseau, L.-M. A priori optimization with recourse for the vehicle routing problem with hard time windows and stochastic service times. *Eur. J. Oper. Res.* **2016**, *249*, 55–66. [CrossRef]
31. Alves, F.; Pereira, A.I.; Barbosa, J.; Leitão, P. Scheduling of Home Health Care Services Based on Multi-agent Systems. In *Highlights Pract Appl Agents Multi-Agent Syst Complex PAAMS Collect*; Bajo, J., Corchado, J.M., Navarro Martínez, E.M., Osaba Icedo, E., Mathieu, P., Hoffa-Dąbrowska, P., del Val, E., Giroux, S., Castro, A.J.M., Sánchez-Pi, N., et al., Eds.; Springer International Publishing: Cham, Switzerland, 2018; pp. 12–23.
32. Marcon, E.; Chaabane, S.; Sallez, Y.; Bonte, T.; Trentesaux, D. A multi-agent system based on reactive decision rules for solving the caregiver routing problem in home health care. *Simul. Model. Pract. Theory* **2017**, *74*, 134–151. [CrossRef]
33. Yuan, B.; Jiang, Z. Disruption Management for the Real-Time Home Caregiver Scheduling and Routing Problem. *Sustainability* **2017**, *9*, 2178. [CrossRef]
34. Mourtzis, D. Simulation in the design and operation of manufacturing systems: State of the art and new trends. *Int. J. Prod. Res.* **2020**, *58*, 1927–1949. [CrossRef]
35. Zhang, L.; Pingaud, H.; Fontanili, F.; Lamine, E.; Martinez, C.; Bortolaso, C.; Derras, M. Balancing the satisfaction of stakeholders in home health care coordination: A novel OptaPlanner CSP model. *Health Syst.* **2023**, 1–21. [CrossRef]
36. Robinson, S. *Simulation: The Practice of Model Development and Use*; Bloomsbury Publishing: London, UK, 2014.

Disclaimer/Publisher's Note: The statements, opinions and data contained in all publications are solely those of the individual author(s) and contributor(s) and not of MDPI and/or the editor(s). MDPI and/or the editor(s) disclaim responsibility for any injury to people or property resulting from any ideas, methods, instructions or products referred to in the content.

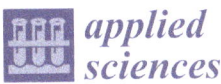

Article

Pareto-Optimized AVQI Assessment of Dysphonia: A Clinical Trial Using Various Smartphones

Rytis Maskeliūnas [1,*], Robertas Damaševičius [1], Tomas Blažauskas [1], Kipras Pribuišis [2], Nora Ulozaitė-Stanienė [2] and Virgilijus Uloza [2]

[1] Faculty of Informatics, Kaunas University of Technology, 44249 Kaunas, Lithuania
[2] Department of Otorhinolaryngology, Academy of Medicine, Lithuanian University of Health Sciences, 44240 Kaunas, Lithuania
* Correspondence: rytis.maskeliunas@ktu.lt

Abstract: Multiparametric indices offer a more comprehensive approach to voice quality assessment by taking into account multiple acoustic parameters. Artificial intelligence technology can be utilized in healthcare to evaluate data and optimize decision-making processes. Mobile devices provide new opportunities for remote speech monitoring, allowing the use of basic mobile devices as screening tools for the early identification and treatment of voice disorders. However, it is necessary to demonstrate equivalence between mobile device signals and gold standard microphone preamplifiers. Despite the increased use and availability of technology, there is still a lack of understanding of the impact of physiological, speech/language, and cultural factors on voice assessment. Challenges to research include accounting for organic speech-related covariables, such as differences in conversing voice sound pressure level (SPL) and fundamental frequency (f0), recognizing the link between sensory and experimental acoustic outcomes, and obtaining a large dataset to understand regular variation between and within voice-disordered individuals. Our study investigated the use of cellphones to estimate the Acoustic Voice Quality Index (AVQI) in a typical clinical setting using a Pareto-optimized approach in the signal processing path. We found that there was a strong correlation between AVQI results obtained from different smartphones and a studio microphone, with no significant differences in mean AVQI scores between different smartphones. The diagnostic accuracy of different smartphones was comparable to that of a professional microphone, with optimal AVQI cut-off values that can effectively distinguish between normal and pathological voice for each smartphone used in the study. All devices met the proposed 0.8 AUC threshold and demonstrated an acceptable Youden index value.

Keywords: AVQI; voice screening; Pareto optimization; voice disorders; dysphonia; voice quality

Citation: Maskeliūnas, R.; Damaševičius, R.; Blažauskas, T.; Pribuišis, K.; Ulozaitė-Stanienė, N.; Uloza, V. Pareto-Optimized AVQI Assessment of Dysphonia: A Clinical Trial Using Various Smartphones. Appl. Sci. 2023, 13, 5363. https://doi.org/10.3390/app13095363

Academic Editors: Chien-Hung Yeh, Wenbin Shi, Xiaojuan Ban, Men-Tzung Lo and Shenghong He

Received: 5 April 2023
Revised: 21 April 2023
Accepted: 21 April 2023
Published: 25 April 2023

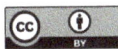

Copyright: © 2023 by the authors. Licensee MDPI, Basel, Switzerland. This article is an open access article distributed under the terms and conditions of the Creative Commons Attribution (CC BY) license (https://creativecommons.org/licenses/by/4.0/).

1. Introduction

A series of voice analysis tools includes many components to evaluate speech functions and voice quality [1,2]. The quantitative evaluation of voice quality using acoustics is advocated [3], and two metrics in this sector are the Acoustic Voice Quality Index (AVQI) and the Acoustic Breathiness Index (ABI) [4]. In the assessment of prolonged phonation and continual speech, multiparametric indexes enable a more robust acoustic analysis of voice quality by taking into account more than one acoustic parameter. However, if continuous speech is included, linguistic discrepancies must be handled [5]. The goal of Grillo's research [6] was to evaluate the acoustic metrics of fundamental frequency, standard deviation, jitter, shimmer, noise-to-harmonic ratio, smoothed cepstral peak prominence (CPPS), and AVQI evaluated invariably by VoiceEvalU8 or manually by two researchers. They discovered that the measurements were of good to exceptional reliability. Furthermore, the human voice is dynamic and evolves over time. The influences of age and sex on acoustic measurements of voice quality are well-known, yet AVQI remains independent of gender [7]. Compared to adults, the AVQI achieved by the pediatric and older adult groups was shown to be substantially higher. AVQI also exhibited significant age effects. Adults' AVQI levels were shown to be more constant than those of children and the elderly. The AVQI scores of elderly adults and children did not differ substantially [8]. Leyns' study examined and contrasted the acoustic short-term effects of pitch elevation training (PET) In transgender women, also focusing on articulation-resonance training (ART), and a combination of both programs. Xirs discovered that fundamental frequencies rose after both PET and ART programs, with a greater increase after PET, but that intensity and voice quality measures did not become altered [9].

Artificial intelligence (AI) approaches can be used to analyze data, reduce computing time, and optimize decision-making processes and forecasts in a variety of industries, including healthcare [10]. Advances in mobile device technology provide new possibilities for remote speech monitoring at home and in clinical settings. A simple mobile device is transformed into a screening tool for the early detection, monitoring, and treatment of voice abnormalities. There is, nevertheless, a necessity to demonstrate equivalence between characteristics generated from mobile device signals and gold-standard microphone preamplifiers. Acoustic speech qualities from Android phone, tablets, and microphone preamplifier records were compared in the study of [11]. Compared to conventional PC-based voice treatment, smartphone voice therapy is less expensive and more flexible for patients and doctors. According to [12], voice quality and patient satisfaction increased in both therapies compared to before therapy, showing recovery. Others discovered that AVQI measures obtained from smartphone microphone voice recordings with experimentally added ambient noise disclosed an amicable settlement with the results of oral microphone recordings, implying that smartphone microphone recordings conducted, even with the existence of acceptable ambient noise, are suitable for estimating AVQI [13]. Pommes wanted to see how standardized mobile phone recordings transferred across a telecom channel affected acoustic indicators of speech quality and how voice specialists perceived it in normophonic speakers [14]. The results reveal that sending a speech signal across a telephone line causes filtering and noise effects, limiting the use of popular acoustic sound quality metrics and indexes. The recording type has a considerable influence on both the AVQI and the ABI. Pitch perturbation (local jitter and periodic standard deviation) and the harmonics-to-noise ratio from Dejonckere and Lebacq appear to be the most reliable acoustic metrics. The study on the end-user mobile app "VoiceScreen" also demonstrated an accurate and robust method for measuring voice quality and the potential to be used in clinical settings as a sensitive assessment of voice alterations throughout the results of phonosurgical treatment [15].

Despite the greater use and availability of technology expertise and equipment, the current study has revealed a lack of awareness of physiological, speech/language and culturally influenced aspects. The primary obstacles to this investigation are the following:

1. Standardization and disclosure of acoustic analysis methods;
2. Recognition of the link between sensory and experimental acoustic outcomes;
3. The obligation to account for organic speech-related covariables, such as distinctions in conversing voice sound pressure level (SPL) and fundamental frequency f0;
4. The requirement for a significant larger dataset to comprehend regular variance between and within voice-disordered individual people.

The results of the studies mentioned above enabled us to presume the feasibility of voice recordings captured with different smartphones in an ordinary clinical setting for the estimation of AVQI. Consequently, the current research was designed to answer the following questions regarding the possibility of a smartphone-based "VoiceScreen" app for AVQI estimation:

1. Are the different estimated average AVQI values for smartphones consistent and comparable?
2. Is the diagnostic accuracy of the estimated AVQIs for different smartphones relevant to differentiate normal and pathological voices?

We hypothesize that the use of different smartphones for voice recordings and the estimation of AVQI in an ordinary clinical environment will be feasible for the quantitative assessment of voice.

Therefore, the present study aimed to develop the universal platform-based application suitable for different smartphones for the estimation of AVQI and evaluate its reliability in the measurements of AVQI and the normal/pathological differentiation of voices.

2. State of the Art Review

2.1. Use of Voice Quality Index Instruments in the Medical Domain

Naturally, the medical domain is the primary field in which impairment and acoustic measures can be used to accurately assess overall voice quality in numerous medical pathologies [16] and therapies [17]. To reduce the danger of voice problems in those who rely heavily on their voices, such as teachers, vocal screening is essential from the start of their professional studies. A dependable and precise screening instrument is required. AVQI has been shown to distinguish between normal and disordered voices and to be a therapy outcome measure. The purpose of the study of [18] was to see whether the AVQI could be used as a screening tool in conjunction with auditory and self-perception of the voice to differentiate between normal and somewhat inferior voices. Enhelt et al. [19] sought to assess the accuracy of AVQI and its isolated acoustic measurements to distinguish voices with varying degrees of deviation in severity of disorder. The results showed that the AVQI is a reliable instrument for distinguishing between different degrees of vocal deviation, and that it is more accurate for voices with moderate and severe abnormalities. When identifying voices with a higher degree of variation, isolated acoustic measurements perform better. Their other investigation [20] discovered that AVQI had the highest accuracy at a length tailored. To improve the reliability of voice analysis, a systematic approach should be followed, along with a specific speech material control that allows comparability between clinics and voice centers. A combination of acoustic measures with the same weight is more accurate in distinguishing different degrees of departure but is inconsistent. In clinical voice practice, outcome measures measuring acoustic voice quality and self-perceived vocal impairment are often utilized. Earlier studies on the link between acoustic and self-perceived measures have indicated relatively minor correlations, but it is unclear whether acoustic measurements connected with voice quality and self-perceived voice handicap become altered in a comparable way throughout voice therapy. As a result, the [21] study looked at the association between the degree of change in AVQI and the Voice Handicap Index (VHI). Voice treatment provided in a community voice clinic to individuals with various diseases was also shown to be successful, as evaluated by improvements in VHI and AVQI [22].

During the COVID-19 pandemic, the use of nose-and-mouth cover respiratory protection masks (RPMs) has become widespread. The effects of wearing RPMs, particularly on the perception and production of spoken communication, are increasingly emerging and their impact on medical voice analysis devices is significant [23]. The effects of face masks on spectral speech acoustics were evaluated in the Keas investigation [24]. Speech intensity, spectral moments, spectral tilt, and energy in mid-range frequencies were among the outcome metrics examined at the utterance level. Although the impact magnitude varied, masks were associated with changes in spectral density characteristics consistent with a low-pass filtering effect. The center of gravity, spectral diversity (in habitual speech), and spectral tilt had greater impacts (in all speech styles). KN95 masks outperformed the surgical masks in terms of speech acoustics. The general pattern of acoustic speech alterations was consistent between the three speaking styles. Compared to habitual speech, loud speech followed by clear speech was successful in removing the filtering effects of masks. In a similar study, Lehnert discovered that wearing COVID-19 protective masks did not significantly degrade the findings of AVQI or ABI based on a selected sample of healthy or minimally impaired voices [25].

According to Parkinson voice research [26], AVQI incorporates acoustics from both vowel and sentence settings and therefore may be preferred to CPPS (vowel) or CPPS (sentence). AVQI has been shown to be a reliable multiparametric measure for assessing the severity of dysphonia, which is often a rare, persistent, and long-term neurological voice problem caused by excessive or incorrect contraction of the laryngeal muscles. Alternatively, the Ulosian technique [27] sought to identify irregularities in the voice affected by PD and build an automated screening tool capable of distinguishing between the voices of patients with PD and healthy volunteers while also generating a voice quality score. The classification accuracy was tested using two speech corpora (the Italian PVS and our own Lithuanian PD voice dataset), and the results were confirmed to be medically adequate. Gale explored the impact of intensive speech therapy that targets the voice or focuses on articulation on the quality of the voice as judged by the AVQI in people with Parkinson's disease [28]. The results show that voice-focused therapy results in significant gains in voice quality in this population.

The growing number of validity studies that evaluate the validity of the AVQI requires a complete synthesis of existing results [29]. AVQI is a contemporary multivariate acoustic measure of dysphonia that assesses overall voice quality. In [30], a comparison of the two groups revealed a considerable difference between them. Consequently, AVQI serves as an excellent diagnostic method for obtaining scores from the dysphonic population and should be investigated in other voice issues. According to Portalete's results [31], while the characteristics detected in the evaluations were similar to those expected from individuals with dysarthria, it is difficult to establish a differential diagnosis of this disorder based solely on auditory and physiological criteria. Similarly, the team of Barsties et al. [32] analyzed two acoustic properties, the cepstral spectral index of dysphonia (CSID) and AVQI, which have gained popularity as valid and reliable multiparametric indicators in the objective evaluation of hoarseness due to their inclusion of continuous speech and sustained vowels. Another multiparametric assessment, ABI, analyzes and detects breathiness mixing during phonation without being unaffected by other features of dysphonia, such as roughness. They discovered that CSID, AVQI, and ABI objectively increase the identification of voice quality problems. Their use is straightforward and their usefulness for physicians is high, in contrast to their demonstrated validity. The authors also reached the same conclusion in a similar study on synthetic voice [33].

The purpose of Gomez's [34] study was to assess the voice in patients with thyroid pathology using two objective indicators with high diagnostic precision. AVQI was used to assess general vocal quality, and ABI was used to assess breathiness, both of which were found to be relevant. Other researchers wanted to use cutting-edge deep learning research to objectively categorize, extract, and assess substitute voicing following laryngeal oncosurgery from audio signals [35]. Their technique had the highest true-positive rate of all of the cutting-edge approaches examined, reaching an acceptable overall accuracy and demonstrating the practical usage of voice quality devices. In a similar study, ASVI was found to be a quick and efficient option after laryngeal oncosurgery [36]. Individuals who have had maxillectomies may have changes in the stomatognathic functions involved in oral communication. Rehabilitative care should prioritize the restoration of these functions by surgical flaps, obturator prosthesis, or both. Improvements in intelligibility and resonance were found in the absence of trans-surgical palatine obturators (TPO) in the vocal evaluation performed by [37], and minor hypernasality was discovered in only one instance in the presence of TPO. In a similar study [38], Sluis found no statistical significance in the VHI-10 scores over time compared to AVQI.

AVQI and comparable instruments were also used in other related areas. For example, the AVQI was also used to determine the effectiveness of the NHS waterpipe as a superficial hydration therapy in healthy young women's voice production. The technique was determined to be useful by the authors, and the perceived phonatory effort decreased significantly at the last assessment point [39]. The authors of [40] attempted to assess the influence of type 1 diabetes mellitus on the voice in pediatric patients using voice quality analysis. The study findings revealed that the AVQI value was higher in the patient group, although not statistically significant. Acoustic measures, such as AVQI and the maximum phonation time (MPT), were used in the study [41] to predict the degree of lung involvement in COVID-19 patients. Each participant created a phonetically balanced sentence with a sustained vowel. In terms of AVQI and MPT, the results demonstrated substantial disparities between COVID-19 patients and healthy persons. Huttenen's study [42] sought to determine the efficacy of a 4-week breathing exercise intervention in patients with voice complaints. The total scores of AVQI and several of its subcomponents (shimmer and harmonic-to-noise ratio), as well as the GRBAS scale's grade, roughness, and strain, showed dramatically enhanced voice quality. However, neither the kind nor frequency of vocal symptoms, nor the perceived phonatory effort, changed as a result of the intervention.

2.2. Measurement of the Effects of Vocal Fatigue and Related Impairments

Measurement of the effects of vocal fatigue and related impairments is another well-established approach. Vocal loading tasks (VLTs) allow researchers to collect acoustic data and study how a healthy speaker alters their voice in response to obstacles. Such instruments can provide detailed voice information and aid speech pathologists in determining whether the vocal activity of instructors at work should be regulated or not [43]. There is a paucity of research on the effect of the talking rate in VLT on acoustic voice characteristics and vocal fatigue [44]. Vocal effort is widespread and frequently leads to decreased respiratory and laryngeal efficiency. However, it is not known whether the respiratory kinematic and acoustic adaptations used during vocal exertion differ between speakers who express vocal fatigue and those who do not. Ref. [45] evaluated respiratory kinematics and acoustic measurements in people with low and high degrees of vocal fatigue while performing a vocal exertion task. Ref. [46] looked at clinically normal voices with no history of vocal problems and assessed weariness. The Vocal Fatigue Index (VFI) was used for the subjective study of vocal loading, while the acoustic and cepstral analysis of voice recordings was used in both circumstances for objective analysis. The results demonstrated that there was a substantial difference in VFI scores between the two circumstances. The acoustic and cepstral properties of the voice also differed significantly between the two circumstances, a result also confirmed in the study [47]. A similar study [48] was conducted with VFI and the Borg vocal effort scale. Before, during and after periods of speaking, they objectively examined fluctuations in relative sound pressure level, frequency response, pitch intensity, averaged cepstral peak amplitude, and AVQI.

AVQI was also used to evaluate the characteristics, vocal complaints, and habits of musicians and students of musical theater. Given the mismatch of high vocal requirements vs. poor vocal education, and hence greater risk for voice issues, choir singers' voice usage remains understudied. With mean scores on the Dysphonia Severity Index and AVQI, choir members demonstrated exceptional voice quality and capabilities [49]. The mean grade score corresponded to a normal to somewhat aberrant voice quality in terms of auditory perception. Patient-reported outcome measures revealed significant deviation scores, indicating significant singing voice impairment. Choir singers appear to be particularly prone to stress, with a high incidence rate. After 15 min of choir singing, the severity index of dysphonia improved considerably compared to the control group, although the self-perceived presence of fatigue and voice complaints increased. In both groups, the fundamental frequency rose. Dheleeser et al. [50] conducted a study on musical theater actors who had comparably good objective voice measurements (DSI, AVQI). There has been an upsurge in the number of VTDs and complaints about the singing voice. The AVQI was used to identify people who were susceptible to stress, vocal misuse, VTD, and pain symptoms. The purpose of [51] was to see if the voices of actors and actresses could be cognitively identified as being more resonant after an intensive Lessac Kinesensic training workshop and to see if AVQI, ABI, and their acoustic measures could indicate classified voices as being more resonant. Unfortunately, statistical analysis that compared perceptual and auditory data for the final samples was not possible. Leyns conducted a similar study and discovered that professional actors had stronger vocal abilities than non-professionals [52]. The voice quality of the dancers is inferior to that of the actors. The findings reveal that one performance has little effect on vocal quality among theater performers and dancers. Nonetheless, the long-term consequences of performance are still being studied. Similar research, which used the AVQI to examine 40-minute vocal loading tests that comprised warm-up, hard singing, and loud reading, found that there were no significant differences in vocal characteristics between female and male conductors [53]. They discovered that the volume of the rehearsal room and the duration of the reverberation had no effect on the characteristics of the acquired voice after vocal loading.

2.3. Language Factors in Voice Quality Analysis

Voice quality metrics have been found to be useful and efficient in the analysis of a variety of very different spoken languages. The purpose of the [54] study was to confirm the impact of different cultural origins and languages (Brazil Portuguese and European Portuguese) on the perception of voice quality. Another goal was to evaluate the relationship between clinical auditory perception assessments and acoustic measures such as AVQI and ABI, as well as their influence on concurrent validity. They discovered that Brazilian raters evaluated voice quality as more deviant and that Brazilian voice samples were less severe (a possible language characteristic). More research is needed to determine whether there was a task or a sample consequence, as well as whether revisions to the AVQI and ABI formulations are needed for Brazilian Portuguese. A similar assessment was made for the Italian speaking population [55]. The auditory perceptual RBH scale (roughness, breathiness, and hoarseness) and acoustical analysis using AVQI validated dysphonia in a study of the Polish population using recorded voice [56]. Jakamarar [57] explored the verification of AVQI in the South Indian population and found it to be superior in terms of diagnostic precision and internal consistency. Kim et al. sought to validate the AVQI version 3.01 and ABI as acoustic analysis tools in Korean [58]. They discovered that AVQI and ABI had good concurrent validity in quantifying the severity of dysphonia with respect to OS and B in a sample of Korean speakers. A further investigation of the Korean population found that each measure had a strong discriminative ability to distinguish the presence or absence of voice difficulties [59]. The findings of this study might be used as an objective criterion to detect voice disorders. According to [60], the AVQI is a robust multiparametric measure that can reliably differentiate between subcategories of severity of perceptual dysphonia with good accuracy in Kannada. Moreover, AVQI has been shown to be useful in analyzing signals with greater degrees of aperiodicity, such as extreme hoarse voice quality [7]. The AVQI was lower (better) in samples with a high degree of strain for Finnish speakers, but the variation was not substantial [61]. Only CPPS distinguished between modest and large degrees of creak. With normophonic speakers, the AVQI does not appear to distinguish between low and high levels of creak and strain. Puzzella [62] investigated the validity (both concurrent and diagnostic) and the test–retest reliability of AVQI in a Turkish speaking community. The link between AVQI scores and auditory perception rating of total voice quality was statistically significant. The dysphonic voice was assigned a necessary threshold by AVQI. Intraclass correlation coefficient values using a two-way mixed effects model, single-measures type, and absolute agreement definition demonstrated high test–retest reliability for the AVQI in Turkish. Furthermore, the considerable values of concurrent validity and diagnostic accuracy of both versions of AVQI-Persian were verified, demonstrating that it can distinguish between normal and diseased voices in Persian speakers [63]. As a conclusion, it is clear that AVQI and similar metrics can be utilized for language-independent screening or diagnosis.

3. Materials and Methods

3.1. Materials

The study comprised 134 adult participants, with 58 men and 77 women, who were evaluated in the Department of Otolaryngology of the Lithuanian University of Health

Sciences, Kaunas, Lithuania. The mean age of the participants was 42.9 (SD 15.26) years. The pathological voice subgroup, which included 86 patients (42 men and 44 women), had a mean age of 50.8 years (SD 14.3) and presented with a variety of laryngeal diseases and associated voice impairments, such as benign and malignant mass lesions of the vocal folds and unilateral paralysis of the vocal fold. Diagnosis was based on clinical examination, including patient complaints and history, voice assessment and video laryngostroboscopy (VLS) using an XION Endo-STROB DX device (XION GmbH, Berlin, Germany) 70° rigid endoscope and/or direct microlaryngoscopy. Five experienced physicians–laryngologists performed the auditory–perceptual evaluations of voice samples. For the purpose of this study, only the evaluation of dysphonia's grade (G) was used from the GRBAS scale (grade, breathiness, roughness, asthenia, and strain). The voice samples were rated into four ordinal severity classes of G on the scale from 0 to 3 points, where 0 = normal voice, 1—mild, 2—moderate, and 3—severe dysphonia [64]. A severity distribution is displayed in Figure 1.

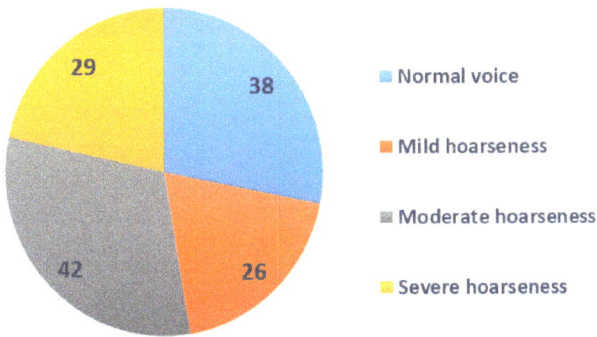

Figure 1. Severity distribution of the patients involved.

The normal voice subgroup consisted of 49 healthy volunteers, 16 men and 33 women, with a mean age of 31.69 (SD 9.89) years. To qualify as vocally healthy, participants were required to have no actual voice complaints, no history of chronic laryngeal diseases or voice disorders, and to self-report their voice as normal. The voices of the participants were evaluated as normal by otolaryngologists specialized in the field of voice, as there were no pathological alterations in the larynx. Demographic data for the study group and diagnoses for the pathological voice subgroup are presented in Table 1.

Voice samples representing five different smartphones were used, namely the iPhone 12 Pro, iPhone 13 Pro Max, Xiaomi Redmi Note 5, iPhone 12 Mini, and Samsung Galaxy S10+. The following processing conditions were applied: smartphones were placed approximately 30.0 cm away from the mouth, at a 90° angle to the mouth, and had internal microphones (bottom) (see Figure 2). The devices were selected from a range of commercial prices. The background noise level averaged 29.61 dB SPL and the signal-to-noise ratio (SNR) was approximately 38.11 dB compared to the voiced recordings, indicating that the environment was suitable for both voice recordings and the extraction of acoustic parameters. The AKG microphone was placed 10.0 cm from the mouth at a comfortable (approximately 90°) microphone-to-mouth angle.

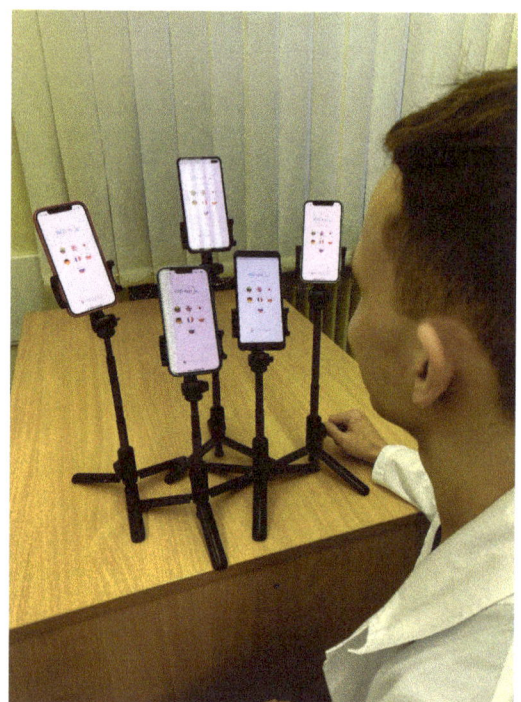

Figure 2. The experimental setup of five different smartphone devices modeled in this study (iPhone SE, iPhone PRO MAX 13, Huawei P50 pro, Samsung S22 Ultra, and OnePlus 9 PRO).

Table 1. Demographic data of the study group.

Diagnosis	Total	Age (mean)	Age (SD)
Normal voice	49	31.69	9.89
Vocal fold nodules	6	42.67	10.86
Vocal fold polyp	21	40.95	12.98
Vocal fold cyst	3	42.67	12.58
Vocal fold cancer	11	65.09	7.71
Vocal fold polypoid hyperplasia	12	53.25	8.07
Vocal fold keratosis	4	56.25	2.63
Vocal fold papilloma	7	41.71	13.67
Unilateral vocal fold paralysis	6	40.83	12.77
Bilateral vocal fold paralysis	4	52.75	12.61
Chronic hyperplastic laryngitis	6	55.67	9.63
Dysphonia	1	22	.
GERD	2	57	15.56
Parkinson's disease	2	71.5	9.19

A phonetically balanced Lithuanian sentence "Turėjo senelė žilą oželį" ("Old granny had a billy goat") was the main utterance used to compare the recordings. The relative frequencies of the phonemes in the sentence are as close as possible to the distribution of speech sounds used in Lithuanian. The examples of spectral analysis results of voice samples are given in Figure 3.

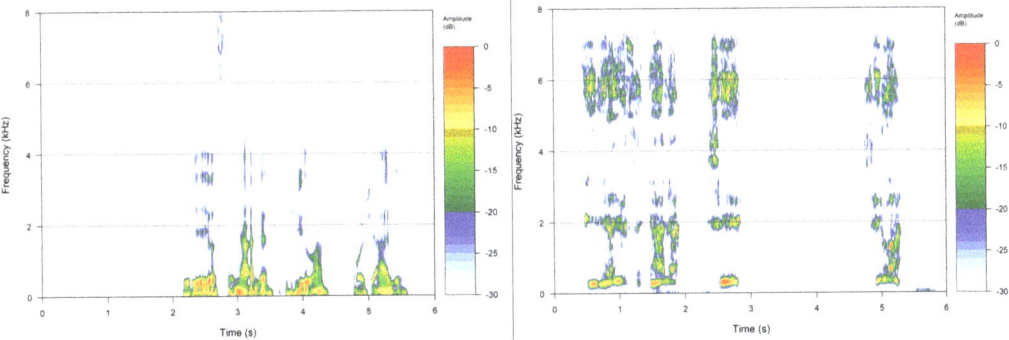

Figure 3. Spectral analysis results of a normal voice (class 0) and voice with severe dysphonia.

3.2. Calculating Required Voice Characteristics

To conduct the clinical research, we built a universal-platform-based version of the "VoiceScreen" software for use with both iOS and Android operating systems, using our Pareto optimized technique. The AVQI and its characteristics are calculated on the server; hence, computationally expensive sound processing is not reliant on the computing capabilities of the user device and may run on any Android or iOS device with a manufacturer-supported version of each respective operating system. The provided smartphone (either iOS or Android) records sound waves obtained while pronouncing given sentences aloud in the first stage. Sound waves are preprocessed in real time. The goal is to remove pauses from the sound waves and to guarantee that only the minimum quantity of sound is available for further processing. Then, that preprocessed sound wave is sent to the server for further analysis. The server runs a Linux operating system and operates our proprietary software to calculate the required characteristics necessary to evaluate the voice. Finally, the AVQI index and related data are sent back to the phone and displayed to the user. Figure 4 shows the structure of the system, while Figure 5 illustrates the operation sequence.

The server-side system performs numerous operations. First, the cepstral peak prominence (CPPS) is calculated (see Figure 6).

Our approach outlines a series of algorithms used to assess impaired voice quality using acoustic measures. The first algorithm resamples and applies pre-emphasis to the sound, then calculates the power cepstrogram. The second algorithm calculates the harmonicity using the cross-correlation technique, while the third algorithm calculates the shimmer, which measures cycle-to-cycle variations in vocal amplitude. The fourth algorithm calculates the long-term average spectrum (LTAS) of the sound waveform. Finally, the AVQI values are calculated, using multiple acoustic measures of voice quality through Pareto optimization. This technique identifies the optimal trade-off between multiple conflicting objectives to find the best solution to improve overall vocal quality while minimizing breathiness, roughness, and strain.

In Algorithm 1, we first resample the sound to twice the value of the maximum frequency and apply pre-emphasis to the resampled sound. Then, for each analysis window, we apply a Gaussian window, calculate the spectrum, transform it into a PowerCepstrum and store the values in the corresponding vertical slice of the PowerCepstrogram matrix. The algorithm returns the resulting PowerCepstrogram. The PowerCepstrogram is a representation of the power spectrum of a signal in the cepstral domain. The algorithm takes as input a sound signal, a pitch floor, a time step, a maximum frequency, and a pre-emphasis coefficient. The output of the algorithm is the PowerCepstrogram.

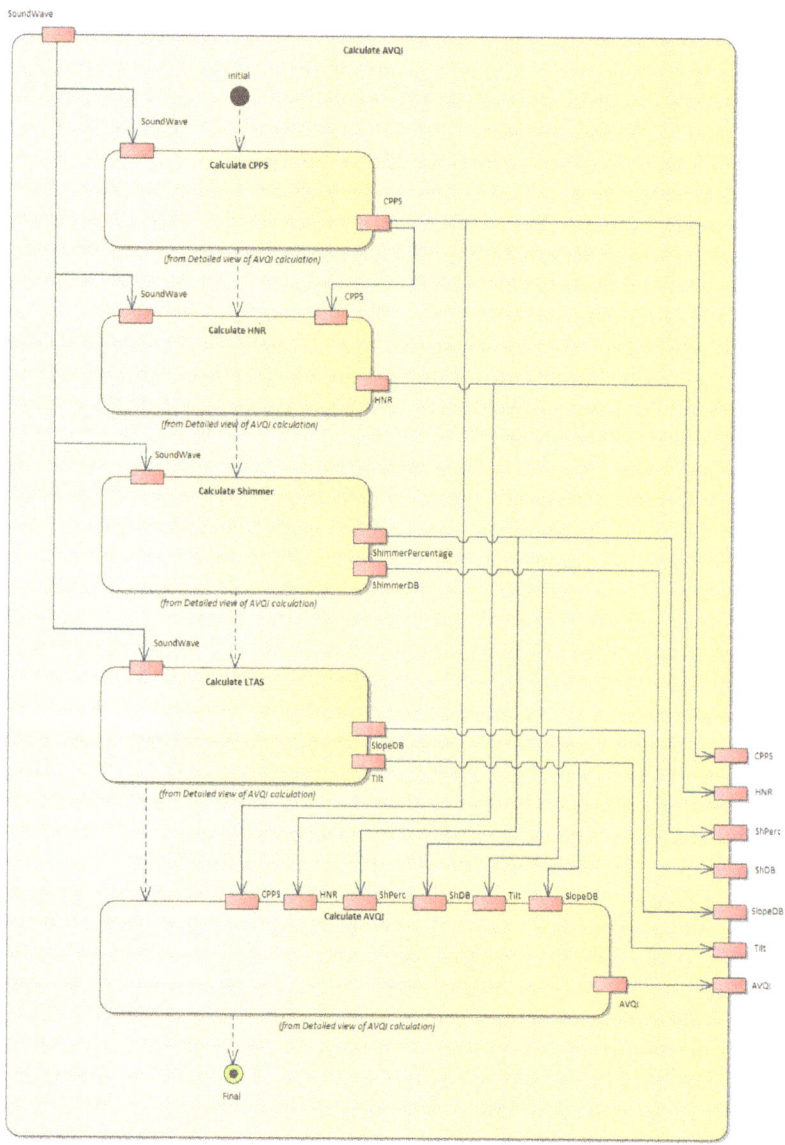

Figure 4. Structure of the system and flow of the operations.

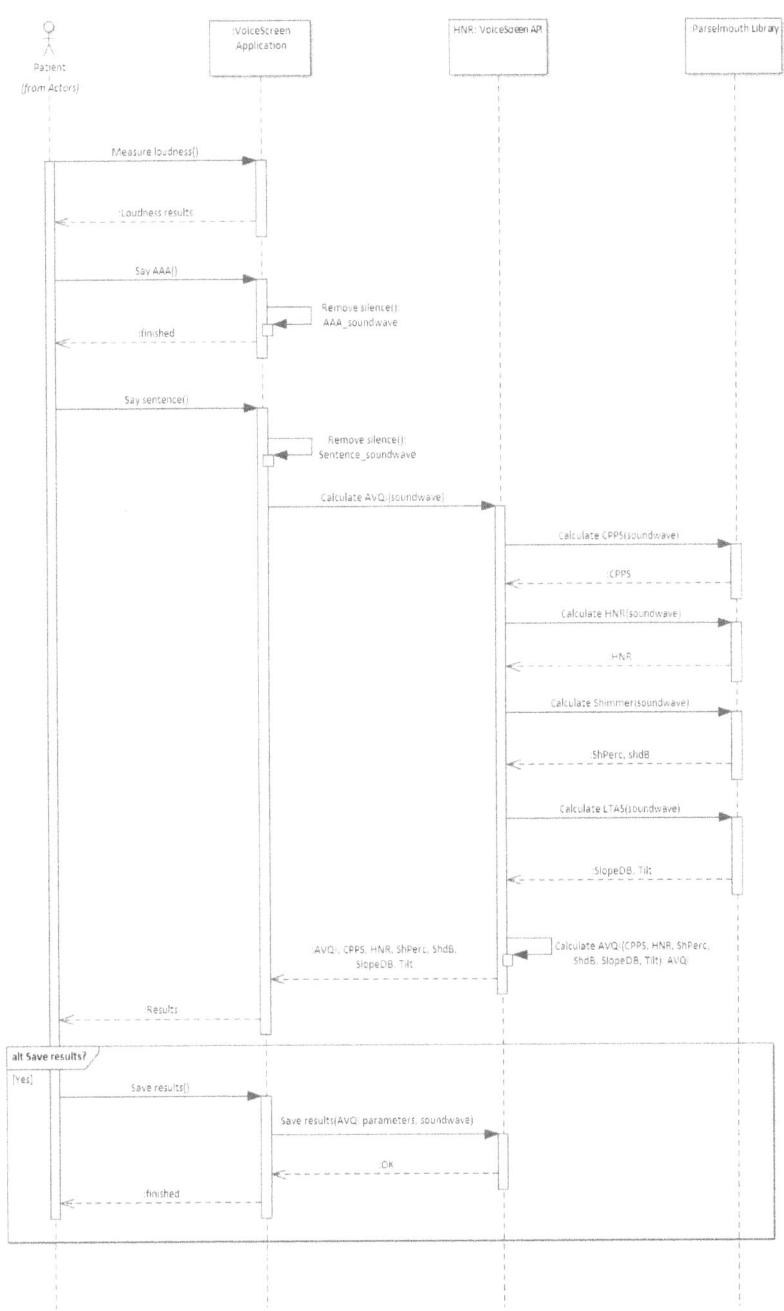

Figure 5. Sequence diagram of operations performed in our approach.

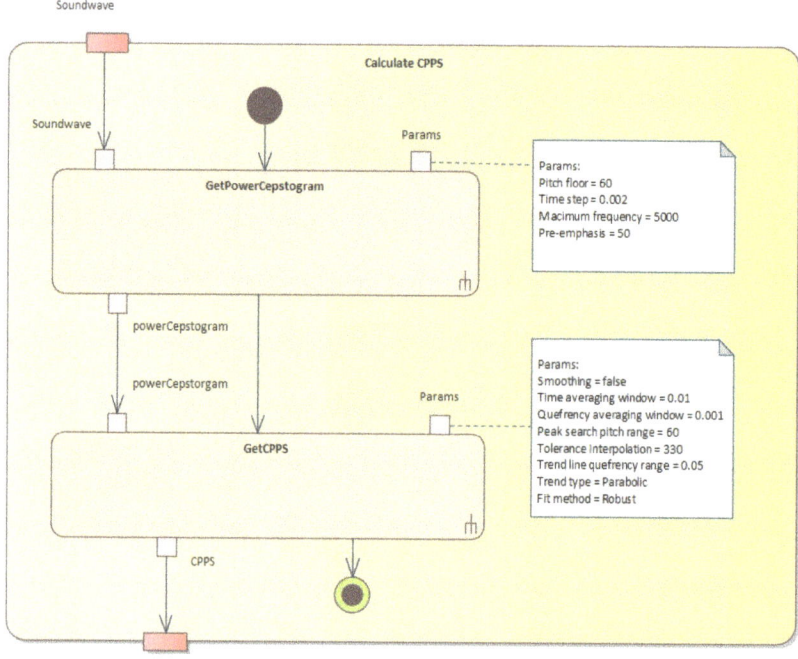

Figure 6. Calculation of the CPPS.

Algorithm 1 PowerCepstogram algorithm.

Require: $sound, pitch\_floor, time\_step, max\_freq, pre\_emphasis\_from$
Ensure: PowerCepstogram
1: **function** POWERCEPSTROGRAM($sound, pitch\_floor, time\_step, max\_freq,$
   $pre\_emphasis\_from$)
2:     $sound \leftarrow$ RESAMPLE($sound, 2 \times max\_freq$)
3:     PRE-EMPHASIZE($sound, pre\_emphasis\_from$)
4:     $window\_length \leftarrow \frac{3}{pitch\_floor}$
5:     $window \leftarrow$ Gaussian window with length $window\_length$
6:     $frame\_length \leftarrow$ length of $window$
7:     $hop\_length \leftarrow time\_step \times 2 \times max\_freq$
8:     $num\_frames \leftarrow \lfloor \frac{length\ of\ sound - frame\_length}{hop\_length} \rfloor$
9:     $power\_cepstrogram \leftarrow$ empty matrix with dimensions ($\lfloor \frac{max\_freq}{pitch\_floor} \rfloor, num\_frames$)
10:    **for** $i \leftarrow 1$ to num_frames **do**
11:        $start \leftarrow (i-1) \times hop\_length + 1$
12:        $end \leftarrow start + frame\_length - 1$
13:        $frame \leftarrow sound[start : end] \times window$
14:        $spectrum \leftarrow$ SPECTRUM($frame$)
15:        $power\_spectrum \leftarrow |spectrum|^2$
16:        $power\_cepstrum \leftarrow$ POWERCEPSTRUM($power\_spectrum$)
17:        $power\_cepstrogram[:, i] \leftarrow$ values from $power\_cepstrum$ up to $\lfloor \frac{max\_freq}{pitch\_floor} \rfloor$
18:    **end for**
19:    **return** $power\_cepstrogram$
20: **end function**

The second step is to perform pitch analysis and calculate harmonicity (see Figure 7 and Algorithm 2).

Algorithm 2 shows an implementation of the pitch analysis method that uses the cross-correlation technique to determine the pitch of a sound signal. The input parameters are the sound signal, the time step, the pitch floor and ceiling, as well as various thresholds and costs that affect the pitch analysis. The algorithm returns a pitch object that contains the pitch measurements and other pitch-related information.

The formant calculation algorithm is presented in Algorithm 3. This algorithm is a partial implementation of a function called "getFormantMean" that calculates the average value of a specified formant for a given time range. The function takes four arguments: "formantNum" specifies which formant to calculate the mean for, "fromTime" and "toTime" specify the time range to consider, and "units" specifies the units of the time range.

Algorithm 4 presents an algorithm to calculate harmonicity using Praat's harmonicity object. This algorithm takes a Praat sound object, a start and end time for the analysis, a time step, a silence threshold, and the number of periods per analysis window. It first creates a Praat harmonicity object from the input sound, with the given time step, silence threshold, and periods per window. It then selects the portion of the harmonicity object corresponding to the specified time range and returns the mean value of the selected portion. Aproach is explained in the Algorithm 4.

Algorithm 2 Pitch analysis based on the cross-correlation method.

1: **function** PITCHANALYSIS(*sound, timeStep, pitchFloor, useGaussianWindow, pitchCeiling, silenceThreshold, voicingThreshold, octaveCost, octaveJumpCost, voicedUnvoicedCost*)
2:    *resampledSound* ← Resample(*sound*, 2 × *pitchCeiling*)
3:    *preEmphasizedSound* ← PreEmphasize(*resampledSound, pitchFloor*)
4:    *windowLength* ← 1/*pitchFloor*
5:    **if** *timeStep* = 0 **then**
6:       *timeStep* ← 0.25/*pitchFloor*
7:    **end if**
8:    **if** *useGaussianWindow* = *True* **then**
9:       *windowLength* ← 2 × *windowLength*
10:   **end if**
11:   *pitch* ← CreateEmptyPitch()
12:   *pitch* ← SetTimeStep(*pitch, timeStep*)
13:   *pitch* ← SetPitchFloor(*pitch, pitchFloor*)
14:   *pitch* ← SetSilenceThreshold(*pitch, silenceThreshold*)
15:   *pitch* ← SetVoicingThreshold(*pitch, voicingThreshold*)
16:   *pitch* ← SetCeiling(*pitch, pitchCeiling*)
17:   *pitch* ← SetOctaveCost(*pitch, octaveCost*)
18:   *pitch* ← SetOctaveJumpCost(*pitch, octaveJumpCost* × 0.01/*timeStep*)
19:   *pitch* ← SetVoicedUnvoicedCost(*pitch, voicedUnvoicedCost* × 0.01/*timeStep*)
20:   **for** *frame* in *preEmphasizedSound* with interval of *timeStep* **do**
21:       *frameLength* ← the length of the analysis window
22:       *window* ← CreateWindow(*frameLength, useGaussianWindow*)
23:       *autocorrelation* ← Autocorrelate(*frame* × *window*)
24:       *candidates* ← ExtractCandidates(*autocorrelation, pitchFloor, pitchCeiling*)
25:       *bestCandidate* ← FindBestCandidate(*candidates, voicingThreshold*)
26:       *pitch* ← AddPitchMeasurement(*pitch, frame, bestCandidate*)
27:   **end for**
28:   *pitch* ← PostProcessPitch(*pitch*)
29:   **return** *pitch*
30: **end function**

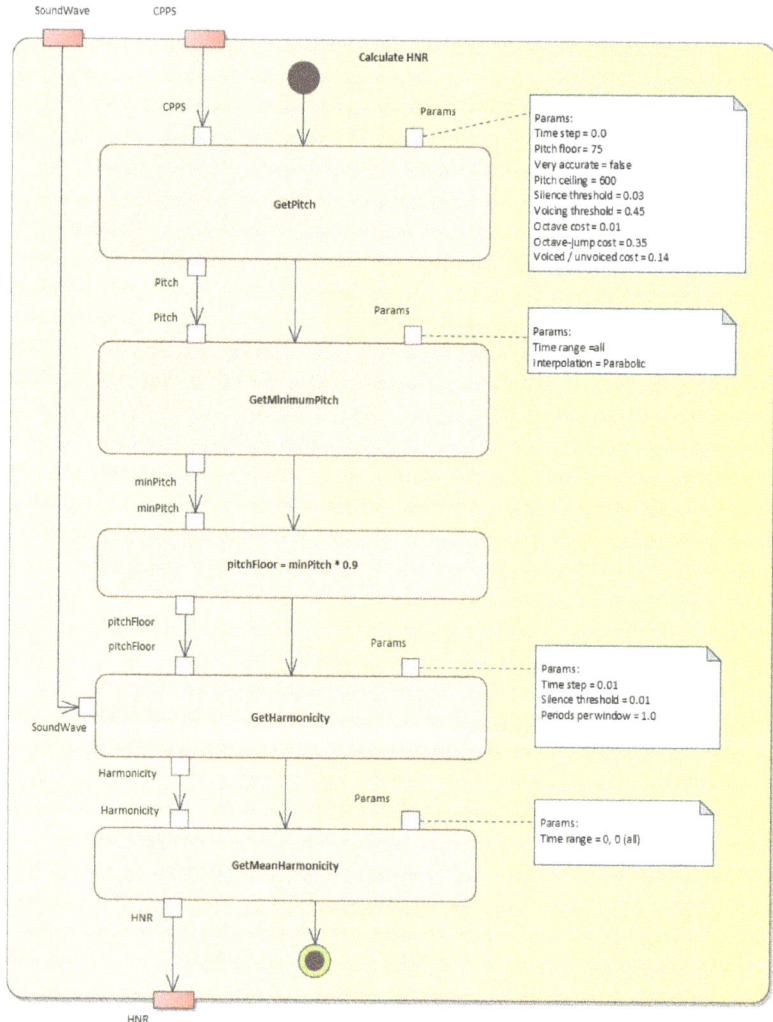

Figure 7. Pitch analysis and harmonicity calculation.

Algorithm 3 Formant calculation.

1: **function** GETFORMANTMEAN($formantNum, fromTime, toTime, units$)
2:     $formantObj \leftarrow$ selected Formant object
3:     $mean \leftarrow 0$
4:     $count \leftarrow 0$
5:     **for** $i \leftarrow 1$ to n **do**
6:         $time \leftarrow$ time at index i of formantObj
7:         **if** $time < fromTime$ or $time > toTime$ **then**
8:             **continue**
9:         **end if**
10:     **end for**
11:     $formantVal \leftarrow$ formant value at index i, formant number $formantNum$ of formantObj
12: **end function**

Algorithm 4 Harmonicity calculation.

1: **function** CALCULATEHARMONICITY(*sound, from_time, to_time, timestep, silence_threshold, periods_per_window*)
2:    *harmonicity* ← TOHARMONICITY(*sound, timestep, silence_threshold, periods_per_window*)
3:    SELECT(*harmonicity, from_time, to_time*)
4:    **return** GET_MEAN (*harmonicity*)
5: **end function**

The third step is to calculate the shimmer (see Figure 8 and Algorithm 5).

This algorithm calculates two measures of shimmer, which is a measure of cycle-to-cycle variations in vocal amplitude. The input is a sound waveform, a point process representing glottal closures, and the start and end times in seconds. The output is the shimmer local value and the shimmer dB value.

Algorithm 5 Shimmer calculation.

Require: *soundWav*, the sound waveform
Require: *pointProcess*, the point process representing glottal closures
Require: *startTime*, the start time in seconds
Require: *endTime*, the end time in seconds
Ensure: *shimmerLocal*, the shimmer local value
Ensure: *shimmerDB*, the shimmer dB value
1: Extract a pitch contour from the sound using the Sound: To Pitch... command with the following settings:
2: - pitch floor: 75 Hz
3: - pitch ceiling: 600 Hz
4: - time step: 0.01 s
5: - range of analysis: *startTime* to *endTime*
6: Convert the pitch contour to a point process using the Pitch: To PointProcess command with the following settings:
7: - silences: unvoiced
8: - voicing threshold: 0.45
9: Initialize a list to store the amplitude differences
10: **for** each period in the point process **do**
11:    Get the start and end times of the period
12:    Calculate the amplitude difference between the two points in the waveform that correspond to the start and end times
13:    Append the absolute value of the amplitude difference to the list
14: **end for**
15: Calculate the average amplitude difference and the average amplitude:
16: - Calculate the mean of the amplitude difference list and store it as *amplitudeDiffAvg*
17: - Calculate the mean of the absolute values of the waveform and store it as *amplitudeAvg*
18: Calculate the shimmer local value:
19: - Divide *amplitudeDiffAvg* by *amplitudeAvg* and multiply by 100
20: - Store the result as *shimmerLocal*
21: Calculate the shimmer dB value:
22: - Calculate the base-10 logarithm of each amplitude difference value in the list and store the result as a new list
23: - Calculate the mean of the new list and multiply by 20
24: - Store the result as *shimmerDB*
25: Return *shimmerLocal* and *shimmerDB*

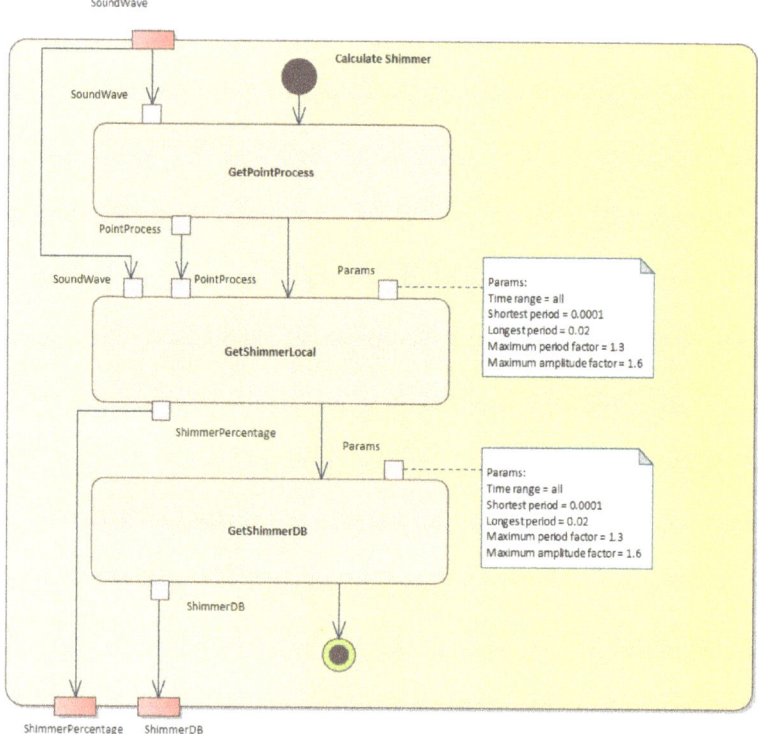

Figure 8. Calculation of the shimmer values.

In the fourth step, we need to calculate the long-term average spectrum (LTAS) (see Figure 9).

The algorithm to calculate the LTAS (long-term average spectrum) is presented in Algorithm 6. This algorithm calculates the LTAS of a given sound waveform and computes the slope and tilt parameters. The LTAS is a smoothed version of the spectrum of the sound waveform, calculated over a long period of time, typically several seconds.

Algorithm 6 LTAS calculation.

Require: *soundWav*: the sound waveform
Ensure: *slope_dB*: the slope in dB and *tilt*: the tilt parameter
  1: *ltas* ← call(soundWav, "To Ltas...", 1)   ▷ Convert sound waveform to Ltas
  2: **for** $i \leftarrow 0$ to $N-1$ **do**   ▷ Calculate power in each band
  3:    s_i ← call(ltas, "Get frequency", i)
  4:    re_si ← call(ltas, "Get real", i)
  5:    im_si ← call(ltas, "Get imaginary", i)
  6:    $b_i \leftarrow 2((re\_si)^2 + (im\_si)^2)/4.0 \cdot 10^{-10}$ ▷ Calculate band power
  7: **end for**
  8: *slope_dB* ← call(ltas, "Get slope...", 0, 1000, 1000, 10000, "energy") ▷ Calculate slope
  9: *ltas_trendline_db* ← call(ltas, "Compute trend line", 1, 10000)   ▷ Compute trendline
10: *tilt* ← call(ltas_trendline_db, "Get slope", 0, 1000, 1000, 10000, "energy") ▷ Calculate tilt parameter
11: **return** *slope_dB*, *tilt*

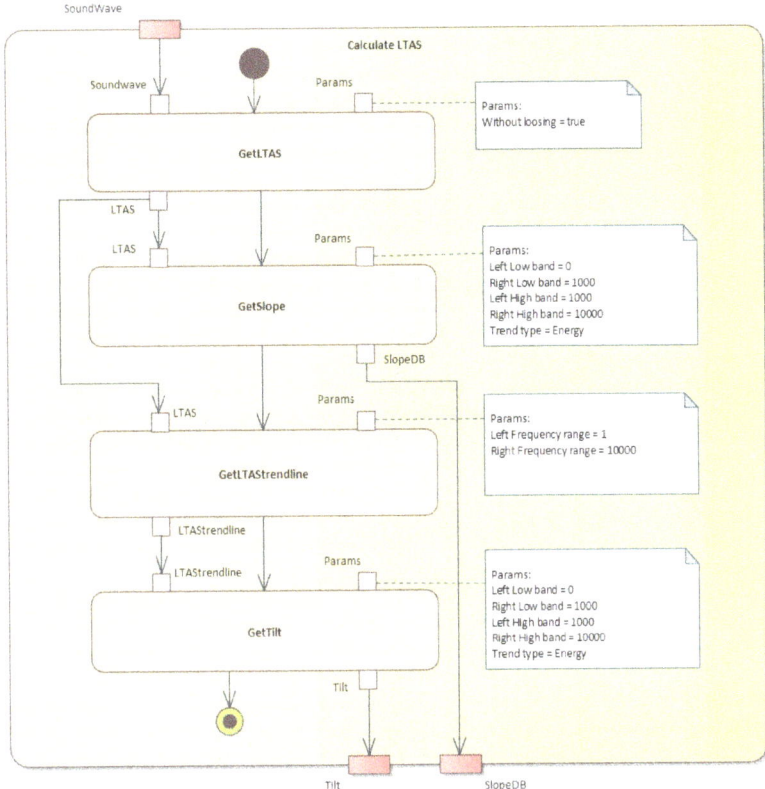

Figure 9. Calculation of the LTAS values.

Finally, we calculate the AVQI values (see Figure 10) given several acoustic measures of voice quality. The calculation algorithm is given in Algorithm 7. The Pareto optimization of AVQI scores is given in Algorithm 8.

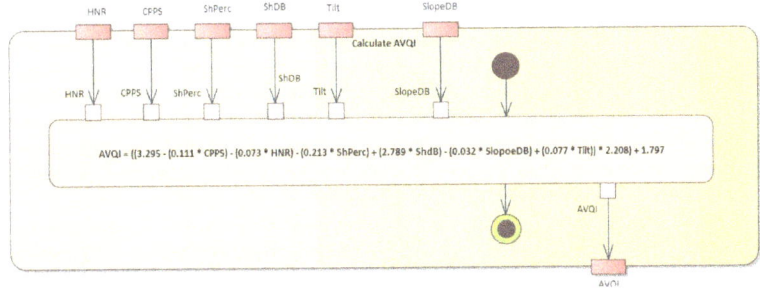

Figure 10. Calculation of the AVQI values.

Algorithm 7 AVQI calculation.

Require: $cpps, hnr, ShPerc, shdB, LtasSlope, LtasTreadTilt$
Ensure: AVQI
1: **function** CALCULATEAVQI($cpps, hnr, ShPerc, shdB, LtasSlope, LtasTreadTilt$)
2: $\quad AVQI \leftarrow ((3.295 - (0.111 \times cpps) - (0.073 \times hnr) - (0.213 \times ShPerc) + (2.789 \times shdB) -$
$(0.032 \times LtasSlope) + (0.077 \times LtasTreadTilt)) \times 2.208) + 1.797$
3: $\quad$ **return** $AVQI$
4: **end function**

Algorithm 8 Pareto optimization of AVQI scores.

1: Define the relevant voice quality parameters and define AVQI score as the objective to be optimized.
2: Select a set of candidate solutions that represent different combinations of the voice quality parameters.
3: Calculate the AVQI scores for each candidate solution using a combination of objective and subjective methods.
4: Plot the candidate solutions on a Pareto front to visualize the trade-off between the objectives.
5: Identify the Pareto optimal solutions on the Pareto front using visual inspection, clustering, or optimization algorithms, such as NSGA-II.
6: Select the Pareto optimal solution that best meets the specific needs and preferences of the AVQI assessment, considering factors such as clinical relevance, patient preference, and ease of implementation.
7: Evaluate the performance of the AVQI algorithm using validation data and feedback from clinicians and patients.
8: Fine-tune the AVQI algorithm and the Pareto optimization parameters based on the validation results and feedback.

Pareto Optimized Assessment of Impaired Voice

Pareto optimization is a technique used to identify the optimal trade-off between multiple conflicting objectives.

Let X be the set of candidate solutions, where each solution $x \in X$ is a vector of n characteristics of voice quality, such as overall voice quality, strain, and pitch. Let $f(x) = (f_1(x), f_2(x), \ldots, f_m(x))$ be a vector of m objective functions that measure the performance of x in each characteristic. The Pareto front is defined as the set of nondominated solutions, i.e., those solutions that cannot be improved in any objective without worsening at least one other objective. Formally, a solution x_1 dominates another solution x_2 if and only if $f_1(x_1) \leq f_1(x_2), f_2(x_1) \leq f_2(x_2)$ and $f_m(x_1) \leq f_m(x_2)$ and there exists at least one objective function f_j such that $f_j(x_1) < f_j(x_2)$. The Pareto front is the set of all nondominated solutions, i.e., $P = \{x \in X | \forall x' \in X, x' \text{ is not dominated by } x\}$. The Pareto optimal solution is any solution $x^* \in P$ that maximizes the trade-off between the objectives, i.e., $\forall x \in P, f(x^*) \leq f(x)$, where $\leq$ denotes Pareto dominance.

In the context of the evaluation of impaired voice by AVQI recorded on the smartphone, Pareto optimization is used to find the best trade-off between different parameters that affect overall vocal quality, such as breathiness, roughness, strain, and pitch. The first step in Pareto optimization is to define the objectives or criteria that need to be optimized. In the case of the AVQI assessment, the objective could be to maximize overall vocal quality while minimizing breathiness, roughness, and strain. Pitch could be considered a separate objective, depending on the specific voice impairment being assessed. The next step is to generate a set of candidate solutions that represent different combinations of objectives. This is done by varying the weights or importance assigned to each objective in the AVQI algorithm. For example, increasing the weight of the overall vocal quality objective would result in a higher score for samples with better overall quality, while decreasing the weight of the breathiness objective would result in a lower score for samples with more breathiness. Once the candidate solutions are generated, Pareto optimization techniques are used to identify the optimal trade-off between the objectives as follows.

Step 1: Calculate the AVQI scores for each candidate solution based on the relevant parameters.

To calculate the AVQI score, we need to first define the relevant parameters that affect voice quality. These could include measures of pitch, loudness, jitter, shimmer, harmonics-to-noise ratio, and other relevant acoustic and perceptual measures. Once the parameters are defined, we can use a combination of objective and subjective methods to calculate the AVQI score. Objective methods use signal processing and machine learning techniques to analyze the acoustic properties of the voice signal and extract relevant features. These features are then combined using a mathematical model to calculate the AVQI score. Examples of objective methods include Praat software, which measures various voice parameters, and the glottal inverse filtering (GIF) method, which estimates the glottal source waveform from the speech signal. Subjective methods use human listeners to rate the quality of the voice based on perceptual criteria, such as clarity, naturalness, and overall acceptability. These ratings are then combined using statistical methods to calculate the AVQI score. Examples of subjective methods include the consensus auditory–perceptual evaluation of voice (CAPE-V), which uses a standardized rating scale to evaluate various aspects of voice quality.

Step 2: Plot the candidate solutions on a Pareto front to visualize the trade-off between the objectives.

To plot the candidate solutions on a Pareto front, we first need to define the objective functions that we want to optimize. For example, we may want to maximize the clarity of the voice while minimizing the jitter and shimmer. We can then calculate the objective values for each candidate solution and plot them on a 2D or 3D graph, where each axis represents an objective function. The Pareto front is the set of candidate solutions that cannot be improved in one objective without sacrificing another objective.

Step 3: Identify the Pareto optimal solutions on the Pareto front that cannot be improved in one objective without sacrificing another objective.

To identify the Pareto optimal solutions, we can use a variety of techniques, such as visual inspection, clustering, or optimization algorithms. Visual inspection involves manually examining the Pareto front and selecting the solutions that best meet the specific needs and preferences of the AVQI assessment. Clustering involves grouping similar solutions together and selecting the representative solutions from each cluster. Optimization algorithms, such as the NSGA-II (non-dominated sorting genetic Algorithm 2) can be used to automatically identify the Pareto optimal solutions.

Step 4: Select the Pareto optimal solution that best meets the specific needs and preferences of the AVQI assessment.

To select the Pareto optimal solution that best meets the specific needs and preferences of the AVQI assessment, we need to consider factors, such as clinical relevance, patient preference, and ease of implementation. We may also want to consult with clinicians and patients to get their feedback and ensure that the selected solution is acceptable and feasible.

Step 5: Fine-tune the AVQI algorithm and the Pareto optimization parameters based on the validation results and feedback from clinicians and patients

To fine-tune the AVQI algorithm and the Pareto optimization parameters, we need to evaluate the performance of the algorithm using validation data and feedback from clinicians and patients. We can use metrics such as accuracy, sensitivity, specificity, and AUC (area under the roc curve) to assess the performance of the AVQI algorithm. We can also ask clinicians and patients to rate the quality of the voice for a subset of the validation data and compare the ratings with the AVQI scores. Based on the validation results and feedback.

4. Results

AVQI Evaluation Outcomes

First, we used two statistical measures to assess the agreement and reliability of the data collected through individual smartphone AVQI evaluations and inter smartphone AVQI measurements. Cronbach's alpha was used as a statistical measure to assess the internal consistency or reliability of AVQI. It ranges from 0 to 1, where 0 indicates no internal consistency or reliability, and 1 indicates perfect internal consistency or reliability. The Cronbach's alpha for individual smartphone AVQI evaluations was calculated to be 0.99, which is an excellent agreement.

Next, we calculated the intraclass correlation coefficient (ICC), which is a statistical measure used to assess the reliability or consistency of the measurements taken by different raters or methods, in our case, different smartphones. It ranges from 0 to 1, where 0 indicates that there is no reliability or consistency, and 1 indicates perfect reliability or consistency. Therefore, the ICC was used to assess the reliability of the intersmartphone AVQI measurements, and we determined the average ICC to be 0.9115, which is an excellent result. The range of ICC values from 0.8885 to 0.9316 suggests that the measurements taken by different smartphones are consistent and reliable throughout the range.

Table 2 displays the mean AVQI scores obtained from various smartphones and a studio microphone.

Table 2. Comparison of the mean results of the AVQI obtained with different smartphones and studio microphones.

Microphone	n	Mean AVQI	Std. Deviation	F	p
AKG Perception 220	134	3.412	1.823	9.03	<0.001
iPhone SE		3.238	1.798		
iPhone PRO MAX 13		3.016	1.735		
Huawei P50 pro		3.581	1.977		
Samsung S22 Ultra		4.407	2.014		
OnePlus 9 PRO		3.736	1.817		

We also performed a one-way ANOVA test to determine whether there are statistically significant differences between the means of three or more independent groups. In our case, a one-way ANOVA was performed to compare the mean AVQI scores obtained from different smartphones. The results of the analysis (presented in Table 2) indicate that there were significant differences in mean AVQI scores between different smartphones ($F = 9.035$; $p \leq 0.001$). Therefore, pairwise comparisons were conducted to determine which smartphones differed significantly from each other. The results of the pairwise comparisons (pairwise analysis) revealed that there were significant differences between AKG Perception 220 (studio microphone) and Samsung S22 Ultra ($p < 0.001$).

We also explored the differences in mean AVQI scores (ranged from 0.17 to 0.99 points) when comparing different smartphones. These indicate that some smartphones performed better than others in terms of producing accurate and high-quality sound recordings.

Table 3 reports that there was a nearly perfect direct linear correlation between the AVQI results obtained from both the studio microphone and different smartphones. This means that the AVQI scores obtained from different smartphones were highly correlated with the AVQI scores obtained from the studio microphone. Pearson's correlation coefficients ranged from 0.976 to 0.99, which is a strong positive correlation.

Table 3. Correlations of AVQI scores obtained with a studio microphone and different smartphones.

Microphones	Criterion	iPhone SE	iPhone	Pro Max 13	Huawei P50 Pro	Samsung S22 Ultra	OnePlus 9 PRO
AKG Perception 220	r	0.9937	0.9904	0.9764	0.9777	0.9895	
	p	0.001	0.001	0.001	0.001	0.001	
	n	134	134	134	134	134	

For analysis, the Bland–Altman plot, often known as the difference plot, is used as a visual way to contrast two measuring methods [65]. The ratios (or disparities, as an alternative) between the two procedures are shown. For all devices compared to the reference microphone, bias and critical difference were computed, and the relevant Bland–Altman graphs are shown in Figure 11.

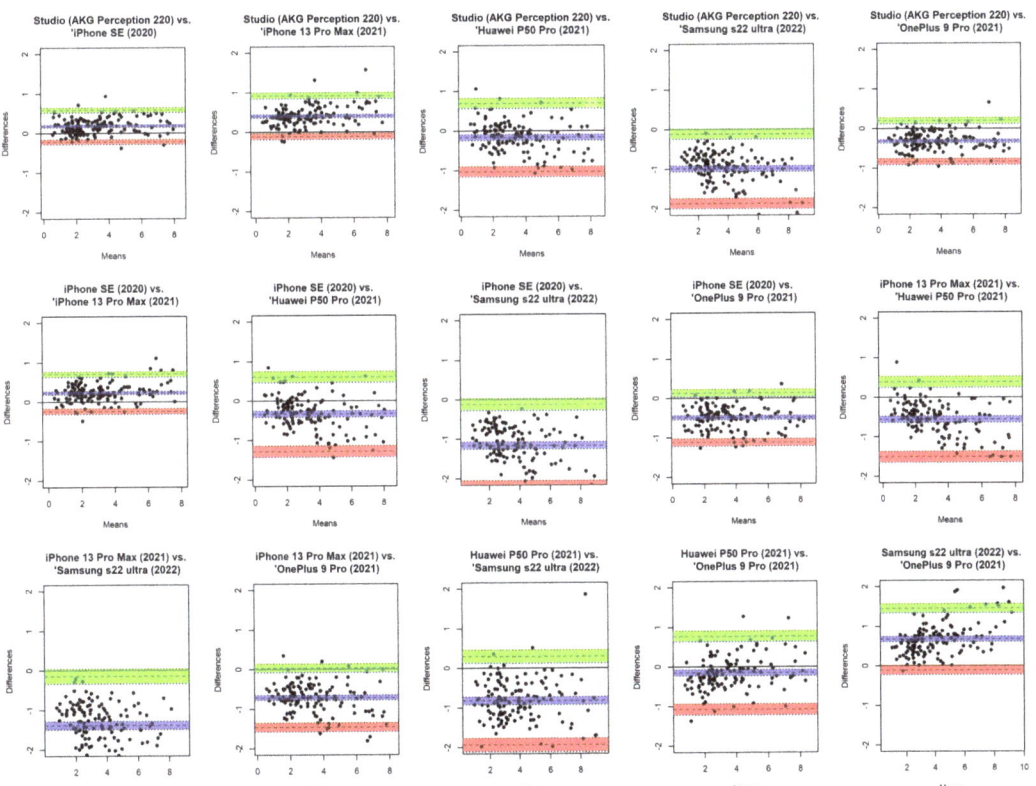

Figure 11. Bland–Altman plot for comparison of AVQI scores obtained from each smartphone device and the reference microphone.

The bias's 95% confidence interval was used. If 0 was omitted from the confidence interval, the bias was considered substantial. To compare the means of the recorded samples from the reference microphone with the means from the five cellphones, we utilized Bland–Altman analysis. Both an absolute number and a percentage of the complete range of the relevant parameter, as determined by the reference microphone, are used to express the amount of the important difference (random error). The results show the crucial difference calculated from studio microphone measurements as a percentage of the parameter's total range and in absolute numbers. For the combined male and female samples, bias and critical difference were computed. In order to determine if gender has any impact on overall bias and crucial difference, the Bland–Altman plots display data points designated by gender. The 95% confidence interval was used in significance testing for bias values, as was previously noted. The correlation between AVQI results obtained from studio using AKG Perception 220 microphone and different smartphones with a 95% confidence interval is illustrated in Figure 12.

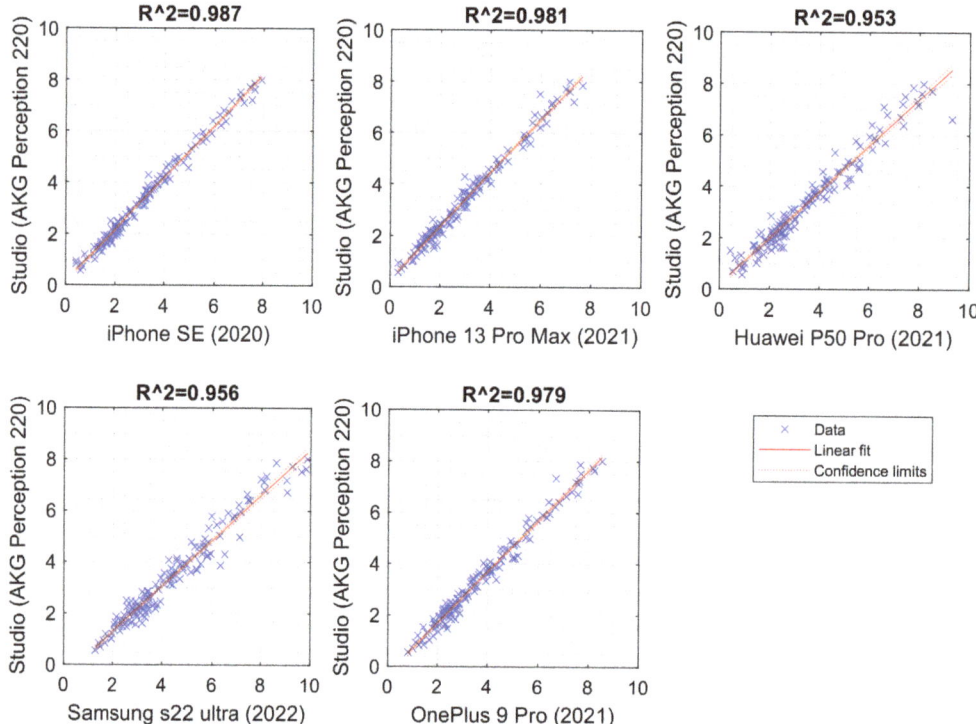

Figure 12. Scatterplot illustrating the correlation between AVQI results obtained from studio using AKG Perception 220 microphone and different smartphones with a 95% confidence interval.

The experimental evaluation continued with the analysis of receiver operating characteristic (ROC) curves using AVQI to determine the diagnostic accuracy of different smartphones compared to a professional microphone (see Figure 13). ROC curves are representations of the relationship between the sensitivity and specificity of a diagnostic test at various cutoff points. They were used to evaluate the performance of diagnostic tests and to determine the optimal cutoff scores for diagnostic accuracy to compare the diagnostic accuracy of different smartphones with a professional microphone.

The diagnostic accuracy of different smartphones was comparable to that of a professional microphone. This suggests that smartphones were able to distinguish between normal and pathological voices with accuracy similar to that of a professional microphone.

To determine the optimal cutoff scores for diagnostic precision, the ROC curves obtained from the studio microphone and different smartphones were visually inspected according to the general interpretation guidelines [66]. This allowed one to identify the best balance between sensitivity and specificity for each smartphone, and the cutoff score was determined accordingly.

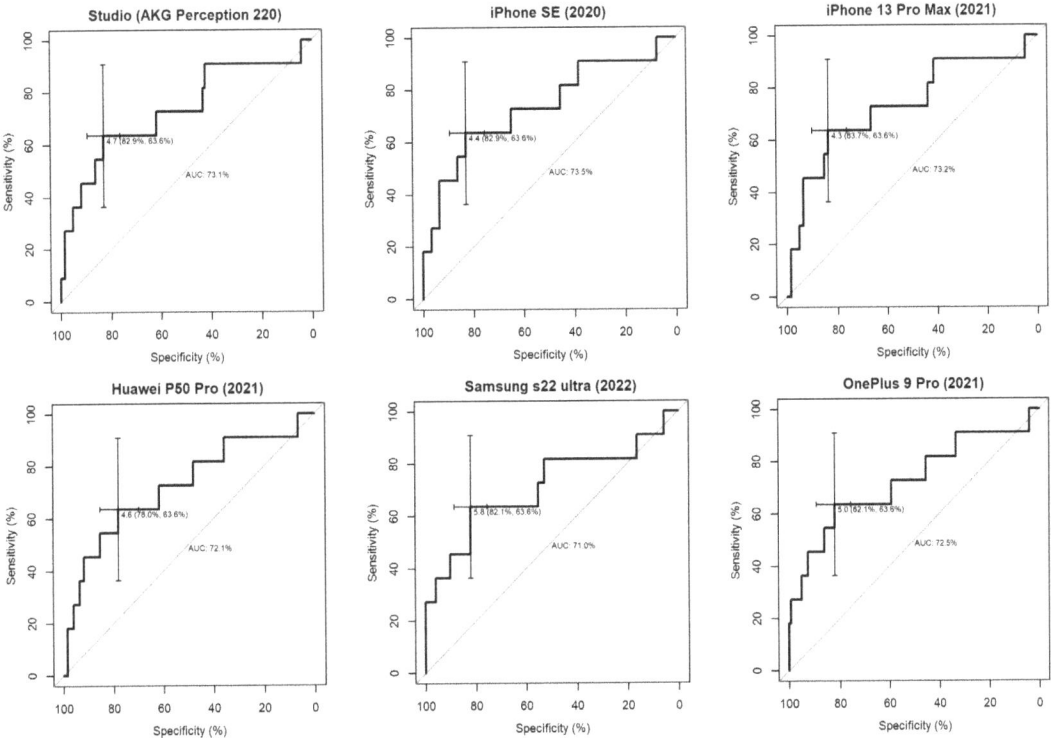

Figure 13. ROC curves illustrating the diagnostic accuracy of studio and different smartphone microphones in discriminating normal/pathological voice.

Furthermore, the AUC statistics analysis demonstrated that AVQI had a high level of precision in distinguishing between normal and pathological voices, as evidenced by the suggested AUC = 0.7 threshold. The findings of the ROC statistical analysis are provided in Table 4.

We also analyzed the area under the curve (AUC) statistics to determine the accuracy of AVQI in distinguishing between normal and pathological voices. This statistical measure was used to evaluate the performance of a diagnostic test. It represents the ability of the test to correctly classify individuals into normal and pathological categories. An AUC of 0.5 indicates that the test is no better than random guessing, whereas an AUC of 1.0 indicates perfect classification. A good level of accuracy was achieved, which means that AVQI was able to correctly classify individuals into normal and pathological categories with a high degree of accuracy (the suggested threshold for high precision was an AUC of 0.7, which means that if the AUC value of AVQI was equal to or greater than 0.7, it could be considered a highly accurate diagnostic test to distinguish between normal and pathological voices).

Through the use of ROC analysis (see Table 4), we determined that there are optimal AVQI cut-off values that can effectively distinguish between normal and pathological voices for each smartphone used in the study. Furthermore, all of these devices met the proposed 0.7 AUC threshold and demonstrated an acceptable Youden index value. These results indicate that AVQI is a reliable tool for distinguishing between normal and pathological voice, be it using a smartphone or professional recording equipment.

Table 4. The findings of the ROC statistical analysis.

AVQI	AUC	Cut-Off	Sensitivity (%)	Specificity (%)	Youden-Index J	F-Score
AKG Perception 220	0.731	4.7	82.9	73.1	0.560	0.777
IPHONE SE	0.735	4.4	82.9	63.6	0.465	0.719
IPHONE PRO MAX 13	0.732	4.3	83.7	63.6	0.473	0.722
Huawei P50 pro	0.721	4.6	78.0	63.6	0.416	0.701
Samsung S22 Ultra	0.710	5.8	82.1	63.6	0.457	0.716
OnePlus 9 PRO	0.725	5.0	82.1	63.6	0.457	0.716

Third, a pairwise comparison of the significance of the differences between the AUCs revealed in the present study is presented in Table 5. We used DeLong's test [67] for two correlated ROC curves, which allows us to statistically compare the AUCs of two dependent ROC curves. This test takes into account the correlation between the ROC curves and provides a more accurate comparison of the AUCs. DeLong's test confirmed that there were no statistically significant differences between the AUCs obtained from AVQI measurements obtained from the studio microphone and different smartphones. This means that the ability of AVQI to distinguish between normal and pathological voices was comparable between the studio microphone and different smartphones. The largest difference observed between the AUCs obtained from the studio microphone and different smartphones was only 0.025. This means that the difference in the ability of AVQI to distinguish between normal and pathological voices between the studio microphone and different smartphones was very small.

Table 5. A pairwise comparison of the significance of differences between AUCs was revealed in the present study.

Phone	AKG Perception 220	iPhone SE	iPhone PRO MAX 13	Huawei P50 Pro	Samsung S22 Ultra	OnePlus 9 PRO
AKG Perception 220	-	0.6176	0.9319	0.4851	0.4534	0.5938
iPhone SE	0.6176	-	0.6991	0.1995	0.2888	0.2478
iPhone PRO MAX 13	0.9319	0.6991	-	0.4851	0.4869	0.6649
Huawei P50 pro	0.4851	0.1995	0.4851	-	0.5978	0.7618
Samsung S22 Ultra	0.4534	0.2888	0.4869	0.5978	-	0.4128
OnePlus 9 PRO	0.5938	0.2478	0.6649	0.7618	0.4128	-

To summarize, across the statistical analysis of the study results, the data demonstrated almost identical and compatible results of AVQI performance between studio microphones and different smartphones. However, it is important to note that differences in the phone operating conditions, microphones within each smartphone series, and version of the operating system software may cause variations in acoustic voice quality measurements between recording systems. Therefore, it is advisable to use the "VoiceScreen" app with caution if tests are being performed using multiple devices. For reliable voice screening purposes, it is recommended to perform AVQI measurements using the same device, preferably with repeated measurements. These considerations should also be taken into account when comparing data from acoustic voice analysis between different recording systems, such as different smartphones or other mobile communication devices, and when using them for diagnostic purposes or monitoring voice treatment results.

5. Discussion and Conclusions

The VoiceScreen algorithm was created for clinical research and can be used on both iOS and Android devices. The AVQI and its characteristics are computed on the server, and the sound waves collected from the provided smartphone are preprocessed to remove pauses and excess sound before being sent to the server for analysis. The evaluation results were found to be reproducible on different smartphone platforms with no statistical differences. Furthermore, there was a nearly perfect direct linear correlation between the AVQI results obtained from the studio microphone and different smartphones, as the individual smartphone AVQI evaluations demonstrated excellent agreement as indicated by a Cronbach alpha of 0.99. Similarly, the inter-smartphone AVQI measurements showed excellent reliability with an average intra-class correlation coefficient (ICC) of 0.9115 (ranging from 0.8885 to 0.9316). The results of the one-way ANOVA analysis did not reveal significant differences in mean AVQI scores between different smartphones, indicating that the results of the AVQI evaluation are reproducible on different smartphone platforms. Similarly, Pearson's correlation coefficients ranged from 0.976 to 0.99, indicating a nearly perfect direct linear correlation between AVQI results obtained from both the studio microphone and different smartphones. Additionally, based on the analysis of ROC curves using AVQI, it was determined that the diagnostic accuracy of different smartphones was comparable to that of a professional microphone. We determined that there are optimal AVQI cut-off values that can effectively distinguish between normal and pathological voices for each smartphone used in the study. Furthermore, all devices met the proposed 0.7 AUC threshold and demonstrated an acceptable Youden index value.

These results confirmed compatible results of the diagnostic accuracy of AVQI in differentiating normal versus pathological voices when using voice recordings from studio microphones and different smartphones, and our approach was found to be a reliable tool for distinguishing between normal and pathological voices, regardless of the device used, with no statistically significant differences between the voice impairment measurements obtained from different devices.

A substantial device effect was detected in a comparable study [68] for low versus high spectral ratio (L/H Ratio) (dB) in both vowel and phrase contexts, as well as for the cepstral spectral index of dysphonia (CSID) in the sentence context. It was discovered that independent of context, the device had a little influence on CPP (dB). The recording distance had a small-to-moderate influence on measurements of CPP and CSID but had no effect on the L/H ratio. The setting was found to have a considerable influence on all three measures, with the exception of the L/H ratio in the vowel context. The range of voice characteristics contained in the voice sample corpus was captured by all devices evaluated.

Author Contributions: Conceptualization, V.U.; Data curation, K.P.; Formal analysis, R.M., R.D., T.B., K.P., N.U.-S. and V.U.; Funding acquisition, V.U.; Investigation, K.P. and N.U.-S.; Methodology, K.P. and V.U.; Project administration, R.M. and V.U.; Resources, R.D., K.P. and V.U.; Software, T.B.; Supervision, R.M.; Validation, R.M., R.D. and K.P.; Visualization, R.D.; Writing—original draft, R.M.; Writing—review and editing, R.M. and R.D. All authors have read and agreed to the published version of the manuscript.

Funding: This project has received funding from European Regional Development Fund (project No. 13.1.1-LMT-K-718-05-0027) under grant agreement with the Research Council of Lithuania (LMTLT). Funded as European Union's measure in response to COVID-19 pandemic.

Institutional Review Board Statement: This study was approved by the Kaunas Regional Ethics Committee for Biomedical Research (2022-04-20 No. BE-2-49) and by Lithuanian State Data Protection Inspectorate for Working with Personal Patient Data (No. 2R-648 (2.6-1)).

Informed Consent Statement: Informed consent was obtained from all subjects involved in the study.

Acknowledgments: The authors acknowledge the use of artificial intelligence tools for grammar checking and language improvement.

Conflicts of Interest: The authors declare no conflict of interest.

Abbreviations

The following abbreviations are used in this manuscript:

SPL	sound pressure level
f0	fundamental frequency
AVQO	Acoustic Voice Quality Index
ABI	Acoustic Breathiness Index
CPPS	smoothed cepstral peak prominence
PET	pitch elevation training
ART	articulation-resonance training
VHI	Voice Handicap Index
RPM	respiratory protection masks
KN95	variant of respiratory protection masks
CSID	cepstral spectral index of dysphonia
TPO	trans-surgical palatine obturators
VHI-10	Voice Handicap Index 10
MPT	maximum phonation time
RBH	roughness, breathiness, hoarseness scale
SD	standard deviation
SNR	signal-to-noise ratio
GRBAS	grade, roughness, breathiness, asthenia, strain scale
iOS	Apple smartphone operating system
HNR	harmonicity
LTAS	long-term average spectrum
ANOVA	analysis of variance
ROC	receiver operating curve
AUC	area under the ROC curve

References

1. McKenna, V.S.; Vojtech, J.M.; Previtera, M.; Kendall, C.L.; Carraro, K.E. A Scoping Literature Review of Relative Fundamental Frequency (RFF) in Individuals with and without Voice Disorders. *Appl. Sci.* **2022**, *12*, 8121. [CrossRef]
2. Jayakumar, T.; Benoy, J.J. Acoustic Voice Quality Index (AVQI) in the Measurement of Voice Quality: A Systematic Review and Meta-Analysis. *J. Voice* **2022**, in press. [CrossRef] [PubMed]
3. Saeedi, S.; Aghajanzadeh, M.; Khatoonabadi, A.R. A Literature Review of Voice Indices Available for Voice Assessment. *J. Rehabil. Sci. Res.* **2022**, *9*, 151–155.
4. Englert, M.; Latoszek, B.B.V.; Behlau, M. Exploring The Validity of Acoustic Measurements and Other Voice Assessments. *J. Voice* **2022**, in press. [CrossRef] [PubMed]
5. Englert, M.; Latoszek, B.B.V.; Maryn, Y.; Behlau, M. Validation of the Acoustic Voice Quality Index, Version 03.01, to the Brazilian Portuguese Language. *J. Voice* **2021**, *35*, 160.e15–160.e21. [CrossRef]
6. Grillo, E.U.; Wolfberg, J. An Assessment of Different Praat Versions for Acoustic Measures Analyzed Automatically by VoiceEvalU8 and Manually by Two Raters. *J. Voice* **2023**, *37*, 17–25. [CrossRef]
7. Shabnam, S.; Pushpavathi, M. Effect of Gender on Acoustic Voice Quality Index 02.03 and Dysphonia Severity Index in Indian Normophonic Adults. *Indian J. Otolaryngol. Head Neck Surg.* **2022**, *74*, 5052–5059. [CrossRef]
8. Jayakumar, T.; Benoy, J.J.; Yasin, H.M. Effect of Age and Gender on Acoustic Voice Quality Index Across Lifespan: A Cross-sectional Study in Indian Population. *J. Voice* **2022**, *36*, 436.e1–436.e8. [CrossRef]
9. Leyns, C.; Daelman, J.; Adriaansen, A.; Tomassen, P.; Morsomme, D.; T'sjoen, G.; D'haeseleer, E. Short-Term Acoustic Effects of Speech Therapy in Transgender Women: A Randomized Controlled Trial. *Am. J. Speech-Lang. Pathol.* **2023**, *32*, 145–168. [CrossRef]
10. Verde, L.; Brancati, N.; De Pietro, G.; Frucci, M.; Sannino, G. A Deep Learning Approach for Voice Disorder Detection for Smart Connected Living Environments. *ACM Trans. Internet Technol.* **2022**, *22*, 1–16. [CrossRef]
11. Fahed, V.S.; Doheny, E.P.; Busse, M.; Hoblyn, J.; Lowery, M.M. Comparison of Acoustic Voice Features Derived From Mobile Devices and Studio Microphone Recordings. *J. Voice* **2022**, in press. [CrossRef] [PubMed]
12. Kim, G.; Lee, Y.; Bae, I.; Park, H.; Kwon, S.. Effect of mobile-based voice therapy on the voice quality of patients with dysphonia. *Clin. Arch. Commun. Disord.* **2021**, *6*, 48–54. [CrossRef]
13. Uloza, V.; Ulozaitė-Stanienė, N.; Petrauskas, T.; Kregždytė, R. Accuracy of Acoustic Voice Quality Index Captured With a Smartphone – Measurements With Added Ambient Noise. *J. Voice* **2021**, in press. [CrossRef] [PubMed]
14. Pommée, T.; Morsomme, D. Voice Quality in Telephone Interviews: A preliminary Acoustic Investigation. *J. Voice* **2022**, in press. [CrossRef]

15. Uloza, V.; Ulozaite-Staniene, N.; Petrauskas, T. An iOS-based VoiceScreen application: Feasibility for use in clinical settings—A pilot study. *Eur. Arch. Oto-Rhino* **2023**, *280*, 277–284. [CrossRef] [PubMed]
16. Brockmann-Bauser, M.; de Paula Soares, M.F. Do We Get What We Need from Clinical Acoustic Voice Measurements? *Appl. Sci.* **2023**, *13*, 941. [CrossRef]
17. Queiroz, M.R.G.; Pernambuco, L.; Leão, R.L.D.S.; Araújo, A.N.; Gomes, A.D.O.C.; da Silva, H.J.; Lucena, J.A. Voice Therapy for Older Adults During the COVID-19 Pandemic in Brazil. *J. Voice* **2022**, *in press*. [CrossRef]
18. Faham, M.; Laukkanen, A.; Ikävalko, T.; Rantala, L.; Geneid, A.; Holmqvist-Jämsén, S.; Ruusuvirta, K.; Pirilä, S. Acoustic Voice Quality Index as a Potential Tool for Voice Screening. *J. Voice* **2021**, *35*, 226–232. [CrossRef]
19. Englert, M.; Lopes, L.; Vieira, V.; Behlau, M. Accuracy of Acoustic Voice Quality Index and Its Isolated Acoustic Measures to Discriminate the Severity of Voice Disorders. *J. Voice* **2022**, *36*, 582.e1–582.e10. [CrossRef]
20. Englert, M.; Lima, L.; Latoszek, B.B.V.; Behlau, M. Influence of the Voice Sample Length in Perceptual and Acoustic Voice Quality Analysis. *J. Voice* **2022**, *36*, 582.e23–582.e32. [CrossRef]
21. Thijs, Z.; Knickerbocker, K.; Watts, C.R. The Degree of Change and Relationship in Self-perceived Handicap and Acoustic Voice Quality Associated With Voice Therapy. *J. Voice* **2022**, *in press*. [CrossRef] [PubMed]
22. Thijs, Z.; Knickerbocker, K.; Watts, C.R. Epidemiological Patterns and Treatment Outcomes in a Private Practice Community Voice Clinic. *J. Voice* **2022**, *36*, 437.e11–437.e20. [CrossRef] [PubMed]
23. Maryn, Y.; Wuyts, F.L.; Zarowski, A. Are Acoustic Markers of Voice and Speech Signals Affected by Nose-and-Mouth-Covering Respiratory Protective Masks? *J. Voice* **2021**, *in press*. [CrossRef] [PubMed]
24. Knowles, T.; Badh, G. The impact of face masks on spectral acoustics of speech: Effect of clear and loud speech styles. *J. Acoust. Soc. Am.* **2022**, *151*, 3359–3368. [CrossRef] [PubMed]
25. Lehnert, B.; Herold, J.; Blaurock, M.; Busch, C. Reliability of the Acoustic Voice Quality Index AVQI and the Acoustic Breathiness Index (ABI) when wearing CoViD-19 protective masks. *Eur. Arch. Oto-Rhino* **2022**, *279*, 4617–4621. [CrossRef]
26. Boutsen, F.R.; Park, E.; Dvorak, J.D. An Efficacy Study of Voice Quality Using Cepstral Analyses of Phonation in Parkinson's Disease before and after SPEAK-OUT!®. *Folia Phoniatr. Logop.* **2023**, *75*, 35–42. [CrossRef]
27. Maskeliūnas, R.; Damaševičius, R.; Kulikajevas, A.; Padervinskis, E.; Pribuišis, K.; Uloza, V. A Hybrid U-Lossian Deep Learning Network for Screening and Evaluating Parkinson's Disease. *Appl. Sci.* **2022**, *12*, 11601. [CrossRef]
28. Moya-Galé, G.; Spielman, J.; Ramig, L.A.; Campanelli, L.; Maryn, Y. The Acoustic Voice Quality Index (AVQI) in People with Parkinson's Disease Before and After Intensive Voice and Articulation Therapies: Secondary Outcome of a Randomized Controlled Trial. *J. Voice* **2022**, *in press*. [CrossRef]
29. Batthyany, C.; Latoszek, B.B.V.; Maryn, Y. Meta-Analysis on the Validity of the Acoustic Voice Quality Index. *J. Voice* **2022**, *in press*. [CrossRef]
30. Bhatt, S.S.; Kabra, S.; Chatterjee, I. A Comparative Study on Acoustic Voice Quality Index Between the Subjects with Spasmodic Dysphonia and Normophonia. *Indian J. Otolaryngol. Head Neck Surg.* **2022**, *74*, 4927–4932. [CrossRef]
31. Portalete, C.R.; Moraes, D.A.D.O.; Pagliarin, K.C.; Keske-Soares, M.; Cielo, C.A. Acoustic and Physiological Voice Assessment And Maximum Phonation Time In Patients With Different Types Of Dysarthria. *J. Voice* **2021**, *in press*. [CrossRef] [PubMed]
32. Latoszek, B.B.V.; Mathmann, P.; Neumann, K. The cepstral spectral index of dysphonia, the acoustic voice quality index and the acoustic breathiness index as novel multiparametric indices for acoustic assessment of voice quality. *Curr. Opin. Otolaryngol. Head Neck Surg.* **2021**, *29*, 451–457. [CrossRef] [PubMed]
33. Latoszek, B.B.V.; Englert, M.; Lucero, J.C.; Behlau, M. The Performance of the Acoustic Voice Quality Index and Acoustic Breathiness Index in Synthesized Voices. *J. Voice* **2021**, *in press*.
34. León Gómez, N.M.; Delgado Hernández, J.; Luis Hernández, J.; Artazkoz del Toro, J.J. Objective Analysis Of Voice Quality In Patients With Thyroid Pathology. *Clin. Otolaryngol.* **2022**, *47*, 81–87. [CrossRef] [PubMed]
35. Maskeliūnas, R.; Kulikajevas, A.; Damaševičius, R.; Pribuišis, K.; Ulozaitė-Stanienė, N.; Uloza, V. Lightweight Deep Learning Model for Assessment of Substitution Voicing and Speech after Laryngeal Carcinoma Surgery. *Cancers* **2022**, *14*, 2366. [CrossRef] [PubMed]
36. Uloza, V.; Maskeliunas, R.; Pribuisis, K.; Vaitkus, S.; Kulikajevas, A.; Damasevicius, R. An Artificial Intelligence-Based Algorithm for the Assessment of Substitution Voicing. *Appl. Sci.* **2022**, *12*, 9748. [CrossRef]
37. Revoredo, E.C.V.; Gomes, A.D.O.C.; Ximenes, C.R.C.; Oliveira, K.G.S.C.D.; Silva, H.J.D.; Leão, J.C. Oropharyngeal Geometry of Maxilectomized Patients Rehabilitated with Palatal Obturators in the Trans-surgical Period: Repercussions on the Voice. *J. Voice* **2022**, *in press*. [CrossRef]
38. van Sluis, K.E.; van Son, R.J.J.H.; van der Molen, L.; MCGuinness, A.J.; Palme, C.E.; Novakovic, D.; Stone, D.; Natsis, L.; Charters, E.; Jones, K.; et al. Multidimensional evaluation of voice outcomes following total laryngectomy: A prospective multicenter cohort study. *Eur. Arch. Oto-Rhino* **2021**, *278*, 1209–1222. [CrossRef]
39. Tattari, N.; Forss, M.; Laukkanen, A.; Rantala, L.; Finland, T. The Efficacy of the NHS Waterpipe in Superficial Hydration for People With Healthy Voices: Effects on Acoustic Voice Quality, Phonation Threshold Pressure and Subjective Sensations. *J. Voice* **2021**, *in press*. [CrossRef]

40. Kara, I.; Temiz, F.; Doganer, A.; Sagıroglu, S.; Yıldız, M.G.; Bilal, N.; Orhan, I. The effect of type 1 diabetes mellitus on voice in pediatric patients. *Eur. Arch. Oto-Rhino* **2023**, *280*, 269–275. [CrossRef]
41. Asiaee, M.; Nourbakhsh, M.; Vahedian-Azimi, A.; Zare, M.; Jafari, R.; Atashi, S.S.; Keramatfar, A. The feasibility of using acoustic measures for predicting the Total Opacity Scores of chest computed tomography scans in patients with COVID-19. *Clin. Linguist. Phon.* **2023** . [CrossRef] [PubMed]
42. Huttunen, K.; Rantala, L. Effects of Humidification of the Vocal Tract and Respiratory Muscle Training in Women With Voice Symptoms—A Pilot Study. *J. Voice* **2021**, *35*, 158.e21–158.e33. [CrossRef] [PubMed]
43. Penido, F.A.; Gama, A.C.C. Accuracy Analysis of the Multiparametric Acoustic Indices AVQI, ABI, and DSI for Speech-Language Pathologist Decision-Making. *J. Voice* **2023**, in press. [CrossRef] [PubMed]
44. Nudelman, C.; Webster, J.; Bottalico, P. The Effects of Reading Speed on Acoustic Voice Parameters and Self-reported Vocal Fatigue in Students. *J. Voice* **2021**, in press. [CrossRef]
45. Fujiki, R.B.; Huber, J.E.; Preeti Sivasankar, M. The effects of vocal exertion on lung volume measurements and acoustics in speakers reporting high and low vocal fatigue. *PLoS ONE* **2022**, *17*, e0268324. [CrossRef]
46. Aishwarya, S.Y.; Narasimhan, S.V. The effect of a prolonged and demanding vocal activity (Divya Prabhandam recitation) on subjective and objective measures of voice among Indian Hindu priests. *Speech Lang. Hear.* **2022**, *25*, 498–506. [CrossRef]
47. Jayakumar, T.; Kalyani, A.; Kashyap Bannuru Nanjundaswamy, R.; Tonni, S.S. A Preliminary Study on the Effect of Bhramari Pranayama on Voice of Prospective Singers. *J. Voice* **2022**, in press. [CrossRef]
48. Anand, S.; Bottalico, P.; Gray, C. Vocal Fatigue in Prospective Vocal Professionals. *J. Voice* **2021**, *35*, 247–258. [CrossRef]
49. Meerschman, I.; D'haeseleer, E.; Cammu, H.; Kissel, I.; Papeleu, T.; Leyns, C.; Daelman, J.; Dannhauer, J.; Vanden Abeele, L.; Konings, V.; et al. Voice Quality of Choir Singers and the Effect of a Performance on the Voice. *J. Voice* **2022**, in press. [CrossRef]
50. D'haeseleer, E.; Quintyn, F.; Kissel, I.; Papeleu, T.; Meerschman, I.; Claeys, S.; Van Lierde, K. Vocal Quality, Symptoms, and Habits in Musical Theater Actors. *J. Voice* **2022**, *36*, 292.e1–292.e9. [CrossRef]
51. Grama, M.; Barrichelo-Lindström, V.; Englert, M.; Kinghorn, D.; Behlau, M. Resonant Voice: Perceptual and Acoustic Analysis After an Intensive Lessac Kinesensic Training Workshop. *J. Voice* **2021**, in press. [CrossRef]
52. Leyns, C.; Daelman, J.; Meerschman, I.; Claeys, S.; Van Lierde, K.; D'haeseleer, E. Vocal Quality After a Performance in Actors Compared to Dancers. *J. Voice* **2022**, *36*, 141.e19–141.e31. [CrossRef] [PubMed]
53. Trinite, B.; Barute, D.; Blauzde, O.; Ivane, M.; Paipare, M.; Sleze, D.; Valce, I. Choral Conductors Vocal Loading in Rehearsal Simulation Conditions. *J. Voice* **2022**, in press. [CrossRef]
54. Englert, M.; Latoszek, B.B.V.; Behlau, M. The Impact of Languages and Cultural Backgrounds on Voice Quality Analyses. *Folia Phoniatr. Logop.* **2022**, *74*, 141–152. [CrossRef] [PubMed]
55. Fantini, M.; Ricci Maccarini, A.; Firino, A.; Gallia, M.; Carlino, V.; Gorris, C.; Spadola Bisetti, M.; Crosetti, E.; Succo, G. Validation of the Acoustic Voice Quality Index (AVQI) Version 03.01 in Italian. *J. Voice* **2021**, in press. [CrossRef] [PubMed]
56. Szklanny, K.; Lachowicz, J. Implementing a Statistical Parametric Speech Synthesis System for a Patient with Laryngeal Cancer. *Sensors* **2022**, *22*, 3188. [CrossRef] [PubMed]
57. Jayakumar, T.; Rajasudhakar, R.; Benoy, J.J. Comparison and Validation of Acoustic Voice Quality Index Version 2 and Version 3 among South Indian Population. *J. Voice* **2022**, in press. [CrossRef] [PubMed]
58. Kim, G.; von Latoszek, B.B.; Lee, Y. Validation of Acoustic Voice Quality Index Version 3.01 and Acoustic Breathiness Index in Korean Population. *J. Voice* **2021**, *35*, 660.e9–660.e18. [CrossRef] [PubMed]
59. Lee, Y.; Kim, G.; Sohn, K.; Lee, B.; Lee, J.; Kwon, S. The Usefulness of Auditory Perceptual Assessment and Acoustic Analysis as a Screening Test for Voice Problems. *Folia Phoniatr. Logop.* **2021**, *73*, 34–41. [CrossRef]
60. Kishore Pebbili, G.; Shabnam, S.; Pushpavathi, M.; Rashmi, J.; Gopi Sankar, R.; Nethra, R.; Shreya, S.; Shashish, G. Diagnostic Accuracy of Acoustic Voice Quality Index Version 02.03 in Discriminating across the Perceptual Degrees of Dysphonia Severity in Kannada Language. *J. Voice* **2021**, *35*, 159.e11–159.e18. [CrossRef]
61. Laukkanen, A.; Rantala, L. Does the Acoustic Voice Quality Index (AVQI) Correlate with Perceived Creak and Strain in Normophonic Young Adult Finnish Females? *Folia Phoniatr. Logop.* **2022**, *74*, 62–69. [CrossRef]
62. Yeşilli-Puzella, G.; Tadıhan-Özkan, E.; Maryn, Y. Validation and Test-Retest Reliability of Acoustic Voice Quality Index Version 02.06 in the Turkish Language. *J. Voice* **2022**, *36*, 736.e25–736.e32. [CrossRef] [PubMed]
63. Zainaee, S.; khadivi, E.; Jamali, J.; Sobhani-Rad, D.; Maryn, Y.; Ghaemi, H. The acoustic voice quality index, version 2.06 and 3.01, for the Persian-speaking population. *J. Commun. Disord.* **2022**, *100*, 106279. [CrossRef] [PubMed]
64. Dejonckere, P.H.; Bradley, P.; Clemente, P.; Cornut, G.; Crevier-Buchman, L.; Friedrich, G.; Heyning, P.V.D.; Remacle, M.; Woisard, V. A basic protocol for functional assessment of voice pathology, especially for investigating the efficacy of (phonosurgical) treatments and evaluating new assessment techniques. *Eur. Arch. Oto-Rhino* **2001**, *258*, 77–82. [CrossRef] [PubMed]
65. Bland, J.; Altman, D. Comparing methods of measurement: Why plotting difference against standard method is misleading. *Lancet* **1995**, *346*, 1085–1087. [CrossRef] [PubMed]
66. Dollaghan, C.A. *The Handbook for Evidence-Based Practice in Communication Disorders*; Brookes Publishing: Baltimore, MD, USA, 2007.

67. DeLong, E.R.; DeLong, D.M.; Clarke-Pearson, D.L. Comparing the Areas under Two or More Correlated Receiver Operating Characteristic Curves: A Nonparametric Approach. *Biometrics* **1988**, *44*, 837. [CrossRef] [PubMed]
68. Awan, S.N.; Shaikh, M.A.; Awan, J.A.; Abdalla, I.; Lim, K.O.; Misono, S. Smartphone Recordings are Comparable to "Gold Standard" Recordings for Acoustic Measurements of Voice. *J. Voice* **2023**. [CrossRef] [PubMed]

Disclaimer/Publisher's Note: The statements, opinions and data contained in all publications are solely those of the individual author(s) and contributor(s) and not of MDPI and/or the editor(s). MDPI and/or the editor(s) disclaim responsibility for any injury to people or property resulting from any ideas, methods, instructions or products referred to in the content.

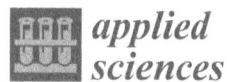

Article

CNN-Based Pill Image Recognition for Retrieval Systems

Khalil Al-Hussaeni [1,*], Ioannis Karamitsos [2], Ezekiel Adewumi [2] and Rema M. Amawi [3]

1. Computing Sciences, Rochester Institute of Technology, Dubai 341055, United Arab Emirates
2. Graduate and Research, Rochester Institute of Technology, Dubai 341055, United Arab Emirates
3. Science and Liberal Arts, Rochester Institute of Technology, Dubai 341055, United Arab Emirates
* Correspondence: kxacad@rit.edu

Abstract: Medication should be consumed as prescribed with little to zero margins for errors, otherwise consequences could be fatal. Due to the pervasiveness of camera-equipped mobile devices, patients and practitioners can easily take photos of unidentified pills to avert erroneous prescriptions or consumption. This area of research goes under the umbrella of information retrieval and, more specifically, image retrieval or recognition. Several studies have been conducted in the area of image retrieval in order to propose accurate models, i.e., accurately matching an input image with stored ones. Recently, neural networks have been shown to be effective in identifying digital images. This study aims to provide an enhancement to image retrieval in terms of accuracy and efficiency through image segmentation and classification. This paper suggests three neural network (CNN) architectures: two models that are hybrid networks paired with a classification method (CNN+SVM and CNN+kNN) and one ResNet-50 network. We perform various preprocessing steps by using several detection techniques on the selected dataset. We conduct extensive experiments using a real-life dataset obtained from the National Library of Medicine database. The results demonstrate that our proposed model is capable of deriving an accuracy of 90.8%. We also provide a comparison of the above-mentioned three models with some existing methods, and we notice that our proposed CNN+kNN architecture improved the pill image retrieval accuracy by 10% compared to existing models.

Keywords: image recognition; pill information retrieval; CNN; CBIR; machine learning; convolutional neural networks

Citation: Al-Hussaeni, K.; Karamitsos, I.; Adewumi, E.; Amawi, R.M. CNN-Based Pill Image Recognition for Retrieval Systems. *Appl. Sci.* **2023**, *13*, 5050. https://doi.org/10.3390/app13085050

Academic Editor: Chien-Hung Yeh

Received: 4 February 2023
Revised: 12 April 2023
Accepted: 13 April 2023
Published: 18 April 2023

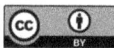

Copyright: © 2023 by the authors. Licensee MDPI, Basel, Switzerland. This article is an open access article distributed under the terms and conditions of the Creative Commons Attribution (CC BY) license (https://creativecommons.org/licenses/by/4.0/).

1. Introduction

Information Retrieval describes the process of sourcing information from a storage system. The retrieved information may be in the format of text, image, sound, or metadata describing a database or data. One interesting area is information retrieval from images, whereby an automated tool is used to identify objects in images. In this day and age, the increased dependency on smartphones has made informational retrieval from mobile phone photos a growing area of research [1].

Traditionally, metadata, such as keywords, captions, or image titles, have helped in information retrieval. However, this manual approach consumes time, effort, and costs. With increasing online activities, including social web applications, research on Content-Based Information Retrieval (CBIR) has become prominent in the field of Information Retrieval. CBIR is the field that describes automated image retrieval techniques that are capable of identifying images based on their "content", i.e., features embedded in the image, such as shape, texture, and color [2–4]. Research is still ongoing to improve the effectiveness of CBIR in terms of extracting primitive features (color and shape) and creating abstraction models to identify the level of relevance. The advances in image retrieval techniques have carved the path to applications in a variety of fields, including medicine, law enforcement, and engineering. Automated pill image recognition remains a significant application of CBIR in the field of medicine.

Given the criticality of medicine consumption, there is little to no room for errors, e.g., mistakenly prescribing or taking the wrong type of medicine. Yet, there is a high possibility of errors occurring while health personnel prescribe, dispense, or administer drugs. Makary and Daniel [5] argued that medical error ranks third on the major causes of death among hospital inpatients in the United States. WHO (the World Health Organization) statistics reveal that approximately 1.3 million patients die annually due to preventable medication blunders in the United States, which comes out to a minimum of one death per day. Moreover, WHO also admits medical error to be one of the top causes of injuries and avoidable harm [6]. Adverse Drug Effects (ADE) can also result in severe ailments, including Stevens–Johnson syndrome and Parkinson's disease [7]. WHO statistics report that health caregivers harm 4 out of every 10 patients globally [8], and Larios Delgado et al. [9] report that 39% of cases are severe enough to cause injury to patients.

Consumers often find it challenging to identify pills; consequently, they run into the risk of harming themselves from either consuming the wrong medication, underdosing, or overdosing. The risk of misidentifying pills is more prominent when pills are moved to different packaging containers, combined into a single container, or shared into pillboxes for ease of administration. Moreover, the financial implications of medication error are alarming: One-seventh of the Canadian budget and about 1% ($42 billion) of the total global health spending are spent on mitigating the effects of medication error [8].

To ensure safe medication consumption, each pill is made to have a distinctive appearance by having a unique combination of size, color, shape, and imprint [10]. An unidentified pill can, therefore, be cross-referenced by health practitioners against a database of prescription drugs. Pharmacists usually help their patients during a brown bag consultation with the drugs they bring in for identification. A manual search can be tedious, exhausting, and time-consuming, particularly when dealing with many pills with large generic variations. Moreover, reading tiny imprints on small drugs can easily introduce human error. Alternatively, automated pill recognition techniques can help identify pills rather quickly, decrease the possibility of pill misidentification, and provide visual assurance to the patient. Examples of such automation are the RxList Pill Identification Tool [11] and the Healthline Pill Identifier [12], which are web-based applications offering pill identification services.

The concept of identifying pills from images has been studied, particularly using deep neural networks, with promising results. However, unlike these studies, our proposed approach does not only use neural networks, but also incorporates the non-parametric classifier known as k-Nearest Neighbors (k-NN) [13,14]. The classifier k-NN is effective in developing arbitrary decision regions and can complete in polynomial time. Moreover, k-NN can obtain more convoluted decision boundaries than the usual mapping technique used in the prediction layer of a generic convolutional neural network. We summarize the contributions of our work as follows:

1. We investigate the challenging problem of image retrieval, specifically targeting pill images.
2. We develop an efficient image retrieval system based on deep learning and the k-Nearest Neighbor (k-NN) classifier.
3. We employ a real-life dataset of pill images to evaluate the proposed system against accuracy and runtime, as well as compare the results with relevant image retrieval systems from the literature.
4. Our proposed model increased the accuracy of identifying pills form images by 10% while maintaining the same runtime as comparable methods.

The paper is organized as follows. Section 2 surveys the literature for related work that has been conducted on information retrieval in general and information identification from images, specifically. The proposed method and architecture are discussed in Section 3. Experimental settings and results are detailed in Section 4. A discussion of the results and comparisons are presented in Section 5. Finally, the paper concludes in Section 6.

2. Related Work

A huge amount of work has been done by researchers over the years to improve information retrieval from stored data. The literature contains various models that significantly contributed to this area of research. In this section, we survey some of the most prominent models and approaches in the area of information retrieval by briefly going over the history and then focusing on work in pill image identification.

Probabilistic information retrieval using weighted indexing was introduced in the 1960s by Maron and Kuhns [15]. The authors of [16] proposed to store and organize information using a tree-like structure, called the Adel'son-Vel'skiy and Landis (AVL) tree. Chang and Liu [17] improved the work done by Foster [18] by proposing a picture indexing and abstraction method, which led to a paradigm shift in image retrieval. Salton and Lesk [19,20] proposed one of the most prominent advancements to retrieval by developing a method called System for the Mechanical Analysis and Retrieval of Text (SMART). Rabitti and Stanchev [21] proposed a non-text based approach for retrieving images from an extensive image database.

The use of color histograms was explored by Wang et al. [22]. They explained that Local Feature Regions (LFR) would be more effective in retrieving images. On the same note of color histograms, Lee et al. [23] utilized Wang et al.'s color histogram approach to propose an automatic pill recognition system based on pill imprint, which encompassed three features: shape, color, and texture. Lee et al. extracted feature vectors based on edge localization and invariant moments of tablets as an identifier. Their experimental results showed 73% matching accuracy over a dataset of 13,000 legal drug pill images.

Deep learning techniques have been introduced in Content-Based Information Retrieval (CBIR). Such techniques are used to enhance feature extraction from input images in order to identify and retrieve similar images from a database [24]. Deep learning has been impressive in its competence in recognizing objects [25,26] and faces [27], and in handling extensive learning problems [28]. Deep learning has also improved clinical workflows by enhancing the experience of both the caregivers and patients [9]. Several deep learning-based models exist in the literature, such as the Convolutional Neural Network (CNN) [24], GoogLeNet [29], AlexNet [30], and the Residual Network (ResNet) [31]. A Convolutional Neural Network (CNN) is a deep learning technique for digital image retrieval. A CNN architecture comprises a sequence of interacting convolutional, pooling, and fully connected layers [24].

Several techniques have been developed for pill image recognition with different accuracy levels and limitations [32,33]. MobileDeepPill [34] is a CNN architecture that integrates pill color, gradients, and shape measurements to compare between consumer and reference images. Guo et al. [35] used a support vector machine (SVM) to study the color property, wherein they achieved a 97.90% overall color classification accuracy. However, the effectiveness of Guo et al.'s technique is limited by certain factors such as the lighting condition, the camera resolution, and the pill and background color contrast. Some pill recognition techniques have been developed to identify a pill based on only a subset of shape, color, and imprint, such as the works in [36–38]. The work in [39] identified pills that had only one of four pre-identified colors and classes.

Recently, Kwon et al. [40], Holtkötter et al. [41], and other similar works proposed neural network-based methods to detect pills from images. Unlike our method that aims to identify a single pill from a pill image, the approaches in [40,42,43] focused on identifying a pill from an image containing a group of pills. The studies in [41,44] aimed to detect the presence of pills in an image of a blister to track oral pill intake. The work by Nguyen et al. [45] utilized external help, namely, extracted information from prescriptions, to learn the potential associations between pills. While the problems in these studies differ from ours, we believe that our study complements the body of work in the literature by proposing an accurate *and* efficient method for identifying pills.

3. Methodology

This study aims to enhance image retrieval accuracy and efficiency to minimize clinical errors when prescribing drugs, particularly pills. Overall, the scenario is as follows: A medical practitioner or patient takes a photo of an unidentified pill. Then, the pill photo (query image) is sent to our proposed system for identification against an existing database of pill images. The challenge lies in the fact that photos may be captured in less-than-ideal environments. For example, the photo could be captured using a low-quality camera, in a room with not enough lighting, from different angles, or with a noisy background.

In order to tackle the above challenge, we propose an image retrieval approach based on two steps: (1) a preprocessing phase with features extraction and (2) classification. The overall proposed methodology is illustrated in Figure 1.

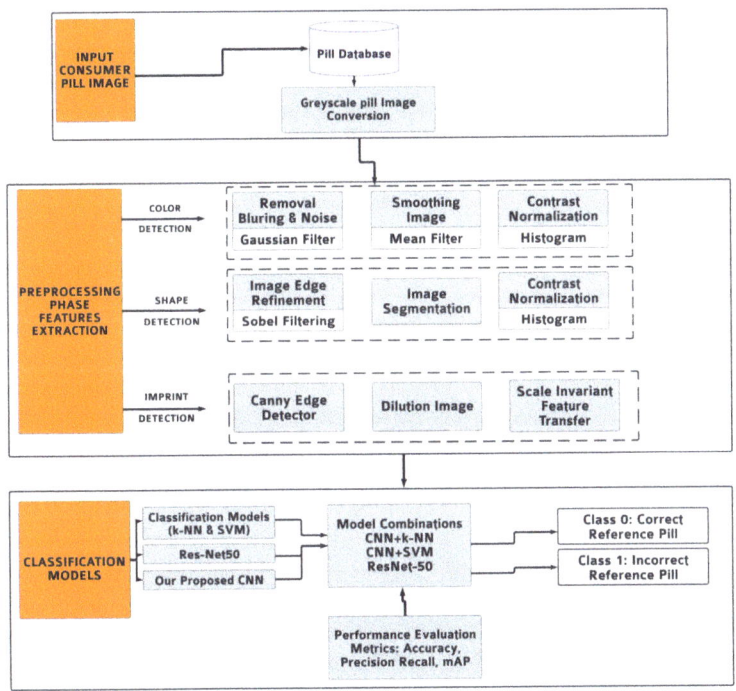

Figure 1. Proposed Approach.

3.1. Preprocessing and Features Extraction

An input pill image (query image) undergoes a series of preprocessing processes in order to make up for the color distortion and identify relevant information. The overall preprocess shows 3 main steps for the detection and extraction of color, shape, and imprint.

Before a pill image undergoes the segmentation steps in Figure 1, the image is converted to a grayscale format. This preprocessing step is used to regulate the intensity of the red, green, and blue (RGB) components in the image. Therefore, it is essential to denote a single intensity value for each pixel. Figure 2 shows an example of a raw input pill image (Figure 2a) and its grayscale version (Figure 2b). We note that all the pill images shown in the various figures in this paper are from the National Library of Medicine (NLM) pill image dataset [46].

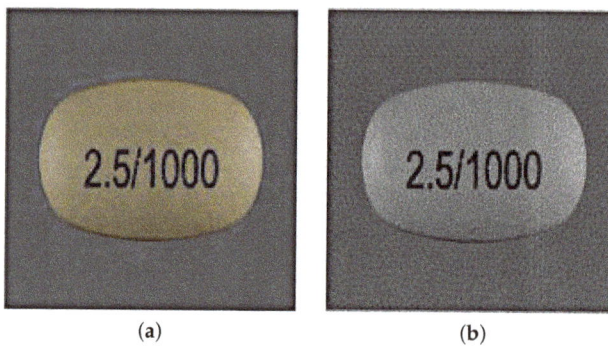

Figure 2. Colored vs. grayscale intensity pill image: (**a**) Raw input pill image; (**b**) pill image after grayscale conversion.

For color detection, a Gaussian filter is applied to the greyscale image to blur the image, thus removing unwanted details and noise. After that, a mean filter is applied to the output of the Gaussian filter to smooth the image. Next, histogram equalization is used to enhance the color contrast and to extract the colors. Figure 3 visualizes the color detection process of the same pill image in Figure 2b. For shape detection and extraction, we use Sobel filtering on the greyscale image to refine the image, which helps reveal the edges and the boundary lines of the drug pill. Figure 4 visualizes the shape detection and extraction process of the same pill image in Figure 2b. Lastly, for imprint extraction, we apply a Canny edge detector to determine all the edges in the image, followed by a dilution operation to soften the image. Clear imprint is finally revealed after applying Scale Invariant Feature Transform (SIFT) and Multi-Scale Local Binary Pattern (MLBP) descriptors. Figure 5 visualizes the imprint extraction process of the same pill image in Figure 2b.

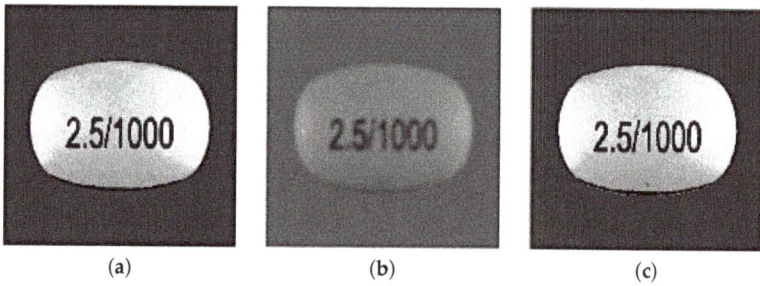

Figure 3. Pill image after applying various filters for color detection: (**a**) Gaussian filter. (**b**) Mean filter. (**c**) Local histogram equalization filter.

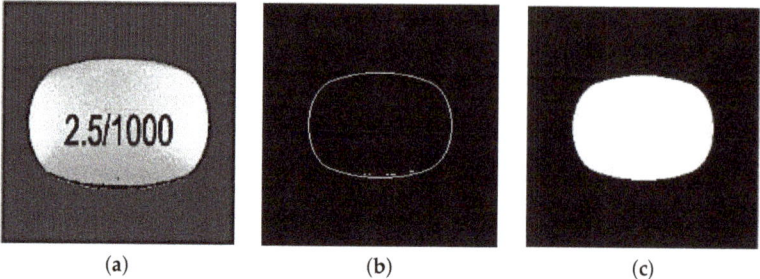

Figure 4. Pill image after applying various filters for shape detection: (**a**) Local histogram equalization filter. (**b**) Sobel filter. (**c**) Segmented shape.

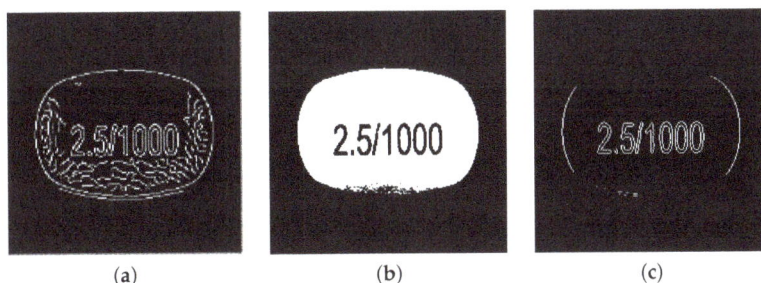

Figure 5. Pill image imprint extraction process: (**a**) Canny edge detector. (**b**) Dilution. (**c**) Scale Invariant Feature Transform.

3.2. Proposed CNN Architecture

The first step constructs a Convolutional Neural Network (CNN) to extract the query image features, namely, shape, color, and imprint. The second step uses a classifier to match the extracted query image features with those of an existing pill image. The overall proposed architecture is illustrated in Figure 6.

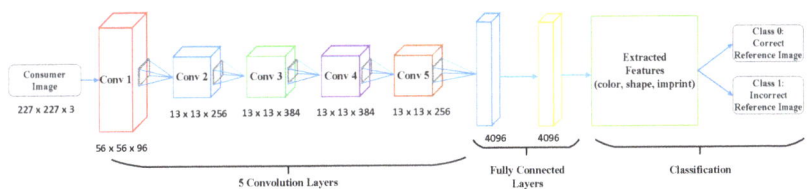

Figure 6. An overview of the proposed CNN model architecture.

The first layer of the proposed CNN network is responsible for accepting the input pill image. In our case, the input layer accepts RGB images of size 227 × 227 pixels. After that, they are fed into the CNN model, which processes them as follows:

- Pill images go through one convolutional layer (Conv1) with 56 × 56 × 96, which means that the input to the layer is a pill image with a height and width of 56 pixels and that has 96 color channels.
- The resulting tensors (images) go through four additional convolution layers with a smaller height and width (13 pixels) than the previous layer, and the number of input channels is increased to 256 color channels.
- The resulting feature maps are converted to a fully connected (FC) layer of 4096 neurons, which is connected to a second fully connected layer of 4096 neurons.
- Then, the extracted features (color, shape, and imprint) are fed into the classification layers; we then employ a k-NN classifier to handle the prediction more accurately and with less runtime.
- Finally, the classification layers output a predicted class, i.e., a matched set of images from a stored database. For more details on the CNN layers and processing, we refer the reader to [30,47].

We also note that we use the terms "prediction" and "identification" interchangeably throughout the paper.

3.3. Classification

After extracting the features of an input raw pill image, the next step is to predict the pill type using a classifier. Classification is a supervised machine learning technique where the class (pill type) to be predicted is known in advance. Several classifiers exist in the literature, though the vary in accuracy and efficiency. Below are some of the most prominent classifiers.

1. k-Nearest Neighbors (k-NN) [13,14] is a non-parametric classifier that assumes similar objects (i.e., data points) are usually "closer" to one another in comparison to dissimilar objects. k-NN measures similarity between data points using distance metrics. One of the most common distance metrics is the Euclidean distance and is measured by the following function:

$$d(X, Y) = \sqrt{\sum_{i=1}^{n}(y_i - x_i)^2}, \quad (1)$$

where X and Y are two data points in the n-dimensional space, and x_i and y_i are Euclidean vectors from the point of origin. When our proposed model receives a query image, the model converts the image to feature vectors, which the classifier will use to predict the pill type in the query image. We set k to 5 for all our experimental analysis in Section 4.

2. The Support Vector Machine (SVM) [48] is a classifier that, when given a set of input objects, creates an imaginary wall that separates dissimilar objects. This imaginary wall is called a *hyperplane*, because it can separate data points represented in spaces beyond three-dimensional. Given a set of input data points, there are several potential hyperplanes that the SVM can create. The SVM creates the best separation between the data points, i.e., it only keeps the hyperplane that minimizes the classification error.

3. Residual Network [31], or otherwise known as ResNet, is a neural network-based model that can be used as a final identifier in a convolutional layout. ResNet can accommodate more than 50 layers and be used to classify and extract features in an image. This technique makes use of skip connections to reduce the training error and help add the output of earlier layers to later layers without losing the image quality.

4. Results

The proposed model was implemented using MATLAB R2018 on an Ubuntu virtual machine with 100 GB of HDD, 24 GB of RAM, and 6 CPUs at 2.5 GHz. After that, we designed a set of experiments to evaluate the performance of our proposed model in terms of accuracy (percentage of correctly predicted pill types) and efficiency (runtime until completion).

4.1. Dataset

The proposed method was evaluated using pill images from the publicly available National Library of Medicine (NLM) dataset [46]. The NLM dataset comprises 7000 pill images from 1000 unique pills. Each pill image is categorized either as a *reference* image or as a *consumer* image. Figure 7 illustrates these two categories; Figure 7a shows a sample pill in a reference image; and Figure 7b shows the same pill in a consumer image. Reference images were taken under regulated conditions, thereby ensuring appropriate control over lighting and background. The NLM dataset contains 2000 reference images that belong to 1000 unique pills (each of which has a front and back image). On the other hand, consumer images were taken in such a way to mimic the quality of images that users would capture using their mobile phone cameras. That is, consumer images vary in quality, focus, and device types. The NLM dataset comprises 5000 consumer images, where each of the 1000 unique reference image has 5 associated consumer images.

Table 1 summarizes the metadata of the reference and consumer images, respectively. Images were shot in a 24 bit-depth jpeg format with a TrueColor color type. The major differences between the reference images and consumer images lie in the camera types, image sizes, and positioning. All the reference images were taken in a centered position, whereas the consumer images were taken in a co-sited position.

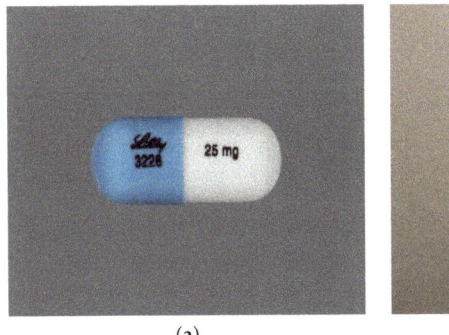
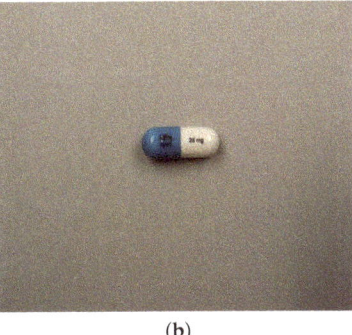

(a) (b)

Figure 7. Sample pill image: (**a**) Reference version. (**b**) Consumer version.

Table 1. Metadata of reference and consumer images.

Features	Reference Image	Consumer Image
Format	jpeg	jpeg
Width	2400	4416
Height	1600	3312
XResolution	72	180
YResolution	72	180
ColorType	TrueColor	TrueColor
BitDepth	24	24
YCbCrPositioning	Centered	Co-Sited

4.2. Performance Analysis

Given an input pill image taken by a consumer, we wished to evaluate how accurate our model was at identifying the corresponding reference pill image based on pill shape, color, and imprint.

Figure 8 visually showcases the result of applying our proposed pill image recognition model using the pill images in the NLM dataset. Each object in Figure 8 is a pill. Matched pills (consumer image and its corresponding reference image) were put next to each other. The objective of this figure is to visually demonstrate the overall accuracy of the proposed model. In the remainder of this section, we will use widely adopted accuracy metrics, namely, mean Average Precision (mAP), confusion matrices to measure True Positives, and Top-k Accuracy. Moreover, we compared our model and labeled *CNN+kNN* with *CNN+SVM* and *ResNet-50* [31].

The above-mentioned three accuracy metrics are based on the notions of Precision and Recall. Precision measures the fraction of correct identifications among all positive identifications. Recall measures the fraction of correct identifications among all the dataset's actual positives. The term "positive" refers to a target class; in this case, a pill. Below are the equations for Precision, Recall, and Accuracy:

$$Precision = \frac{TP}{TP + FP} \qquad (2)$$

$$Recall = \frac{TP}{TP + FN} \qquad (3)$$

$$Accuracy = \frac{TP + TN}{TP + FN + FP + TN}, \qquad (4)$$

where *TP* (True Positive) is the number of correct predictions of a target class, *FN* (False Negative) is the number of wrong predictions of a target class, *FP* (False Positive) is the number of wrong predictions of a non-target class, and TN (True Negative) is the number of correct predictions of a target class.

Figure 8. Matching the NLM dataset consumer pill images with reference pill images using the proposed model.

For a classifier to correctly predict a target class, the classifier must find an "acceptable" match between a query image (consumer pill image) and a target image (reference pill image). This match is numerically defined by a *threshold* that measures the fraction of the overlapping area between the query image and the target image. Based on this threshold, the values of Precision and Recall vary.

Another performance metric that is commonly used in the evaluation of information retrieval and object detection systems is the mean Average Precision (mAP). The mAP metric measures the average precision values of a classifier across different Recall values. A higher mAP score indicates better performance of the model in retrieving relevant information or detecting objects accurately. The mAP incorporates the trade-off between Precision and Recall, and it considers both false positives (FP) and false negatives (FN). This measurement provides a broader understanding of the classifier accuracy in identifying pills. The mAP is calculated as follows:

- For each object class, calculate the Average Precision (AP) as:

$$AP = \frac{1}{n} * \sum_{k=1}^{n} Precision\_at\_each\_k\text{-}object \quad (5)$$

where (n) is the total number of relevant items in the dataset for the given object class, and the Precision at each relevant k-object is the Precision calculated at the position of the relevant item in the ranked list of predicted items.
- Calculate the mAP as the mean of the AP scores for all object classes:

$$mAP = \frac{1}{N} * \sum_{k=1}^{N} AP_k \quad (6)$$

where (N) is the total number of object classes in the dataset.

Given the pill images in the NLM dataset, we calculated the *mAP* performance metric for *ResNet-50*, *CNN+SVM*, and *CNN+kNN* (our proposed model), for a $0.1 \leq$ threshold ≤ 0.9. The mAP metric comparison is illustrated in Table 2. Moreover, we plotted the Precision–Recall curves of the three models. A Precision–Recall curve of a prediction model visualizes the accuracy of the model. The larger the area under the curve is, the better the prediction quality (reflecting both good Prediction and Recall). Figure 9 shows three Prediction–Recall curves for the above-mentioned three models, respectively.

Table 2. mAP Comparison Models.

Models	Mean Average Precision (mAP)
ResNet-50	80%
CNN+SVM	86.3%
CNN+kNN (our proposed model)	90.8%

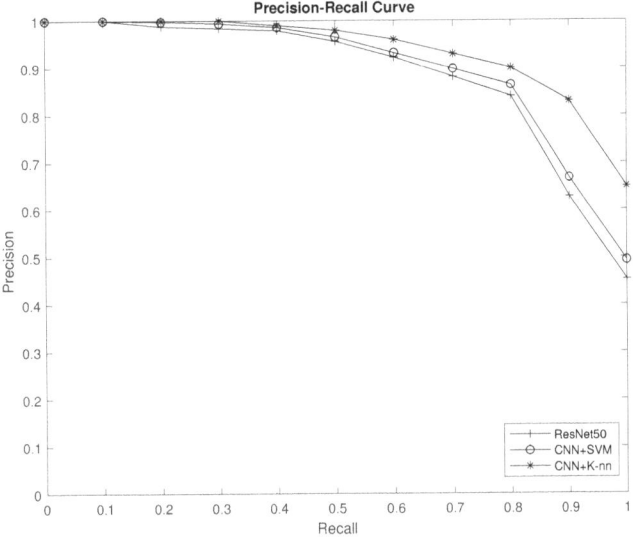

Figure 9. Precision–Recall curves of three pill identification models: *ResNet-50*, *CNN+SVM*, and *CNN+kNN*.

The Precision in Equation (2) is computed upon determining the TP and FP values of a target class in a prediction task. These values can be determined after running the prediction model against a dataset of images. For example, if a query image contains a round pill shape, then is the model able to predict that the shape of the query image is in fact round? In other words, we would like to know how many round-shaped pills the model successfully predicted as round-shaped (as opposed to any other shape).

In the above example, the target class was *Round*, which belongs to the "shape" property of a pill. Our model extracts three features from any query pill image: shape, color, and imprint (see Figure 6).

To help us evaluate the performance of our model in terms of correctly identifying target classes, we constructed a confusion matrix for each pill feature. Figure 10 represents three confusion matrices for shape, color, and imprint, respectively. The x-axis and y-axis arbitrarily list values (or target classes) of a specific feature (e.g., *Round*, *Capsule* and *Oval* are values of the shape property). The x-axis represents the known target class, whereas the y-axis represents the predicted class. An intersection between any pair of values (c_x, c_y)

on the x-axis and y-axis, respectively, represents the number of times (or percentage) that the model predicted c_y given a pill of a target class of c_x.

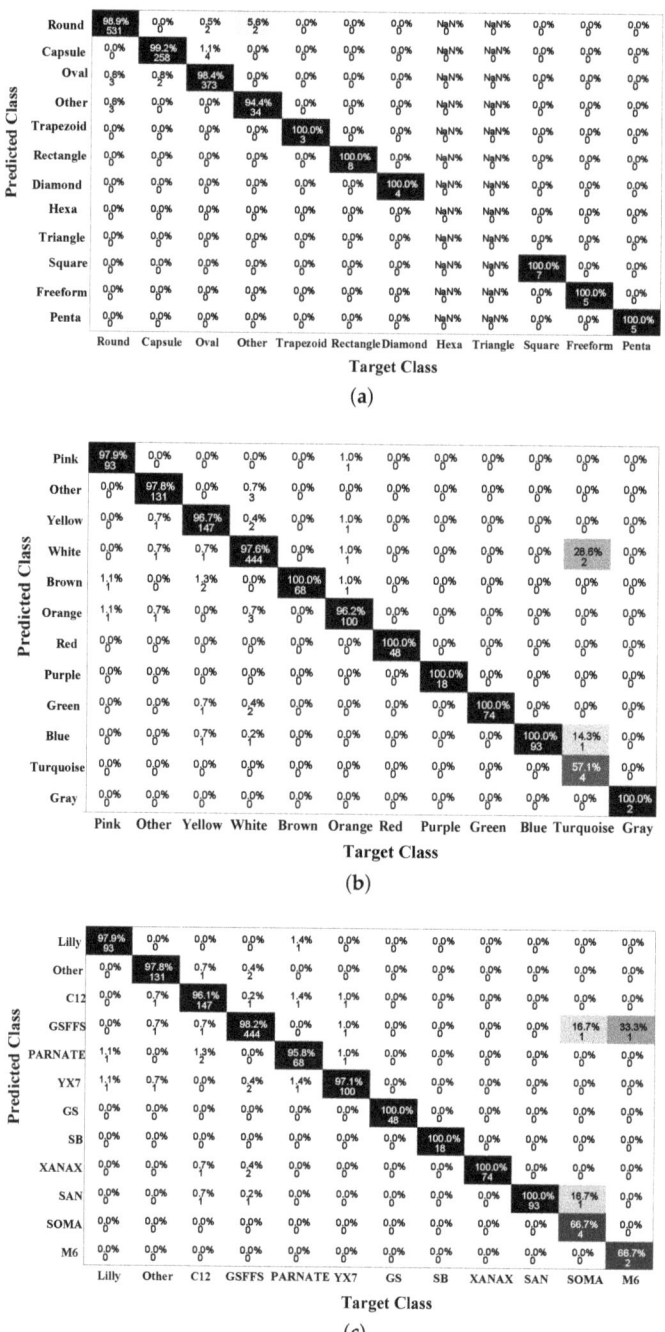

Figure 10. Confusion matrices reporting our model accuracies w.r.t. predicting pill: (**a**) shape, (**b**) colors, and (**c**) imprints.

For example, Figure 10 demonstrates the ability of the proposed model to understand the shape of the query pill. Looking at the *Round* target class on the x-axis, the model predicted *Round* as *Round* 98.9% of the times, but predicted *Round* as *Oval* 0.6% of the times.

The Top-k Accuracy metric considers a model's prediction to be correct if the target class exists among the top k predictions. For example, given a query pill image I_q from the NLM dataset and k = 5, if the model matches I_q with an ordered set of n images $\langle I_1, I_2, I_3, \ldots, I_n \rangle$, where $I_q \in \{I_1, I_2, I_3, I_4, I_5\}$, then the Top-k Accuracy metric considers this match to be a correct prediction. It stands to reason that, as k increases, the Top-k Accuracy is expected to increase, because the metric considers a larger pool of potential matches. For k = 1 and 5, Table 3 reports the results of the Top-k Accuracy of the four related models.

Table 3. Top-k Accuracy in Related Models (%).

Method	Top-1	Top-5
SqueezeNet [49]	49.0%	76.8%
AlexNet [30]	62.5%	83.0%
ResNet-50 [31]	71.7%	85.5%
MobileNet [50]	71.7%	92.0%
MobileDeepPill [34]	73.7%	95.6%
InceptionV3 [51]	74.4%	93.3%
CNN+SVM (our suggested model)	76.5%	92.0%
CNN+kNN (our proposed model)	80.5%	96.1%

Based on the evaluations performed by Larios Delgado [9], *ResNet-50* [31] performed the best among all the other models. Next, we performed further comparisons between *ResNet-50*, *CNN+SVM*, and *CNN+kNN* (our proposed model). Table 4 varies k in the Top-k Accuracy measure between $1 \leq k \leq 15$, and reports the finding for *ResNet-50*, *CNN+SVM*, and *CNN+kNN*.

Table 4. Top-k Accuracy Comparison (%).

k-Value	ResNet-50	CNN+SVM	CNN+kNN
k = 1	71.7%	76.5%	80.5%
k = 2	74.5%	82.1%	86.1%
k = 3	82.0%	89.0%	94.0%
k = 4	83.0%	90.5%	95.5%
k = 5	85.5%	92.0%	96.1%
k = 6	86.5%	92.2%	96.5%
k = 7	88.0%	92.5%	97.0%
k = 8	89.0%	92.7%	97.5%
k = 9	89.8%	93.0%	97.8%
k = 10	90.5%	93.0%	97.9%
k = 11	90.8%	93.0%	98.0%
k = 12	91.0%	93.0%	98.0%
k = 13	91.0%	93.0%	98.0%
k = 14	91.0%	93.0%	98.0%
k = 15	91.0%	93.0%	98.0%

We noticed that, as k increased, the Top-k Accuracy result in Table 4 also increased, since the set of potential matched images expanded. Our proposed *CNN+kNN* model maintained a consistently higher Top-k Accuracy result across all values of k, followed by *CNN+SVM* and *ResNet-50*.

4.3. Efficiency

We would like to evaluate the performance of our proposed model in terms of runtime and compare it to similar models. Runtime is measured as the start from the moment the user submits a query pill image to the moment the model returns matched images. Runtime is averaged over all the NLM dataset images. Table 5 reports the total execution time of each of the three models, *ResNet-50*, *CNN+SVM*, and *CNN+kNN*, in milliseconds. All the three models achieved nearly the same runtime.

Table 5. Runtime Comparison (ms).

ResNet-50 (Best Performing (Table 3)	CNN+SVM	CNN+kNN (Our Proposed Model)
1.25 ms	1.05 ms	1.02 ms

5. Discussion

The experimental results in Section 4 suggest that our proposed *CNN+kNN* model architecture outperformed the closely-related *ResNet-50* model and the *CNN+SVM* model. Although all three classification techniques (k-NN, SVM, and ResNet-50) performed well, the proposed *CNN+kNN* model was able to achieve the highest accuracy.

Table 2 compares the mAP values of *ResNet-50*, *CNN+SVM*, and *CNN+kNN* using the NLM dataset. With regard to the mAP values, applying the *CNN+kNN* successfully increased the prediction Precision from 80% to 91%. This finding implies that, if the *CNN+kNN* model predicts a target class (i.e., finds a pill type of a query pill image), then there is a 91% chance that the prediction will be correct.

In Figure 9, we compared between the three models to evaluate the "goodness" of the prediction model. Each line in the figure represents the model's Precision–Recall curve. A larger area under the curve implies better Precision and Recall. That is, the more the curve pushes to the top-right corner of the plot, the better the model is. Out of all the three models, *CNN+kNN* had the largest area, thus implying a higher prediction quality.

Figure 10 provides us with an idea of how well (or bad) the model understands the different features of a pill in order to make a decision about the pill type. Figure 10a suggests that the model was successfully able to differentiate between all distinct shapes. However, Figure 10b,c suggest that the model struggled in making a decision when the pill color was *Turquoise* and imprint was *SOMA* and *M6*, respectively. The low Precision values for these target classes (e.g., 57.1% for predicting *Turquoise*) may be due to the low number of training images with pills having these target classes.

Table 4 suggests that using a Convolutional Neural Network with the k-Nearest Neighbor classifier improves pill identification accuracy by about 10%, which is considered a significant improvement. For sensitive applications or diseases, we suggest considering Top-1 Accuracy. If Top-5 Accuracy is to be considered, albeit at 96% accuracy, we suggest consulting an expert for confirmation.

The runtime experiment, as reported in Table 5, suggests that using the k-NN classifier does not compromise the efficiency of the overall image retrieval system. This finding implies that a pill image retrieval system's accuracy can be improved without compromising its runtime.

Although our experiments suggest higher pill image retrieval success than comparable methods, we encountered some challenges pertaining to consumer image quality. Conflicting light conditions, placement of the pills, and the distance from the camera used in the consumer images negatively impacted the shape extraction process. Thus, the presence of high noise in images may incur high classification error if the image retrieval model is not equipped with adequate filters to account for such noise.

Lastly, we would like to mention that, for the performance evaluation of our proposed model, we used the NLM dataset [46]. This dataset was published by the National Institutes of Health for an open research competition, and it has since been widely used by various seminal exiting works in the area of pill identification from images. For the sake of performance comparison with existing studies in the same area (see Table 3, we adopted the NLM dataset in our evaluations. That said, we plan on using more datasets in our future work that builds on this study to further validate our findings.

6. Conclusions

The impact of consuming the wrong medication can be lethal. This paper proposes a method for identifying pills from images. The proposed method studies the impact of combining widely-known classifiers, namely k-NN and SVM, with neural networks. The classifier is placed between the fully connected feature layer and the output layer to handle prediction. Experimental evaluation was conducted on a real-life dataset called the NLM dataset, and results were compared with those obtained from comparable models. We have examined three deep learning models for the classification of pill images; two are hybrid models (a combination of proposed CNN with SVM and k-NN classifiers), and the third is the ResNet-50 model. Results show that using the k-NN classifier in a Convolutional Neural Network architecture (our proposed model) increased pill identification accuracy by around 10% while maintaining almost the same runtime as in the compared methods (nearly 1 ms per execution).

For future work, the proposed method can be improved to account for some inherent drawbacks in consumer-grade pill images. For example, the model may not be able to accurately determine the shape of a pill if the pill image was taken under conflicting lighting conditions. One naïve solution to this problem could be constructing a 3D model of the query pill by having more than one image showing the pill from multiple angles.

Author Contributions: Conceptualization, E.A. and R.M.A.; Methodology, K.A.-H. and I.K.; Software, E.A.; Validation, K.A.-H., E.A. and I.K.; Formal analysis, K.A.-H., E.A. and I.K.; Investigation, E.A.; Resources, K.A.-H. and R.M.A.; Data curation, E.A.; Writing—original draft, E.A. and K.A.-H. and R.M.A.; Writing—review and editing, K.A.-H., I.K. and R.M.A.; Visualization, E.A. and R.M.A.; Supervision, K.A.-H. and R.M.A.; Project administration, K.A.-H. All authors have read and agreed to the published version of the manuscript.

Funding: This research is supported in part by the DSO-RIT Dubai Research Fund (2022-23-1003) from the Rochester Institute of Technology—Dubai.

Institutional Review Board Statement: Not applicable.

Informed Consent Statement: Not applicable.

Data Availability Statement: All the pill images used in this study are publicly available through the National Library of Medicine [46].

Acknowledgments: The authors would like to thank the TDRA-ICT Fund for providing high-end computing machines for our experiments through the Digital Transformation Lab at Rochester Institute of Technology—Dubai (RIT-Dubai).

Conflicts of Interest: The authors have no competing interests to declare that are relevant to the content of this article.

Abbreviations

The following abbreviations are used in this manuscript:

CBIR	Content-Based Information Retrieval
WHO	World Health Organization
CNN	Convolutional Neural Network
ResNet	Residual Network
SVM	Support Vector Machine
NLM	National Library of Medicine
NIH	National Institutes of Health
k-NN	k-Nearest Neighbor

References

1. Crestani, F.; Mizzaro, S.; Scagnetto, I. *Mobile Information Retrieval*, 1st ed.; Springer International Publishing: Cham, Switzerland, 2017.
2. Celik, C.; Bilge, H.S. Content based image retrieval with sparse representations and local feature descriptors: A comparative study. *Pattern Recognit.* **2017**, *68*, 1–13. [CrossRef]
3. Madduri, A. Content based Image Retrieval System using Local Feature Extraction Techniques. *Int. J. Comput. Appl.* **2021**, *183*, 16–20. [CrossRef]
4. Dubey, S.R. A Decade Survey of Content Based Image Retrieval Using Deep Learning. *IEEE Trans. Circuits Syst. Video Technol.* **2022**, *32*, 2687–2704. [CrossRef]
5. Makary, M.A.; Daniel, M. Medical error—the third leading cause of death in the US. *BMJ* **2016**, *353*, i2139. [CrossRef] [PubMed]
6. World Health Assembly. *Patient Safety: Global Action on Patient Safety: Report by the Director-Genera*; World Health Assembly: Geneva, Switzerland, 2019; p. 8.
7. WHO. *Medication Without Harm: Real-Life Stories*; WHO: Geneva, Switzerland, 2017.
8. WHO. 10 Facts on Patient Safety. 2019. Available online: https://www.who.int/news-room/photo-story/photo-story-detail/10-facts-on-patient-safety (accessed on 31 July 2022).
9. Larios Delgado, N.; Usuyama, N.; Hall, A.K.; Hazen, R.J.; Ma, M.; Sahu, S.; Lundin, J. Fast and accurate medication identification. *NPJ Digit. Med.* **2019**, *2*, 10. [CrossRef]
10. Yu, J.; Chen, Z.; Kamata, S.i. Pill Recognition Using Imprint Information by Two-Step Sampling Distance Sets. In Proceedings of the 2014 22nd International Conference on Pattern Recognition, Stockholm, Sweden, 24–28 August 2014; pp. 3156–3161. [CrossRef]
11. RxList. Pill Identifier (Pill Finder Wizard). 2022. Available online: https://www.rxlist.com/pill-identification-tool/article.htm (accessed on 31 July 2022).
12. Healthline. Medication Safety: Pill Identification, Storage, and More. 2021. Available online: https://www.healthline.com/health/pill-identification (accessed on 31 July 2022).
13. Guo, G.; Wang, H.; Bell, D.; Bi, Y.; Greer, K. KNN Model-based Approach in Classification. In *On The Move to Meaningful Internet Systems 2003: CoopIS, DOA, and ODBASE*; Springer: Berlin/Heidelberg, Germany, 2003; pp. 986–996, Volume 2888. [CrossRef]
14. Altman, N.S. An Introduction to Kernel and Nearest-Neighbor Nonparametric Regression. *Am. Stat.* **1992**, *46*, 175–185.
15. Maron, M.E.; Kuhns, J.L. On Relevance, Probabilistic Indexing and Information Retrieval. *J. ACM* **1960**, *7*, 216–244. [CrossRef]
16. Adel'son-Vel'skii, G.M.; Landis, E.M. An algorithm for organization of information. *Dokl. Akad. Nauk.* **1962**, *146*, 263–266.
17. Chang, S.K.; Liu, S.H. Picture indexing and abstraction techniques for pictorial databases. *IEEE Trans. Pattern Anal. Mach. Intell.* **1984**, *4*, 475–484. [CrossRef]
18. Foster, C.C. Information Retrieval: Information Storage and Retrieval Using AVL Trees. In Proceedings of the 1965 20th National Conference, Cleveland, OH, USA, 24–26 August 1965; Association for Computing Machinery: New York, NY, USA, 1965; pp. 192–205. [CrossRef]
19. Salton, G.; Lesk, M.E. The SMART Automatic Document Retrieval Systems-an Illustration. *Commun. ACM* **1965**, *8*, 391–398. [CrossRef]
20. Salton, G. *The SMART Retrieval System-Experiments in Automatic Document Processing*; Prentice-Hall, Inc.: Upper Saddle River, NJ, USA, 1971.
21. Rabitti, F.; Stanchev, P. An Approach to Image Retrieval from Large Image Databases. In Proceedings of the 10th Annual International ACM SIGIR Conference on Research and Development in Information Retrieval, New Orleans, LA, USA, 3–5 June 1987; Association for Computing Machinery: New York, NY, USA, 1987; pp. 284–295. [CrossRef]
22. Wang, X.Y.; Wu, J.F.; Yang, H.Y. Robust image retrieval based on color histogram of local feature regions. *Multimed. Tools Appl.* **2010**, *49*, 323–345. [CrossRef]
23. Lee, Y.B.; Park, U.; Jain, A.K.; Lee, S.W. Pill-ID: Matching and retrieval of drug pill images. *Pattern Recognit. Lett.* **2012**, *33*, 904–910. [CrossRef]
24. Maji, S.; Bose, S. CBIR using features derived by deep learning. *ACM/IMS Trans. Data Sci.* **2021**, *2*, 1–24. [CrossRef]
25. Srivastava, N.; Hinton, G.; Krizhevsky, A.; Sutskever, I.; Salakhutdinov, R. Dropout: A Simple Way to Prevent Neural Networks from Overfitting. *J. Mach. Learn. Res.* **2014**, *15*, 1929–1958.
26. Razavian, A.S.; Azizpour, H.; Sullivan, J.; Carlsson, S. CNN Features Off-the-Shelf: An Astounding Baseline for Recognition. In Proceedings of the IEEE Conference on Computer Vision and Pattern Recognition Workshops, Columbus, OH, USA, 23–28 June 2014; pp. 512–519. [CrossRef]
27. Taigman, Y.; Yang, M.; Ranzato, M.; Wolf, L. DeepFace: Closing the Gap to Human-Level Performance in Face Verification. In Proceedings of the IEEE Conference on Computer Vision and Pattern Recognition, Columbus, OH, USA, 23–28 June 2014; pp. 1701–1708. [CrossRef]
28. LeCun, Y.; Bengio, Y.; Hinton, G. Deep learning. *Nature* **2015**, *521*, 436–444. [CrossRef]
29. Szegedy, C.; Liu, W.; Jia, Y.; Sermanet, P.; Reed, S.; Anguelov, D.; Erhan, D.; Vanhoucke, V.; Rabinovich, A. Going deeper with convolutions. In Proceedings of the 2015 IEEE Conference on Computer Vision and Pattern Recognition (CVPR), Boston, MA, USA, 7–12 June 2015; pp. 1–9. [CrossRef]

30. Krizhevsky, A.; Sutskever, I.; Hinton, G.E. ImageNet Classification with Deep Convolutional Neural Networks. *Commun. ACM* **2017**, *60*, 84–90. [CrossRef]
31. He, K.; Zhang, X.; Ren, S.; Sun, J. Deep Residual Learning for Image Recognition. In Proceedings of the IEEE Conference on Computer Vision and Pattern Recognition (CVPR), Las Vegas, NV, USA, 27–30 June 2016; pp. 770–778. [CrossRef]
32. Wang, Y.; Ribera, J.; Liu, C.; Yarlagadda, S.; Zhu, F. Pill Recognition Using Minimal Labeled Data. In Proceedings of the IEEE Third International Conference on Multimedia Big Data (BigMM), Laguna Hills, CA, USA, 19–21 April 2017; pp. 346–353. [CrossRef]
33. Ou, Y.Y.; Tsai, A.C.; Zhou, X.P.; Wang, J.F. Automatic drug pills detection based on enhanced feature pyramid network and convolution neural networks. *IET Comput. Vis.* **2020**, *14*, 9–17. [CrossRef]
34. Zeng, X.; Cao, K.; Zhang, M. MobileDeepPill: A Small-Footprint Mobile Deep Learning System for Recognizing Unconstrained Pill Images. In Proceedings of the 15th Annual International Conference on Mobile Systems, Applications, and Services, Niagara Falls, NY, USA, 19–23 June 2017; Association for Computing Machinery: New York, NY, USA, 2017; pp. 56–67. [CrossRef]
35. Guo, P.; Stanley, R.; Cole, J.G.; Hagerty, J.; Stoecker, W. Color Feature-based Pillbox Image Color Recognition. In Proceedings of the 12th International Joint Conference on Computer Vision, Imaging and Computer Graphics Theory and Applications—Volume 4: VISAPP, (VISIGRAPP 2017), Porto, Portugal, 27 February–1 March 2017; pp. 188–194. [CrossRef]
36. Cordeiro, L.S.; Lima, J.S.; Rocha Ribeiro, A.I.; Bezerra, F.N.; Rebouças Filho, P.P.; Rocha Neto, A.R. Pill Image Classification using Machine Learning. In Proceedings of the 2019 8th Brazilian Conference on Intelligent Systems (BRACIS), Salvador, Brazil, 15–18 October 2019; pp. 556–561. [CrossRef]
37. Suksawatchon, U.; Srikamdee, S.; Suksawatchon, J.; Werapan, W. Shape Recognition Using Unconstrained Pill Images Based on Deep Convolution Network. In Proceedings of the 2022 6th International Conference on Information Technology (InCIT), Nonthaburi, Thailand, 10–11 November 2022; pp. 309–313. [CrossRef]
38. Proma, T.P.; Hossan, M.Z.; Amin, M.A. *Medicine Recognition from Colors and Text*; Association for Computing Machinery: New York, NY, USA, 2019; ICGSP '19. [CrossRef]
39. Swastika, W.; Prilianti, K.; Stefanus, A.; Setiawan, H.; Arfianto, A.Z.; Santosa, A.W.B.; Rahmat, M.B.; Setiawan, E. Preliminary Study of Multi Convolution Neural Network-Based Model To Identify Pills Image Using Classification Rules. In Proceedings of the 2019 International Seminar on Intelligent Technology and Its Applications (ISITIA), Surabaya, Indonesia, 28–29 August 2019; pp. 376–380. [CrossRef]
40. Kwon, H.J.; Kim, H.G.; Lee, S.H. Pill Detection Model for Medicine Inspection Based on Deep Learning. *Chemosensors* **2022**, *10*, 4. [CrossRef]
41. Holtkötter, J.; Amaral, R.; Almeida, R.; Jácome, C.; Cardoso, R.; Pereira, A.; Pereira, M.; Chon, K.H.; Fonseca, J.A. Development and Validation of a Digital Image Processing-Based Pill Detection Tool for an Oral Medication Self-Monitoring System. *Sensors* **2022**, *22*, 2958. [CrossRef]
42. Nguyen, A.D.; Pham, H.H.; Trung, H.T.; Nguyen, Q.V.H.; Truong, T.N.; Nguyen, P.L. High Accurate and Explainable Multi-Pill Detection Framework with Graph Neural Network-Assisted Multimodal Data Fusion. *arXiv* **2023**, arXiv:2303.09782.
43. Chang, W.J.; Chen, L.B.; Hsu, C.H.; Lin, C.P.; Yang, T.C. A Deep Learning-Based Intelligent Medicine Recognition System for Chronic Patients. *IEEE Access* **2019**, *7*, 44441–44458. [CrossRef]
44. Ting, H.W.; Chung, S.L.; Chen, C.F.; Chiu, H.Y.; Hsieh, Y.W. A drug identification model developed using deep learning technologies: Experience of a medical center in Taiwan. *BMC Health Serv. Res.* **2019**, *20*, 312. [CrossRef] [PubMed]
45. Nguyen, A.D.; Nguyen, T.D.; Pham, H.H.; Nguyen, T.H.; Nguyen, P.L. Image-based Contextual Pill Recognition with Medical Knowledge Graph Assistance. In Proceedings of the Asian Conference on Intelligent Information and Database Systems, Ho Chi Minh City, Vietnam, 28–30 November 2022.
46. National Library of Medicine. Pill Identification Challenge. 2016. Available online: https://www.nlm.nih.gov/databases/download/pill_image.html (accessed on 31 July 2022).
47. Stanford. CS231n: Convolutional Neural Networks for Visual Recognition. 2022. Available online: http://cs231n.stanford.edu/ (accessed on 31 July 2022).
48. Vapnik, V.N. *Statistical Learning Theory*; Wiley-Interscience: Hoboken, NJ, USA, 1998.
49. Iandola, F.N.; Han, S.; Moskewicz, M.W.; Ashraf, K.; Dally, W.J.; Keutzer, K. SqueezeNet: AlexNet-level accuracy with 50x fewer parameters and <0.5MB model size. *arXiv* **2016**, arXiv:1602.07360.
50. Howard, A.G.; Zhu, M.; Chen, B.; Kalenichenko, D.; Wang, W.; Weyand, T.; Andreetto, M.; Adam, H. MobileNets: Efficient Convolutional Neural Networks for Mobile Vision Applications. *arXiv* **2017**, arXiv:1704.04861.
51. Szegedy, C.; Vanhoucke, V.; Ioffe, S.; Shlens, J.; Wojna, Z. Rethinking the Inception Architecture for Computer Vision. In Proceedings of the 2016 IEEE Conference on Computer Vision and Pattern Recognition (CVPR), Las Vegas, NV, USA, 27–30 June 2016; pp. 2818–2826. [CrossRef]

Disclaimer/Publisher's Note: The statements, opinions and data contained in all publications are solely those of the individual author(s) and contributor(s) and not of MDPI and/or the editor(s). MDPI and/or the editor(s) disclaim responsibility for any injury to people or property resulting from any ideas, methods, instructions or products referred to in the content.

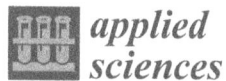

Article

Cross-Platform Gait Analysis and Fall Detection Wearable Device

Ming-Hung Chang [1], Yi-Chao Wu [2,*], Hsi-Yu Niu [3], Yi-Ting Chen [4] and Shu-Han Juang [5]

[1] Department of Electrical Engineering, Lunghwa University of Science and Technology, Taoyuan 333326, Taiwan
[2] Department of Electronic Engineering, National Yunlin University of Science and Technology, Yunlin 540301, Taiwan
[3] Department of Electrical Engineering, National Kaohsiung University of Science and Technology, Kaohsiung 807618, Taiwan
[4] Department of Computer Science and Engineering, National Taiwan Ocean University, Keelung 202301, Taiwan
[5] Institute of Materials Science and Engineering, National Taipei University of Technology, Taipei 106344, Taiwan
* Correspondence: alanwu@yuntech.edu.tw; Tel.: +886-5-5342601 (ext. 4330)

Abstract: Since the fall was often occurred in elders daily, this paper focused on gait analysis with fall detection to develop a wearable device. To ensure that the mobile application, APP, could be used in different platform of mobile phone, such Android or iOS, the designed wearable device also could be used in cross-platform in mobile phone. Therefore, a cross-platform gait analysis and fall detection wearable device (CPGAFDWD) was proposed. Since CPGAFDWD APP was used in web browser without limiting to platform, it could be used for different platforms of mobile phone. The gait analysis could be detected at home. The fall detection also could be executed in any place immediately. The patients and medical staff all could query the status of rehabilitation in any place and any time via the Internet. The experimental results showed that the correct rate of gait analysis and fall detection could be up to 90% in cross-platform of mobile phone. In the future, CPGAFDWD will be planned to be verified by Institutional Review Board, IRB, for clinical treatment.

Keywords: gait analysis; fall detection; wearable device; cross-platform; Institutional Review Board

1. Introduction

In Taiwan, an analysis report from the Health Promotion Administration, HPA, showed that the rehabilitation treatment is more important in modern medicine. It also showed that the fall accident becomes the second accident among all accidents for the elders more than sixty-five years in Taiwan due to significant decline for controlling and balancing muscle, such as gait analysis [1–5].

In Ref. [6], it developed a wearable Freezing of Gait (FOG) collection device for wavelet analysis on shank sagittal velocity signals and a synchronization of loss threshold (SLT) for prediction of FOG in people with Parkinson's Disease (PD).

In Ref. [7], it proposed a wearable foot gait collection device with step direction algorithm for motion state and direction of feet exercising. By using this wearable device, the burnt calories could be calculated. The health state of user also could be observed at any time and place by using this wearable foot gait collection device.

In Ref. [8], a piecewise linear labeling was proposed to calculate the angular positions and velocities of thigh and torso segments as the training model data based on the variable toe-off onset with different walking speed. By the proposed piecewise linear labeling, the speed adaptability of gait phase estimation could be improved. Estimation accuracy of gait phase could be improved.

In Ref. [9], it showed that the risk of fatal falls for elderly people is getting important. The Centers for Disease Control and Prevention (CDC) also showed that the serious injuries of elderly people may be occurred even if the falling is innocent. Hence, a system with wearable fall detection devices for tracking patient's whole activity by accelerometer sensors was proposed. The patient's predetermined alert could be identified and the corresponding alerts could be sent to the patients. Devices for tracking motion with high performance, low power, and low cost included the smart wearable sensors. Data could be decided based on data processing unit.

In Ref. [10], it showed that the fatality may be occurred by fall, especially for elderly people who live alone. Hence, this paper aimed to detect fall by supervised machine learning (ML) algorithms, such as decision tree (DT), k-Nearest Neighbour (k-NN), and support vector machine (SVM). The experimental results showed that the sensitivity and accuracy of DT is better than *those* of k-NN and SVM.

In Ref. [11], it addressed the necessity of human fall elements by wearable devices regrading falls included signals acquired, features extracted, and algorithms, jointly. In Ref. [12], it proposed a new data augmentation application for different rotation errors in wearable fall detection sensors.

The above mention showed the importance of gait analysis and fall detection. Most of gait analysis was suggested to be executed in any place, such as home, by medical staff to save time and money for patients. Although the gait analysis at home could reduce the time, money, and manpower for patients and medical institutions, how to ensure the motion of gait analysis is correct becomes the first important issue without any medical staff. Moreover, how to upload the data of gait analysis to cloud database and detect the fall accident in real time by APP was another issue.

A cross-platform gait analysis and fall detection wearable device (CPGAFDWD) was thus proposed firstly in this paper. Most of wearable devices were used by APP in mobile device, such as mobile phone. Since the platform of mobile phone may be different, such as iOS and Android, to ensure the APP we designed could be applied for different kinds of platforms is needed. Hence, a cross-platform APP was proposed to be integrated for CPGAFDWD in this paper.

Therefore, a cross-platform gait analysis and fall detection wearable device (CP-GAFDWD) was proposed to address the above issues in this paper. The architecture of CPGAFDWD was shown in Figure 1. The user interface of cross-platform APP was shown in Figure 2.

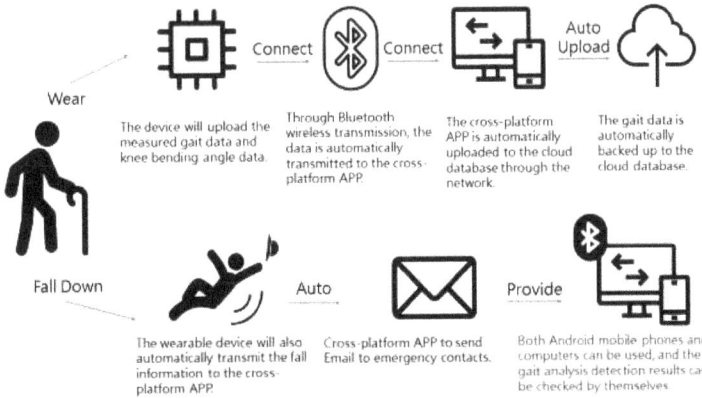

Figure 1. Architecture of CPGAFDWD.

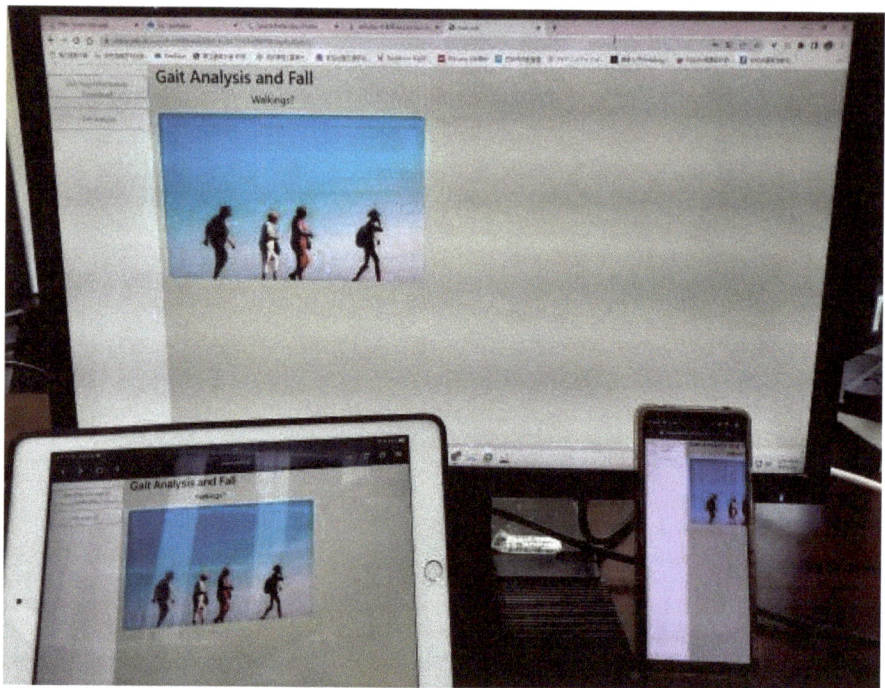

Figure 2. User interface of CPGAFDWD in different platform.

In CPGAFDWD, the development board was used as Arduino board. The sensing modules, such as gyroscope and three-axis accelerometer, were used. The communication modules, such as Bluetooth and WiFi, were used. CPGAFDWD was integrated the Arduino board with the gyroscope, three-axis accelerometer, Bluetooth, and WiFi to detect the gait analysis and fall accident. The sensed data of gait analysis and fall accident from CPGAFDWD were transmitted to APP in real time.

CPGAFDWD collected the sensed data via Bluetooth immediately. Then CPGAFDWD uploaded these data to cloud database called MongoDB, via WiFi or 4G in real time. In CPGAFDWD, a web APP was designed by Node.js. Since web APP was used by browser without constraining to any platform, CPGAFDWD could be used in multi-platform of mobile phone. The users could track the status of gait analysis and receive the alarm of fall accident by CPGAFDWD.

The experiments of gait analysis included the step, length, and angle of pace. In ths statistical treatment with relevant comparisons, our pace step measurement was compared with the actual pace step of laboratory members on walking. Our pace angle measurement was compared with the actual pace angle of laboratory members by using protractor. For the fall detection, it was compared with the actual fall simulated by laboratory members. The experimental results showed that the rate of correct pace step measurement, the rate of correct pace length measurement, and the rate of correct pace angle measurement all could be up to 90%. For the fall detection, the experimental results showed that the detection rate of fall accident could be up to 100%. In the above results, it proved that CPGAFDWD could be applied for gait analysis and fall detection applications.

In CPGAFDWD, the experimental results showed that the user could track the status of gait analysis and receive the alarm of fall accident via the Internet in real time. Moreover, the above results were used in both of iOS and Android to prove that CPGAFDWD could be applied in cross-platform of mobile phone.

The remainder of this paper was arranged in the following sections. Section 2 presented the related work. Section 3 stated our proposed CPGAFDWD. Section 4 stated our experimental results. Section 5 showed the discussion. Finally, Section 6 concluded this paper.

2. Related Work

In Refs. [1,2], it described the importance of fall detection for elders due to deterioration of foot function. To address this issue, a wearable device composed of three-axis accelerometer, gyroscope, and GPS was designed. Hence, the date time and location of fall could be detected by this wearable device.

A multi-condition adaptive step detection algorithm was proposed to improve the pedestrian dead reckoning system for increasing the measurement precision of the stride, step, and heading better than the existed traditional algorithms [3].

In Ref. [4], a linear mixed model was used to determine differences between spatial gait and non-motor symptoms, such as freezing in the levodopa-medicated-state (ON-state) called Parkinson's disease. The levodopa-medicated-state was divided into non-freezers, freezing with only OFF-levodopa, and freezing with both ON- and OFF-levodopa. The experimental results proved that the variability for intra-patient in spatial gait features in ONOFF-FOG was much higher than those in others.

In Ref. [5], the rehabilitation of balance and gait between sensory retraining (ESR) and implicit repeated exposure (IRE) was evaluated, such as balance, mobility, assessed sensation, and participation. It showed that both of ESR and IRE are all prone to implement for outpatient clinic.

In Ref. [13], it compared the traditional approaches with inertial sensors for the measurement of hip and knee osteoarthritis in remote health care. It showed that the inertial sensors are more suitable for remote health care with extremity osteoarthritis.

The generalizability of deep learning models for predicting outdoor irregular walking surfaces was proposed to show that the results of laboratory-based gait analysis could not be used in real situation. Although the inertial measurement units may be used for real situation, the gait analysis may be still inaccurate since the behavior of walking was more complex in real world. Hence, this paper evaluated the surface classification performance with different data splitting, sensor location, and count by different machine learning models [14].

In the above motion, it showed that the inertial measurement was often used in real situation for gait analysis. It also showed the importance of gait analysis and fall detection. However, none of them could measure the step count, step length, and angle of knee joint measurements with fall detection. Moreover, the wearable with cross-platform APP was not addressed since the cross-platform APP was required recently, such as Android and iOS. Therefore, a cross-platform gait analysis and fall detection wearable device (CPGAFDWD) was proposed to address these issues in this paper.

3. Methods

In this section, it was divided into "Cross-Platform Gait Analysis and Fall Detection Wearable Device" and "Cross-Platform APP" to be depicted.

3.1. Cross-Platform Gait Analysis and Fall Detection Wearable Device

In modern medical, the gait analysis, such as knee joint rehabilitation, and fall detection were getting important, especially for elders [1]. In the existed gait analysis, some of them could be executed at home to save time and money for patients and medical staff. Hence, how to combine health care with technology for residential gait analysis becomes an important issue gradually [3–5,13,14].

Although the residential gait analysis could reduce the time money, and manpower, how to judge the correct motion of gait analysis without any help of medical staff becomes an important issue [15,16]. In the same condition, to detect the fall accident correctly was another important issue. Hence, we integrated the Arduino board with gyroscope, three-axis accelerometer, and Bluetooth to develop a gait analysis and fall detection wearable device, GAFDWD, to address the above issues. Compared with [9–12], the existed fall detection wearable device only focused on fall detection without considering gait analysis. They often aimed to improve the accuracy of fall detection, low power, and low cost. None of them addressed the APP in mobile devices. Moreover, they addressed nothing for cross-platform in mobile devices, such as Android and iOS. Compared with other software, there is no way to call the emergency contact directly, and the emergency contact cannot receive the notification in time. Hence, the above mention was the advantages of CPGAFDWD compared to other software. Since CPGAFDWD included wearable, cross-platform APP, and cloud database, the remote accessing by the Internet was needed. It is also the limitation of CPGAFDWD.

To upload the detected data from GAFDWD to cloud database in real time, to design an APP for GAFDWD was required. Since the APP was depended on the platform of mobile device to be used, how to ensure the APP we designed could be applied for different platforms was an important issue. Hence, a cross-platform APP, CPAPP, was proposed for GAFDWD in this paper. In CPAPP, it received the sensed data captured from CPAPP via Bluetooth, and then sent these data to cloud database, such as MongoDB, via the Internet in real time. The users could track the status of gait analysis and receive the alarm of fall detection by CPAPP immediately.

In GAFDWD, the hardware included gyroscope, three-axis accelerometer, and Bluetooth, as shown in Figure 3. The gyroscope and three-axis accelerometer were used as GY-521. The captured signal from GY-521 was transferred into the sensed data of gait analysis and fall detection by fusion calculation, such as rotation matrix, quaternion, and Euler angle format, respectively. The Bluetooth was used as HM-10 to transmit the sensed data after fusion calculation to CPAPP via Bluetooth. Then CPAPP uploaded the data to cloud database as MongoDB in real time. Figure 4 showed the mechanism for GAFDWD.

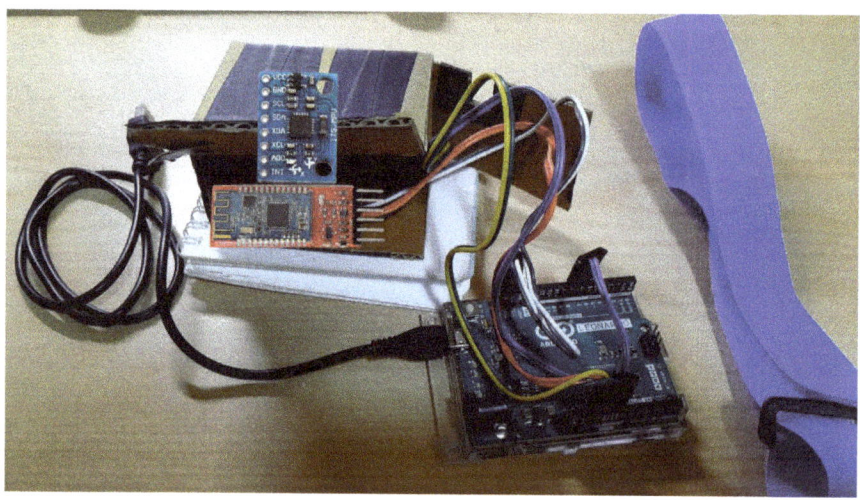

Figure 3. Hardware of CPGAFDWD.

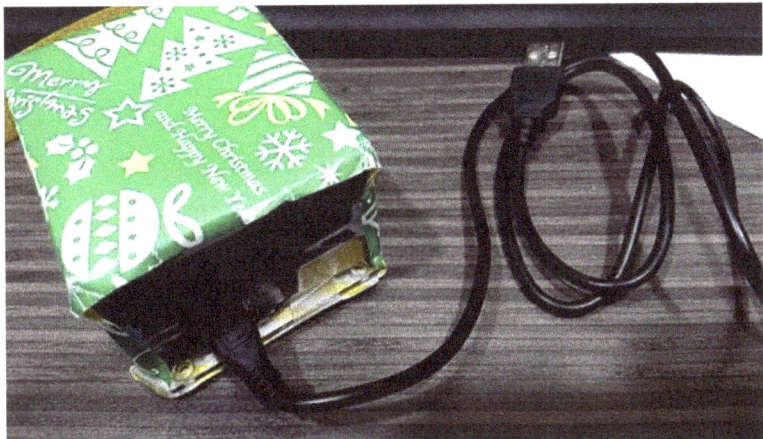

Figure 4. Case of CPGAFDWD.

3.2. Cross-Platform APP

In cross-platform APP, CPAPP, a web APP by Node.js with MongoDB was designed here. To ensure APP used in Android, the APP is often designed by App Inventor or Android Studio. To ensure APP used in iOS, the APP is often designed by Swift. However, App Inventor and Android Studio only could be developed on Android device. In the same way, Swift only could be developed on Android device. In the above mention, it showed that the cost of R&D, software, and hardware for APP designing in cross-platform is high. Since the web APP is executed by browser, it could not be constrained to different platforms of mobile device. Hence, CPAPP could be applied in multiple platforms, such iOS and Android. In CPAPP, it transmitted the data to cloud database via the Internet immediately while it received the sensed data from GAFDWD via Bluetooth. The data of gait analysis and the alarm of fall detection all could be query and notified by CPAPP in any time and place. A block diagram of the software and the ways of communication between the individual elements of the software was shown in Figure 5.

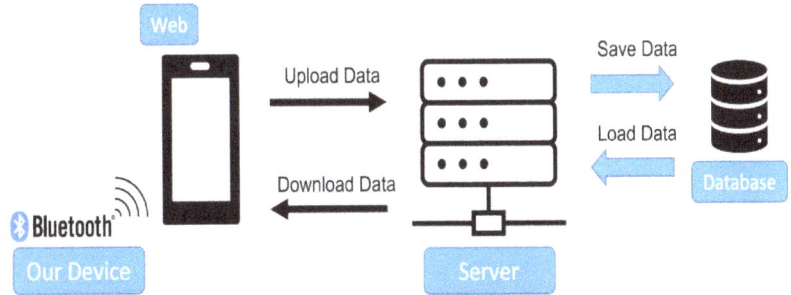

Figure 5. Block diagram of the software.

In this section, it showed the different user interfaces and the corresponding functions of CPAPP, such as login, measurement of pace step, measurement of pace length, measurement of pace angle, and fall detection in both of iOS and Android. Figure 2 had showed the login of CPAPP in both of iOS and Android. In Figures 6 and 7, it showed the measurement of pace step in both of iOS and Android. In Figures 8 and 9, it showed the measurement of pace length in both of iOS and Android. In Figures 10 and 11, it showed the measurement of pace angle in both of iOS and Android. Figures 12 and 13 showed the measurement of fall detection. From Figures 2 and 6–13, it proved that CPAPP designed in this paper could be applied for cross-platform of mobile device.

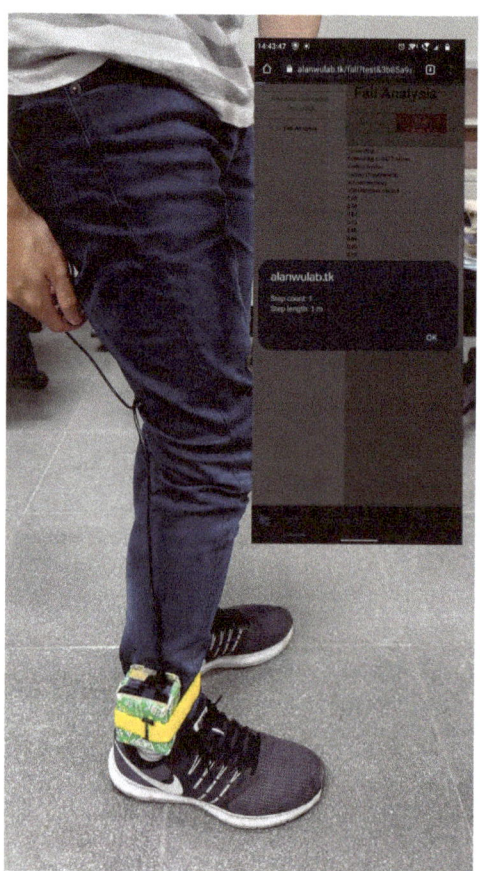

Figure 6. Step count detection of CPGAFDWD in Android.

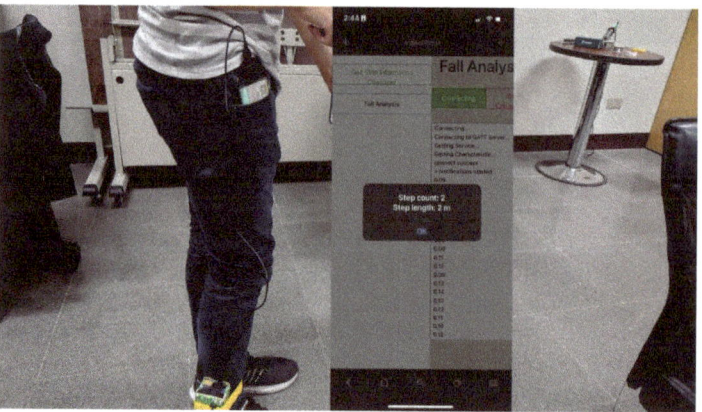

Figure 7. Step count detection of CPGAFDWD in iOS.

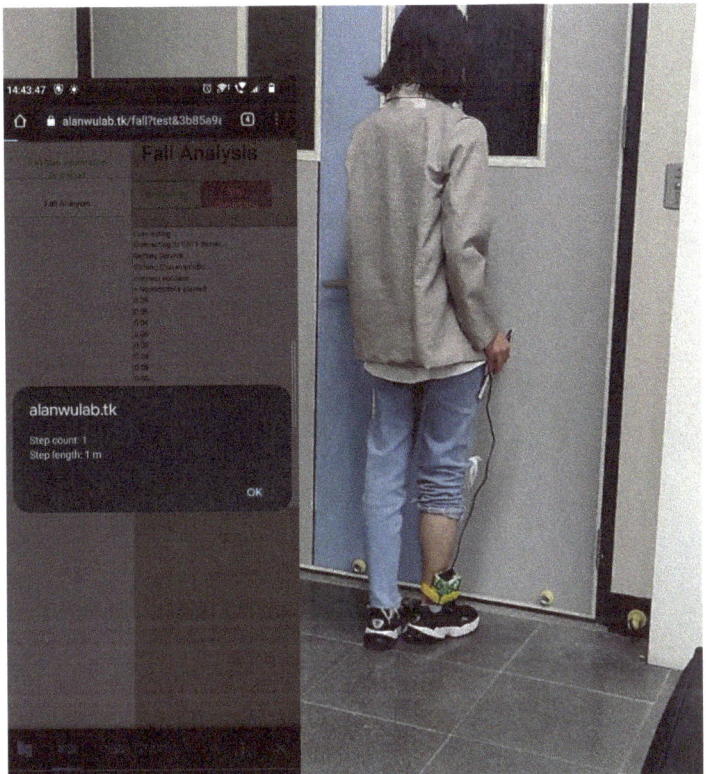

Figure 8. Step length detection of CPGAFDWD in Android.

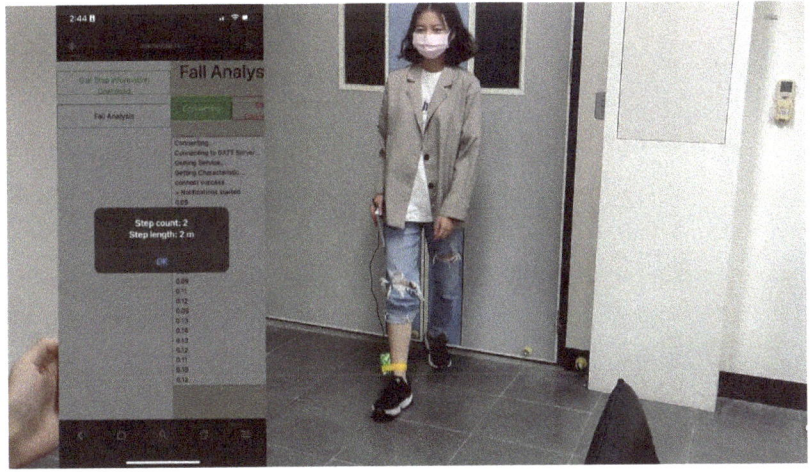

Figure 9. Step length detection of CPGAFDWD in iOS.

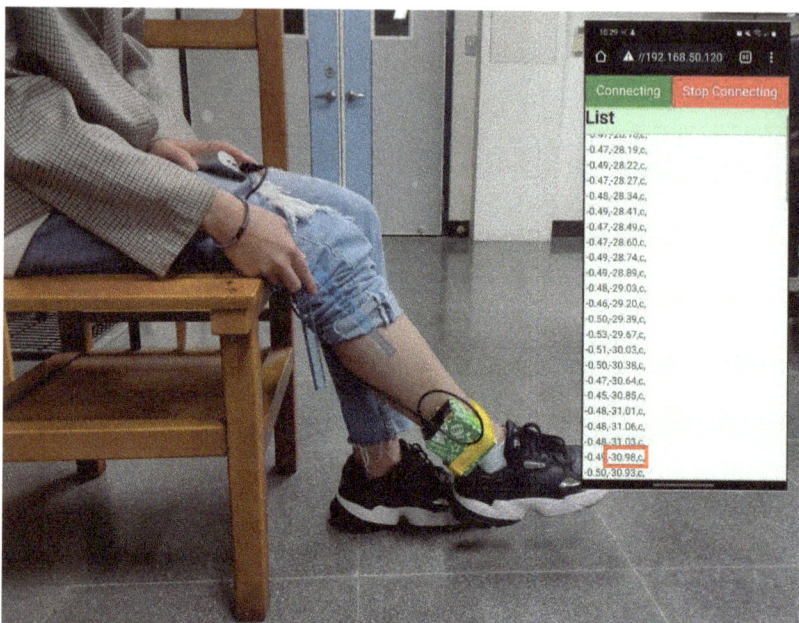

Figure 10. Angle detection of CPGAFDWD in Android.

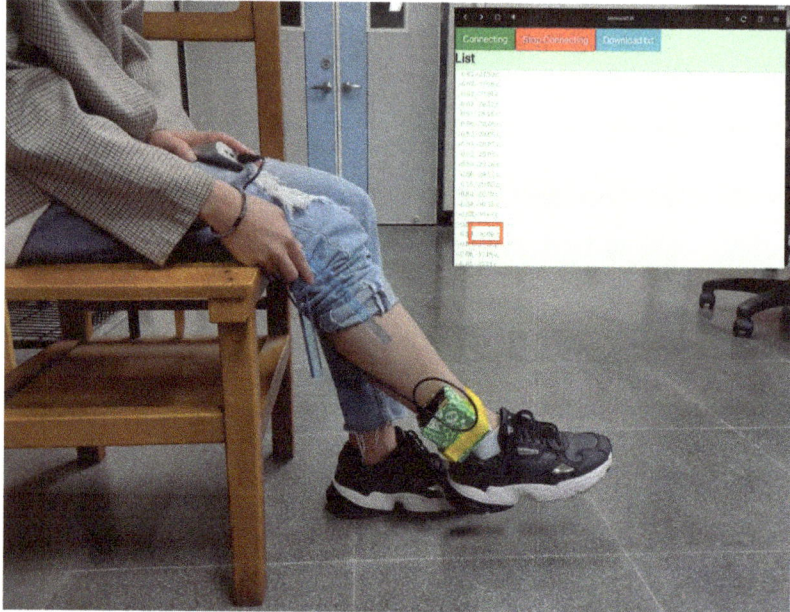

Figure 11. Angle detection of CPGAFDWD in iOS.

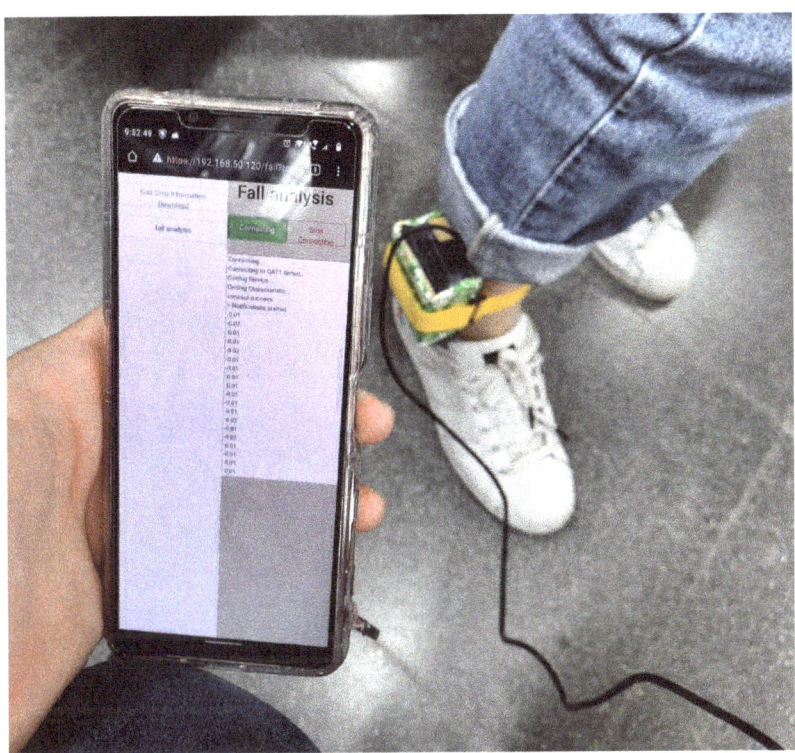

Figure 12. Fall detection of CPGAFDWD in Android.

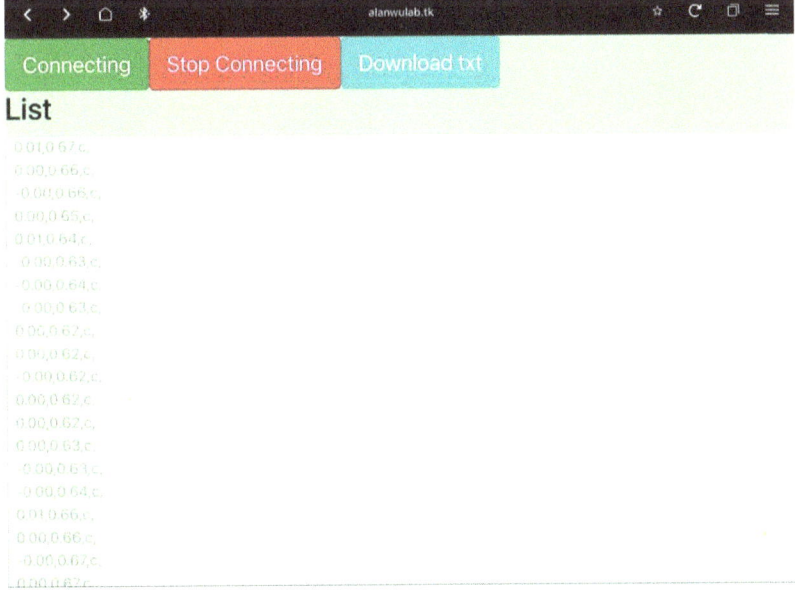

Figure 13. Fall detection of CPGAFDWD in iOS.

Therefore, a cross-platform gait analysis and fall detection wearable device (CP-GAFDWD) proposed in this paper could be applied for the real-time residential gait analysis and fall detection in cross-platform of mobile device. The time, money, and manpower could be reduced for patients and medical institutions by CPGAFDWD.

4. Results

To avoid the ethical permission in our experiment, the experimental results were executed by the laboratory members not the real patients and the wearable device should be attached at the ankle [17–25]. The number of laboratory members was more than 20. In the step count (*SC*), the range of acceleration value was calculated by the first quartile and third quartile values based on quartile method firstly [17–19]. After excluding outlier value, the range of acceleration was calculated from −0.28 to 0.17, as shown in Figure 14. Once the value of acceleration was between −0.28 and 0.17, the step count was increased by 1. It showed that the cross-platform gait analysis and fall detection wearable device (CPGAFDWD) we proposed could calculate the step count (*SC*), accurately. The units of measurement along the x-axes of Figure 14 was microsecond. The units of measurement along the y-axes of Figure 14 was the *y* value of three-axis acceleration.

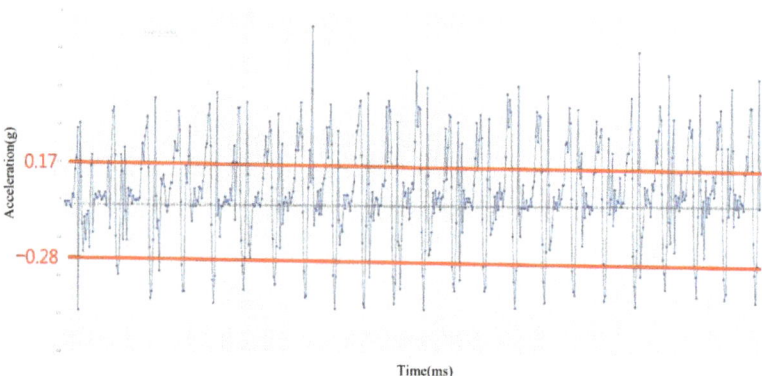

Figure 14. Acceleration for step count.

The step distance (*SD*) was calculated by the maximal and minimal acceleration values of one step count with 4th root calculation as in Equation (1), where A_{max} and A_{min} were denoted as the maximal and minimal acceleration values, and n was denoted as the total step count [20].

$$SD = \sqrt[4]{A_{max} - A_{min}} \times n \qquad (1)$$

The fall detection (*FD*) was determined by the maximal and minimal acceleration values. After the experimental results executed by the laboratory members with the wearable device we designed at the ankle, the maximal and minimal acceleration values were −2 and 2. Once the value of acceleration was below −2 or over 2, the alarm of *FD* was triggered. As shown in Figure 15, the value of acceleration from time unit 191 to 210 was below −2 or over 2. In this situation, the alarm of *FD* was triggered. It proved that CPGAFDWD could detect the fall detection (*FD*), accurately.

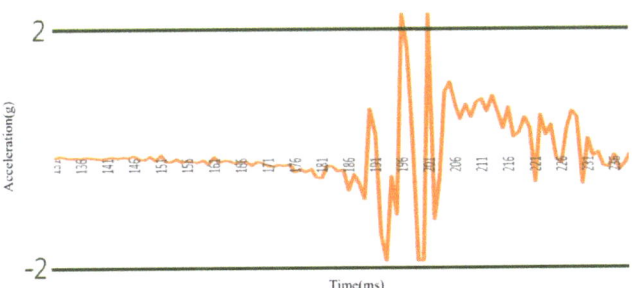

Figure 15. Acceleration for fall detection.

The accurate rate of SC, AR_{SC}, was defined as in Equation (2), where N_{SC}^D was defined as the number of detected SC and N_{SC}^C was defined as the number of actual correct SC. The error rate of SD, ER_{SD}, was defined as in Equation (3), where N_{SD}^D was defined as the number of detected SD and N_{SD}^C was defined as the number of actual correct SD. The accurate rate of angle estimation, AR_{Angle}, was defined as in Equation (4), where N_{Angle}^D was defined as the number of angle estimation and N_{Angle}^C was defined as the number of actual angle. The accurate rate of FD, AR_{FD}, was defined as in Equation (5), where N_{FD}^D was defined as the number of detected FD and N_{FD}^C was defined as the number of actual correct FD. In each performance metric, such as AR_{SC}, ER_{SD}, AR_{Angle}, and AR_{FD}, was 20 times in a round. Each experimental result was 10 rounds. Hence, it showed that CPGAFDWD we proposed could calculate the angle, accurately. Moreover, it also showed that CPGAFDWD we proposed could detect the fall, accurately.

$$AR_{SC} = \frac{N_{SC}^D}{N_{SC}^C} \times 100\% \qquad (2)$$

$$ER_{SD} = \frac{|N_{SD}^C - N_{SD}^D|}{N_{SD}^C} \times 100\% \qquad (3)$$

$$AR_{Angle} = \frac{N_{Angle}^D}{N_{Angle}^C} \times 100\% \qquad (4)$$

$$AR_{FD} = \frac{N_{FD}^D}{N_{FD}^C} \times 100\% \qquad (5)$$

In the experimental results, the units of measurement along the x-axes of Figure 15 was microsecond. The units of measurement along the y-axes of Figure 15 was the y value of three-axis acceleration. It showed that AR_{SC} was up to 92%, 95%, and 89%, while N_{SC}^C was 10, 15, and 20, respectively. The average AR_{SC} by CPGAFDWD was higher than the average AR_{SC} by SVM step classifier [7,20]. ER_{SD} was up to 4%, 8%, and 4%, while N_{SC}^C was 10, 15, and 20, respectively. The average ER_{SD} was below 6%. AR_{Angle} was up to 92%, 95%, and 95%, while N_{Angle}^C was 30, 60, and 90, respectively. The average AR_{Angle} was up to 92%. ER_{SD} was up to 100%, where N_{SC}^C was set to 500 and N_{FD}^C was set to 10 in each round. The average AR_{FD} was up to 90%.

5. Discussion

In this section, it focused on Cross-Platform APP, CPAPP, such as the different user interfaces and the corresponding functions, firstly. The login of CPAPP in both of iOS and Android was showed in Figure 3. The measurement of pace step in both of iOS and Android was showed in Figures 6 and 7. The measurement of pace length in both of iOS and Android was showed in Figures 8 and 9. The measurement of pace angle in both of iOS and Android was showed in Figures 10 and 11. the measurement of fall detection was showed in Figures 12 and 13. In Figures 6–13, it proved that CPAPP designed in this paper could be applied for cross-platform of mobile device, such as Android and iOS.

The basis of reported percentages was calculated based on Equations (1)–(5) and the experimental results were obtained by laboratory members on walking and falling. In the experimental result of gait analysis and fall detection wearable device, GAFDWD, AR_{SC}, ER_{SD}, AR_{Angle}, and AR_{FD} were the performance metrics. AR_{SC} was up to 92%, 95%, and 89%, while N_{SC}^C was 10, 15, and 20, respectively. In Refs. [7,20], it used SVM to classify in the walking gait test by a wearable foot gait collection device with step direction algorithm at any time and place as same as our GAFDWD. The experimental results showed that the accuracy rate of SVM is 86%, and only 86 steps are judged for every 100 steps. However, our GAFDWD in walking gait accuracy could reach about 90%.

The average AR_{SC} by CPGAFDWD was higher than the average AR_{SC} by SVM step classifier [7,20]. ER_{SD} was up to 4%, 8%, and 4%, while N_{SC}^C was 10, 15, and 20, respectively. The average ER_{SD} was below 6%. AR_{Angle} was up to 92%, 95%, and 95%, while N_{Angle}^C was 30, 60, and 90, respectively. The average ER_{SD} was below 6% and the average AR_{Angle} was up to 92%. ER_{SD} was up to 100%, where N_{SC}^C was set to 500 and N_{FD}^C was set to 10 in each round. The minimum ER_{SD} was 4% and the maximal AR_{Angle} was up to 95%. The average AR_{FD} was up to 90%.

The above results showed that the cross-platform gait analysis and fall detection wearable device (CPGAFDWD) proposed in this paper could be applied for gait analysis and fall detection and also could be applied for cross-platform mobile devices. In the future work, the accuracy will be improved in clinical work in the later stage.

6. Conclusions

Due to the progress in medical technology and the advent of an aging society, the rehabilitation treatment gets attention gradually. The rehabilitation methods are different according to different parts of the body and symptoms.

In this paper, it focused on gait analysis, such as step count, step length, and angle of knee joint measurements, since the gait analysis was often needed for elderly. In addition to gait analysis, fall accident was also often occurred for elderly.

In the above mention, it showed the importance for gait analysis and fall detection in modern rehabilitation medicine. However, the existed gait analysis in hospital was still executed by specific medical instruments. In this way, the time and money for patients must increase. The feasibility of gait analysis thus decreased, since the gait analysis could not be executed in any place and any time. For medical institutions, the manpower also increased.

Hence, how to ensure that gait analysis could be executed in any place and any time becomes an important issue. However, how to ensure that the gait analysis was correct at home becomes another important issue, since the incorrect gait analysis may lead to incorrect rehabilitation. The rehabilitation treatments may be discounted.

Therefore, a cross-platform gait analysis and fall detection wearable device, CP-GAFDWD, was proposed to address the above issues in this paper. In CPGAFDWD, it aimed to ensure that the gait analysis could be correct without limiting to any time and place for patients. The experimental results also showed that the correct rate of gait analysis was over 90% and the correct rate of fall detection was close to 100%. It proved that CPGAFDWD we proposed could be applied for gait analysis and fall detection in any time and place. The time, money, and manpower thus could be reduced for patients and medical institutions. In the future, we will apply IRB for CPGAFDWD used in clinical medicine.

Author Contributions: M.-H.C. was responsible for Supervision and Project Administration. Y.-C.W. was responsible for Conceptualization, Methodology, Investigation, Writing—Original Draft, and Writing—Review & Editing. H.-Y.N. was responsible for Resources and Software. Y.-T.C. was responsible for Validation and Formal analysis. S.-H.J. was responsible for Data Curation and Visualization. All authors have read and agreed to the published version of the manuscript.

Funding: APC was funded by National Science and Technology Council (NSTC) of Taiwan to National Yunlin University of Science and Technology under 111-2221-E-143-002.

Institutional Review Board Statement: Not applicable.

Informed Consent Statement: Not applicable.

Data Availability Statement: Not applicable.

Acknowledgments: This paper was supported by the National Science and Technology Council (NSTC) of Taiwan to National Yunlin University of Science and Technology under 111-2221-E-143-002.

Conflicts of Interest: The authors declare no conflict of interest.

References

1. Kumar, H.R.; Janardhan, S.; Prakash, D.; Kumar, M.K.P. Fall Detection System using Tri-Axial Accelerometer. In Proceedings of the IEEE International Conference on Recent Trends in Electronics, Information & Communication Technology, Bangalore, India, 18–19 May 2018; pp. 1846–1850.
2. Jefiza, A.; Pramunanto, E.; Boedinoegroho, H.; Purnomo, M. Fall Detection Based on Accelerometer and Gyroscope using Back Propagation. In Proceedings of the IEEE International Conference on Electrical Engineering, Computer Science and Informatics, Yogyakarta, Indonesia, 19–21 September 2017; pp. 1–6.
3. Zhang, Y.; Zhu, Z.; Wang, S. Multi-Condition Constraint Adaptive Step Detection Method Based on the Characteristics of Gait. In Proceedings of the IEEE International Conference on Ubiquitous Positioning, Indoor Navigation and Location-Based Services, Wuhan, China, 22–23 March 2018; pp. 1–5.
4. Bridenbaug, S.A.; Kressig, R.W. Laboratory Review: The Role of Gait Analysis in Sensors' Mobility and Fall Prevention. *Gerontology* **2011**, *57*, 256–264. [CrossRef] [PubMed]
5. Tong, L.; Chen, W.; Song, Q.; Ge, Y. A Research on Automatic Human Fall Detection Method Based on Wearable Inertial Force Information Acquisition System. In Proceedings of the IEEE International Conference on Robotics and Biomimetics, Guilin, China, 19–23 December 2009; pp. 949–953.
6. Tal, K.; Benedetta, H.; Or, K.; Noam, G.; Sharon, H.-B.; Gabi, Z.; Meir, P. Bilateral Leg Stepping Coherence as a Predictor of Freezing of Gait in Patients With Parkinson's Disease Walking With Wearable Sensors. *IEEE Trans. Neural Syst. Rehabil. Eng.* **2022**, *31*, 798–805.
7. Lai, Y.X.; Ma, Y.W.; Huang, Y.M.; Chen, J.L.; Mukhopadhyay, S.C. Ubiquitous Motion Sensing Service Using Wearable Shoe Module and Mobile Device. In Proceedings of the IEEE International Conference on Instrumentation and Measurement Technology, Minneapolis, MN, USA, 6–9 May 2013; pp. 1–4.
8. Hong, W.; Lee, J.; Hur, P. Piecewise Linear Labeling Method for Speed-Adaptability Enhancement in Human Gait Phase Estimation. *IEEE Trans. Neural Syst. Rehabil. Eng.* **2022**, *31*, 628–635. [CrossRef]
9. Janardhan, K.; Parthasarathi, P.; Karyemsetty, N.; Arunkumar, K.; Krishnamoorthy, R.; Umapathy, K. Device Free Human Body Fall Detection to Aid Senior Citizen. In Proceedings of the IEEE International Conference on Electronics, Communication and Aerospace Technology, Coimbatore, India, 1–3 December 2022; pp. 1158–1162.
10. Wasi, M.W.I.; Dziyauddin, R.A.; Amir, N.I.M.; Ahmad, R. Machine Learning Algorithm for Fall Classification Using Wearable Device. In Proceedings of the IEEE International Conference on Future Telecommunication Technologies, Johor Baharu, Malaysia, 14–16 November 2022; pp. 62–66.
11. Edna, A.-R.; Rosero, E. Multimodal Wearable Technology Approaches to Human Falls. In Proceedings of the IEEE International Conference on Humanitarian Technology Conference, Ottawa, ON, Canada, 2–4 December 2022; pp. 86–92.
12. Yu, X.; Ma, T.; Jang, J.; Xiong, S. Data Augmentation to Address Various Rotation Errors of Wearable Sensors for Robust Pre-impact Fall Detection. *IEEE J. Biomed. Health Inf.* **2022**, 1–11. [CrossRef]
13. Landes, R.D.; Glover, A.; Pillai, L.; Doerhoff, S.; Virmani, T. Levodopa ONOFF-state freezing of gait: Defining the gait and non-motor phenotype. *PLoS ONE* **2022**, *17*, e0269227. [CrossRef] [PubMed]
14. Ofek, H.; Alperin, M.; Knoll, T.; Livne, D.; Laufer, Y. Explicit versus implicit lower extremity sensory retraining for post-stroke chronic sensory deficits: A randomized controlled trial. *Disabil. Rehabil.* **2022**, 1–7. [CrossRef] [PubMed]
15. Rose, M.J.; Costello, K.E.; Eigenbrot, S.; Torabian, K.; Kumar, D. Inertial Measurement Units and Application for Remote Health Care in Hip and Knee Osteoarthritis: Narrative Review. *JMIR Rehabil. Assist. Technol.* **2022**, *9*, e33521. [CrossRef] [PubMed]
16. Shah, V.; Flood, M.W.; Grimm, B.; Dixon, P.C. Generalizability of Deep Learning Models for Predicting Outdoor Irregular Walking Surfaces. *J. Biomech.* **2022**, *139*, 111159. [CrossRef] [PubMed]

17. Auvinet, B.; Berrut, G.; Touzard, C.; Moutel, L.; Collet, N.; Chaleil, D.; Barrey, E. Reference data for normal subjects obtained with an accelerometric device. *Gait Posture* **2002**, *16*, 124–134. [CrossRef] [PubMed]
18. Bonomi, A.G.; Goris, A.H.; Yin, B.; Westerterp, K.R. Detection of Type, Duration, and Intensity of Physical Activity Using An Accelerometer. *Med. Sci. Sport. Exerc.* **2009**, *41*, 1770–1777. [CrossRef] [PubMed]
19. Espy, D.; Yang, F.; Bhatt, T.; Pai, Y.-C. Independent influence of gait speed and step length on stability and fall risk. *Gait Posture* **2010**, *32*, 378–382. [CrossRef] [PubMed]
20. Ambrose, A.F.; Paul, G.; Hausdorff, J.M. Risk factors for falls among older adults: A review of the literature. *Maturitas* **2013**, *75*, 51–61. [CrossRef] [PubMed]
21. Xing, H.; Li, J.; Hou, B.; Zhang, Y.; Guo, M. Pedestrian Stride Length Estimation from IMU Measurements and ANN Based Algorithm. *J. Sens.* **2017**, *2017*, 6091261. [CrossRef]
22. Riehle, T.H.; Anderson, S.M.; Lichter, P.A.; Whalen, W.E.; Giudice, N.A. Indoor Inertial Waypoint Navigation for the Blind. In Proceedings of the IEEE International Conference on Medicine and Biology Society, Osaka, Japan, 3–7 July 2013; pp. 5187–5190.
23. Tumkur, K.; Subbiah, S. Modeling Human Walking for Step Detection and Stride Determination by 3-Axis Accelerometer Readings in Pedometer. In Proceedings of the IEEE International Conference on Computational Intelligence, Modelling and Simulation, Kuantan, Malaysia, 25–27 September 2012; pp. 199–204.
24. Weinberg, H. Using the ADXL 202 in Pedometer and Personal Navigation Applications. *Analog Device*, AN-602 APPLICATION NOTE. 2002. Available online: https://www.semanticscholar.org/paper/Using-the-ADXL-202-in-Pedometer-and-Personal-Weinberg/96383a5f1008740f213e2ab48161a65b265f16f6 (accessed on 1 February 2023).
25. Webster, B.J.; Darter, B.J. Principles of Normal and Pathologic Gait. In *Atlas of Orthoses and Assistive Devices*, 5th ed.; Elsevier: Amsterdam, The Netherlands, 2019; pp. 49–62.

Disclaimer/Publisher's Note: The statements, opinions and data contained in all publications are solely those of the individual author(s) and contributor(s) and not of MDPI and/or the editor(s). MDPI and/or the editor(s) disclaim responsibility for any injury to people or property resulting from any ideas, methods, instructions or products referred to in the content.

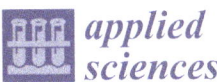

Article

Trust Components: An Analysis in The Development of Type 2 Diabetic Mellitus Mobile Application

Salaki Reynaldo Joshua [1], Wasim Abbas [1], Je-Hoon Lee [1,*] and Seong Kun Kim [2,*]

1 Department of Electronics, Information and Communication Engineering, Kangwon National University, Samcheok-si 25913, Republic of Korea
2 Department of Liberal Studies, Kangwon National University, Samcheok-si 25913, Republic of Korea
* Correspondence: jehoon.lee@kangwon.ac.kr (J.-H.L.); kimseong@kangwon.ac.kr (S.K.K.)

Abstract: Trust in information and communication technology devices is an important factor, considering the role of technology in carrying out supporting tasks in everyday human activities. The level of trust in technology will influence its application and adoption. Recognizing the importance of trust in technology, researchers in this study will examine trust components for the development of a type 2 diabetes mobile application. The results of this study resulted in three major focuses, namely the application design (consisting of architecture), UI design, and evaluation of trust factors of the application: functionality, ease of use, usefulness, security and privacy, and cost. This analysis of trust components will be useful for the application or adoption by users of a type 2 diabetes mellitus mobile application so that users will trust the application both in terms of functionality and the generated information.

Keywords: mobile application; diabetes; architecture; trust components; testing

1. Introduction

1.1. Mobile Health Application for Diabetes Mellitus

Mobile health applications are software tools that help users monitor their health conditions via smartphones and tablets [1]. Their functionality ranges from simple diaries, medication reminders, and tracking health progress to more complex programs certified as medical devices by health authorities. Currently, mobile health applications with a large number of users have a high potential for improving healthcare [2]. The reliability of these applications remains in doubt, limiting their widespread adoption [3]. Extensive research on trust in technology and the role of user trust in the selection of various information technology (IT) artifacts have yet to be conducted [4].

Diabetes mellitus is a genetically and clinically heterogeneous metabolic disorder characterized by carbohydrate tolerance loss [5]. Diabetes mellitus is clinically characterized by fasting and postprandial hyperglycemia, atherosclerosis, and microangiopathic vascular disease [6].

Diabetes mellitus is classified into two types: type 1 and type 2 diabetes. Type 1 diabetes is characterized by the pancreas, the body's insulin factory, being unable or less able to produce insulin [7]. As a result, the body's insulin is lacking or not present at all, and sugar accumulates in the blood circulation because it cannot be transported into cells [8]. Type 2 diabetes mellitus (T2DM) is the most common type [9]. The pancreas can still produce insulin in type 2 diabetes, but the quality of the insulin is poor, and it cannot properly function, causing blood glucose levels to rise [10]. Patients with this type of diabetes usually do not need additional insulin injections in their treatment but do need drugs that work to improve insulin function, lower glucose, improve sugar processing in the liver, and perform several alternative treatments for support [11]. Age, sex, family history, physical activity, and eating habits are the risk factors that have the greatest association

---

Citation: Joshua, S.R.; Abbas, W.; Lee, J.-H.; Kim, S.K. Trust Components: An Analysis in The Development of Type 2 Diabetic Mellitus Mobile Application. *Appl. Sci.* **2023**, *13*, 1251. https://doi.org/10.3390/app13031251

Academic Editors: Chien-Hung Yeh, Wenbin Shi, Xiaojuan Ban, Men-Tzung Lo and Shenghong He

Received: 30 November 2022
Revised: 4 January 2023
Accepted: 5 January 2023
Published: 17 January 2023

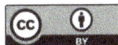

Copyright: © 2023 by the authors. Licensee MDPI, Basel, Switzerland. This article is an open access article distributed under the terms and conditions of the Creative Commons Attribution (CC BY) license (https://creativecommons.org/licenses/by/4.0/).

with the incidence of type 2 diabetes mellitus (T2DM) among the many factors that cause diabetes mellitus [12].

All types of diabetes can cause many complications in the body and increase the risk of premature death. Heart attack, kidney failure, stroke, leg amputation, vision loss, and nerve damage are all possible complications. Type 2 diabetes mellitus (T2DM) is a chronic disease that requires ongoing therapy and patient education to prevent acute complications and lower the risk of long-term complications [13].

Type 2 diabetes mellitus (T2DM) problems can be overcome in various ways, including pharmacologically and non-pharmacologically. Non-pharmacological therapy includes lifestyle changes by adjusting diet (medical nutrition therapy), therapy using fruit juice, increasing physical activity, and education on various problems related to diabetes, all of which are continuously carried out. Pharmacological therapy includes oral anti-diabetic administration and insulin injections. Pharmacological therapy should be used in conjunction with non-pharmacological therapy [14].

1.2. Usability Test

Usability has a word for "usable", which is defined as being useful. To be considered good, something must minimize failure while also providing satisfaction and benefits to application users [15]. Usability is the ease of using something. In this case, it is intended that the developed application be simple to use and testing be conducted to determine the success of the developed application by focusing on ease, effectiveness, efficiency, and satisfaction of users [16].

Usability is a factor that determines whether an application is good or not. There are five main components of usability [17]. The five components are learnability (easiness to learn), efficiency (efficiency), memorability (ease for users to remember), errors (error rate), and satisfaction (satisfaction) [18].

Usability testing is a process that involves people as test participants, representing targets, to evaluate the extent to which a product meets usability criteria [19]. Usability testing can be performed by interviewing or giving questionnaires to users [20]. In testing the user groups, it is recommended to use 3–4 users from each category if there are two groups. However, if there are three or more groups of users, then use three users from each category for the usability level measurement listed in Table 1 [21].

Table 1. Usability Level Measurement.

No.	Usability Level Measurement	
	Level	Description
1	Learnability	It is defined as the speed with which the user can use the system, the ease of use in the performance of a function, and the wishes of the user.
2	Efficiency	It is defined as a resource instrument that has a function to achieve better goals.
3	Memorability	Users are tested to see how long they can remember using the application.
4	Errors and security	How many problems are caused by errors that are inconsistent with what users expect from the system?
5	Satisfaction	The application's freedom of expression and user comfort are both subjective measures of the user's perception of the system.

1.3. Trust in the Mobile Application

The idea of competence is that an agent will safely, dependably, and consistently operate in a particular situation, which underlines how crucial trust is to the deployment of any online ecosystem. That is, whether an entity decides to do business with another firm is heavily influenced by trust in the original firm. The authors argue that, before using or providing services in an electronic market, both the consumers and providers must have trust in one another. If there is no mutual trust between them, then resources will not be fully shared, and there may be a lot of fraudulent transactions. Such a situation would be detrimental to honest buyers and sellers, preventing them from taking advantage of the benefits of the online world [22].

Trust, as it is in the online system, is critical to the success of mobile applications. Customers must constantly choose which mobile apps to download and/or use because there are hundreds of thousands of them available in application stores. When several mobile apps with comparable functionalities begin to appear in application stores, the decision becomes even more difficult because users must choose the most reliable application. Customers will always prefer to download and use a mobile app that is useful, dependable, and of high quality. However, it can be difficult to choose a mobile app that is thus practical, trustworthy, and high quality. This is evident from the numerous comments left by users who downloaded poor-quality mobile applications and expressed their frustration with them in the application shops. Therefore, it is essential to establish early confidence in mobile apps before users download and use them [23].

From a security and privacy standpoint, the emergence of mobile apps poses additional threats to the confidentiality of information and data. There have been several instances where mobile apps have grabbed and mined private information from users, including address books, photographs, and more. Such occurrences blatantly expose the invasion of the client's privacy and further harm the consumers. Unfortunately, it reveals that more than half of the popular mobile applications for Android and iOS under consideration send user data to third-party servers. Aside from the issue of individual privacy, an increasing number of organizations and businesses are also opposed to their employees using mobile devices [24]. They are extremely concerned about the possibility of mobile apps accessing and gathering sensitive and important company documents (e.g., through business emails on mobile devices).

Installing security measures and policies can reduce the risk of sensitive business information being leaked to the public, but these must be supplemented and improved by the use of trust measurement. The majority of security experts agree that the best strategy for reducing the risk of document leakage in mobile apps is to prevent applications from being installed in the first place. However, such a strategy could not be advantageous for both employees and enterprises, especially in light of the fact that mobile apps increase employee productivity and benefit companies. Therefore, there are only two options left for protecting crucial corporate data: teach staff how to choose legitimate mobile apps and provide them tools for evaluating the reliability of mobile apps before installing and using them. Measuring trust in mobile apps is critical as the primary and additional layer of security and privacy protection. Trust also improves security by better-securing resources and information [25].

1.4. Previous Research

Initially, the development of an Android mobile application was focused on controlling type 2 diabetes. At this point, the research team had 20 people, ten with diabetes and ten without, participate in the use of diabetes mobile applications with supporting hardware, such as a wearable band, glucose meter, and treadmill [26]. The results of the initial research are used as reference material for the development of the second stage. At this stage, the researchers evaluate some of the functionality and accessibility of the application by conducting tests involving 40 people, consisting of twenty with diabetes and twenty without diabetes. The results of the second stage of research conclude that there is a need for changes and adaptation of applications for users, especially related to user registration for applications, as well as glucometer and wearable band (smartwatch) connectivity with various versions [27]. Previous researchers have conducted preliminary research through two previous studies, which are shown in Table 2.

Table 2. Previous Research.

No.	Research		
	Title	Year	Publisher
1	"Therapeutic Exercise Platform for Type 2 Diabetic Mellitus" [26]	2021	Journal of Electronics, MDPI
2	"Self-Care IoT Platform for Diabetic Mellitus" [27]	2021	Journal of Applied Sciences, MDPI

2. Analysis

2.1. Mobile Application in Healthcare

Smartphone users continue to increase as mobile phones become more sophisticated, efficient, and portable. The use of smartphones has become an important item and a lifestyle in society. A mobile application is one that enables mobility through the use of equipment, such as a cell phone (mobile phone), a PDA (personal digital assistant), or a smartphone [28]. Mobile applications can wirelessly access and use a web application using a mobile device, where the data obtained is only in the form of text and does not require much bandwidth. The use of the mobile application only requires a mobile phone that is equipped with General Packet Radio Service (GPRS) facilities and its connection. There are several aspects that must be considered to build a mobile application, especially the hardware. In terms of bandwidth, the current network conditions have made it possible to obtain a large enough bandwidth for the cellular network [28]. Table 3 summarizes the application classification in healthcare.

Several mobile-based applications in the healthcare sector have been developed with a variety of operating systems, depending on user needs, such as Android, iOS, Windows Mobile, Blackberry OS, and Symbian. Android is a mobile device software collection that includes an operating system, middleware, and the main mobile applications [29]. Android has four distinct features (Table 4) [30,31].

Table 3. Application Classification in Healthcare.

No.	Application Classification		
	Researcher	Classification	Description
1	B. D. A. Pititto	Disease prediction	A disease prediction application is an application that is used to help patients or application users find out the prediction of disease along with the overall results of the obtained diagnosis based on the symptoms felt. This application was developed using certain methods according to the scope of the case study (disease) to be analyzed by calculating all parameters related to the symptoms of the disease. The development of this disease prediction application is useful to help doctors and also provide recommendations to patients or users who have difficulty knowing the disease they are suffering from but only know the symptoms they feel.
2	J. H. Park	Clinical communication	A clinical communication application is the development of technology in the health sector that helps achieve a state or health status as a whole, both physically, mentally, and socially. This application focuses on communication-related health. The database in this application will store and process the existing data so that it can be useful for later use. Several clinical communication applications provide real-time communication services between patients and doctors to conduct health consultations. Doctors will collect information about the patient's health status, or they can access a database to view the patient's medical history.

Table 3. Cont.

No.	Application Classification		
	Researcher	Classification	Description
3	Adu, U. H. Malabu	Medication	The lack of information about treatment and drugs is the basis for developing health applications in this field. If it is not handled properly, the patient or customer will self-regulate the drug therapy they receive, which will lead to an increase in cases of drug administration errors that are not in accordance with the patient's needs. The medication health application focuses on education about drug information, assisting in health consultations on drug administration based on symptoms, and viewing the history of purchasing and using drugs stored in the database.
4	Lee, J.-H.	Exercise	Exercise health applications (also called health and fitness applications) are applications that can provide information to users without limitations of place or time and help them achieve their health and fitness targets. Some exercise applications provide features that are able to connect applications with other supporting devices to collect health information more comprehensively, for example, by connecting applications with treadmills, cycles, smartwatches, or other supporting devices.
5	R. K Więckowska	Nutrition	The nutrition application is an application that helps patients and users find out their nutritional needs and status by referring to nutrition and health sciences efficiently, cheaply, and accurately when each country has different nutritional guidelines. This is extremely useful because food consumption has an impact on a person's nutritional status. Good nutritional status, also known as optimal nutritional status, occurs when the body receives and uses enough nutrients to support physical growth, brain development, workability, and overall health to the greatest extent possible. The nutrition application already has a nutritional value based on a calculated formula (nutritional standards). By accessing the database, the application can find specific numbers (foods or beverages) that will be or have been consumed.

Table 4. Android Characteristics.

No.	Android Characteristics	
	Characteristic	Description
1	Open source	Android is designed to be completely open, allowing any app to access any of the phone's core functions, such as making calls, sending text messages, using the camera, and so on. To optimize the device's memory and hardware resources, Android employs a specially designed virtual machine. Because Android is open source, it can be freely expanded to include newer, more advanced technologies as they become available. This platform will continue to evolve, allowing for the development of innovative mobile applications.
2	Accessibility	Android makes no distinction between the phone's main application and third-party applications. All applications can be designed to have equal access to a phone's capabilities to provide a diverse range of services and applications to users.
3	Reliability	Android removes barriers to developing new and innovative apps. A developer, for example, can combine web information with data on a person's phone, such as the user's contacts, calendar, or geographic location.

Table 4. Cont.

No.	Android Characteristics	
	Characteristic	Description
4	Easy to develop	Android provides a wide range of libraries and tools for developing better applications. Android includes a set of tools that can be used to help developers increase productivity when developing Google Inc. applications. Google has rebuilt Android from the ground up and made it open source, allowing developers to use it without paying Google for a license and build Android without restrictions. The Android Software Development Kit (SDK) includes the tools and Application Programming Interface (API) required to begin developing applications for the Android platform in Java.

2.2. Telehealth

As a part of telehealth, telemedicine focuses on the therapeutic side, while telemedicine covers the prophylactic, preventive, and therapeutic aspects. One of the functions of telehealth and a major requirement for providing health services is patient monitoring and scheduling [32]. The coverage of telehealth, telemedicine, and electronic health (e-health), as well as telecare and m-health, is described by Totten AM et al. (Table 5) [33].

Table 5. Telehealth Operational Definition.

No.	Telehealth Operational Definition	
	Objective	Description
1	Synchronous	Provides services or remote health services at the same time as consultations via video call (Zoom, Skype, etc.) or telephone
2	Asynchronous	Provides health services via emote/not concurrently (email or online chat consultation).
3	Mobile health	A mobile-based health service, such as health education and consultation, can be delivered through smartphones or mobile-based applications.
4	Virtual agent	Remote health service delivery through certain chatbots or applications that can help patients or users conduct 24 h health consultations
5	Artificial intelligence	Remote health services with artificial intelligence technology, such as being able to measure heart rate, make drug recommendations based on symptoms, and calculate or monitor sleep hours

3. Research Methodology

3.1. Research Method

This study was carried out at Kangwon National University's Circuit and System Design Laboratory with several systematic stages in order to produce research reports and products (a mobile application) that were in accordance with the objectives of the research implementation. The research method includes four stages (Figure 1), starting with system requirements, designing system architecture, developing a prototype, and implementing it.

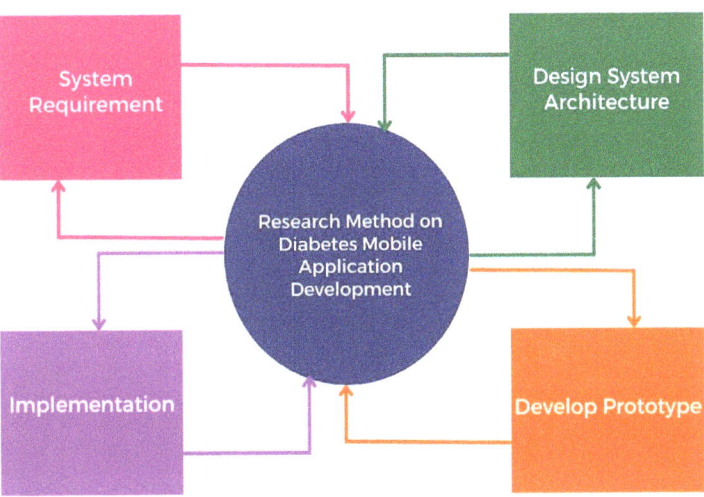

Figure 1. Research Method.

3.2. Software Development Methodology

A "framework" is a software development method that is used to structure, plan, and control the process of developing an information system. Over the years, many different frameworks have been developed, each with its own set of strengths and weaknesses. The prototype model is suitable for exploring customer requirements and specifications in more detail, but it has a high risk of increasing project costs and time. The software development model used is a prototype model [34].

In developing this application, we use the prototype model as an approach to mobile application development. We undergo three stages: creating and revising the mockup, conducting customer test drives, and listening to customers. All steps in this prototype model were chosen because they are in accordance with the project being developed, which does not have many stages, and the parties or teams involved can also be maximized in the three existing stages (Figure 2). The details of each process are summarized in Table 6.

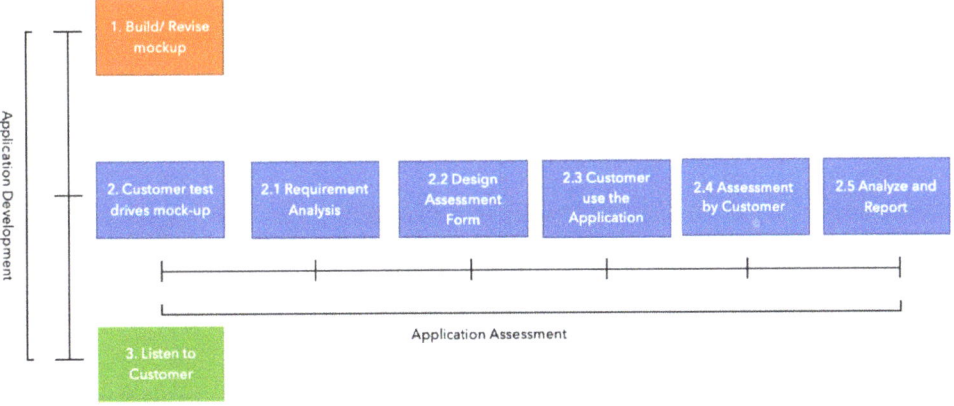

Figure 2. Application Development and Assessment Process.

Table 6. Application Development and Assessment.

No.	Process	Description
	Application Development and Assessment	
1	Build/Revise mockup	The prototype model begins by gathering customer requirements for the software that will be created. At this stage, we researchers are gathering information about the needs of type 2 diabetes mellitus (T2DM) patients, which is poured in the form of features and services that monitor medication, food intake, exercise, and sleep.
2	The customer test drives the mockup	After listening to customer needs, a prototype program is created to give customers a better idea of what they truly want. The prototype program is typically an unfinished (but fully functional) program that simulates the software flow so that it appears to be completely finished. In this study, our researchers focused on four customer needs as functions or features in the application: medication monitoring, food intake monitoring, exercise monitoring, and sleep monitoring features.
2.1	Requirement analysis	The requirement analysis stage is characterized by an intense interaction between the system analysts and the system user community (end-users), during which the system development team demonstrates its expertise in order to gain user feedback and trust and obtain good participation. Because users may have had previous information system failures, it is difficult to persuade them to agree (being skeptical) about their information system requirements.
2.2	Design assessment form	Assessment in application development is an effort to obtain data or information from the processes and results that have been carried out. Before conducting an assessment, an assessment form is created, which includes several indicators to ensure that the information the users seek is accurate.
2.3	The customer uses the application	At this stage, the customer will use the mobile application that has been developed, where the application to be used is the latest updated version (version 2) with several changes from the previous version (version 1).
2.4	Assessment by the customer	The previous stage's assessment form is distributed to customers in order to gather information about the application's use on both the performance of version 1 and version 2 of the application.
2.5	Analyze and report	The assessment form that has been distributed will be collected and analyzed for data, and after that, it will be made into a report.
3	Listen to the customer	The customer or user evaluates this prototype program until specifications that match their wishes or needs are found. At this stage, the researcher will conduct a test involving 40 users who are participants (diabetic patients or non-patients) who are involved in using a mobile-based diabetes application.

4. System Design

4.1. User Interface

The user interface (UI) is the part of the experience with which the user interacts [35]. UI is not just about colors and shapes but about providing users with the right tools to achieve their goals. In addition, UI is more than just buttons, menus, and forms that the user must fill out. A "user interface" is used when the system and users can interact with each other through commands, such as using the content or entering data. The user interface is one of the most important aspects of application development because it is visible, audible, and touchable. At this point, the researchers have created (Table 7) a user interface for the type 2 diabetes mellitus mobile application based on the appropriate needs.

Table 7. Design of the Application.

No.	Page	Mockup (Design)	User Interface (Implementation)
1	**Login** On the login page, the user will fill in data in the form of an ID and password (if you have previously registered), while for new users, the application provides services to register by filling in detailed data or automatically using a Google account.		
2	**Personal information** Users are asked to enter information, such as their nickname, sex (male or female), date of birth, height, and weight, on the personal information page.		
3	**Home** On the home page, the application briefly displays features that can be explored by users in the form of icon visualization, such as statistics to view the results of health data calculations, Bluetooth connections to devices, surveys, sugar levels, medicine, exercise, and a calendar.		
4	**Register IoT pack** Users use the Register to IoT Pack page to connect applications to devices they own, such as wearable bands, glucometers, treadmills, and so on.		

Table 7. *Cont.*

No.	Design of the Application		
	Page	Mockup (Design)	User Interface (Implementation)
5	**Monitoring medication** The medication monitoring page enables users to view or control the medication intake schedule as recommended, or it can be entered manually by the user.	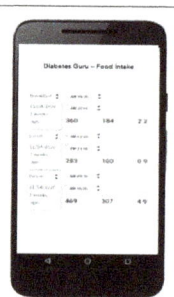	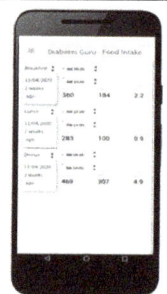
6	**Monitoring food intake** The food intake monitoring page allows users to directly control food intake by making direct adjustments at the specified time, which is divided into three parts: breakfast, lunch, and dinner.	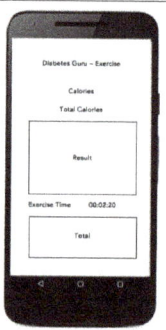	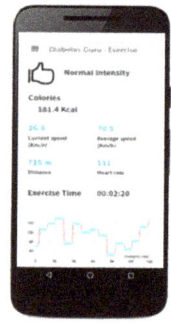
7	**Monitoring exercise** The exercise monitoring page helps users see the exercise that has been completed. The results of the exercise are in the form of current speed, average speed, distance, and heart rate.	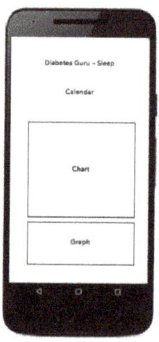	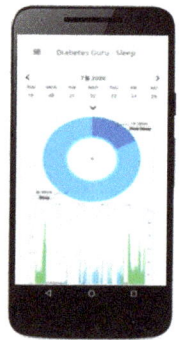
8	**Monitoring sleep** The sleep monitoring page is visualized in the form of charts and calendars to make it easier for users to see the results of the evaluation and monitoring of sleep. The user can see the total presentation as well as the average rest and sleep hours of the user.		

4.2. Benefits of Application and Trustworthiness

In application development, there must be benefits that are expected to be the goal of developing the application. The following are the potential benefits of the type 2 diabetes mellitus mobile application. Table 8 summarizes the potential benefits of the application.

Table 8. Potential Benefits of the Application.

No.	Benefits
1	Patients can accurately determine the level of risk of type 2 diabetes mellitus
2	Increase patient capacity for self-management of type 2 diabetes mellitus
3	Facilitates the decision-making process for optimal insulin dosage
4	Help maintain and manage a healthy lifestyle
5	Doctors will be more helpful in diagnosing type 2 diabetes mellitus and its complications
6	Nutritionists will be more helpful in determining the daily menu and physical exercise for people with type 2 diabetes mellitus
7	Improve communication between patients and healthcare professionals

Trust components in the development of an application are an important factor (Table 9). An application user will feel comfortable using the application if it has a good level of trust. The development of the type 2 diabetes mellitus mobile application includes the following trust components.

Table 9. Trust Components in Mobile Application Development.

No.	Trust Components	Description
1	Convenience	Basically, users use the application because its functionality fulfills their needs. The development of this diabetes mobile application was made with the aim of helping users meet their needs and providing users with an easy and efficient way to find out their needs related to diabetes treatment/prevention. Convenience, in this case, includes several parts, namely: - Access to mobile applications This is marked by the development of Android applications that can be run online/offline. Easy access anywhere and anytime. - Searching applications The convenience of searching for applications is provided to users by providing access to download applications for free which can be found through the Playstore or other online platforms. - Decision The convenience of the decision is given to the user through the provision of various features that can complement the needs of the user. This shows that the development team provides the flexibility of access to users to decide what services they want to use according to user needs. - Using the application Users will be able to understand the features available in the mobile application thanks to the user-friendly user interface design. This is evident in several designs on the mobile application page that makes use of icons to help users understand the available features.

Table 9. Cont.

No.	Trust Components	Description
2	Attractiveness	Diabetes mobile application development has an attraction that can make customers want to use this application in the form of: - User interface design Landing page elements in diabetes mobile app development; - Price Users do not need to spend money to buy applications because the applications provided are free to install on their mobile devices; - Accessibility Users can access and monitor personal information contained in the history of the diabetes mobile application; - Connectivity The developed application can be connected to a glucometer and other supporting devices, such as a wearable band with a Bluetooth connection.
3	Simplicity	Simplicity is an important indicator that acts as one of the benefits of diabetes mobile applications, including: - Easy to remember The design of the application interface makes it easy for users to remember every feature available in the diabetes mobile application; - Directional Users can easily navigate the application. The application can guide users step by step using menus available in the application, namely through procedures that are easy to learn and understand; - Continuity Consistency is needed in an application. The point is so that users, especially novice users, can still recognize that the page they are viewing is still within the scope or has a relationship with the application being used.
4	Information quality	The quality of information is one of the important advantages for users, especially diabetic users. The results/information available can be the result of evaluation and even referrals for doctors to know in order to effectively and efficiently prevent/control diabetes. The following is the quality of the information contained in the diabetes mobile application: - Informative Informative is the ease and completeness of access to information that allows users to fulfill their information needs. This informative research covers the fulfillment of user information needs on a diabetes mobile application; - Comprehensiveness A mobile device application must have an orientation as the purpose of developing the application. The diabetes mobile application is able to answer the needs of users, both diabetic and non-diabetic. This is indicated by the features/services provided, which are able to adapt to the divinity of the user.

4.3. Unified Modeling Language and Design Testing

Software testing is critical because everyone makes mistakes when developing software. Each software program's errors will be distinct. Therefore, it is necessary to conduct software testing to verify and validate that the program or application created meets the requirement. If it is not the same as what is needed, it is necessary to evaluate it so that improvements can be made to the software.

- Use Case Diagram

The Use Case diagram in the development of diabetes mobile applications will describe the interaction relationship between the system (diabetes mobile application) and the actors involved in the system. The diagram will fully and sequentially describe existing business processes and activities and describe the contents of the diabetes mobile application, where in this diabetes mobile application, the Use Case Diagram is formed from (Figure 3):

1. Actor (two actors): The actor (User) is the user of the diabetes mobile application, and the other actor (Software Engineer) is the application developer;
2. Use case (10 use cases): Create an Account, Register to IoT Pack, Notification, Alert Setting, Monitoring Medication, Monitoring Food Intake, Monitoring Exercise, Monitoring Sleep, View and Manage, and Access System;
3. Association (18 associations): Association between the actor (User) and Use Case, Create an Account, Register to IoT Pack, Notification, Alert Setting, Monitoring Medication, Monitoring Food Intake, Monitoring Exercise, and Monitoring Sleep. Association between the actor (Software Engineer) to Use Case Access System, View and Manage, Create Account, Register to IoT Pack, Notification, Alert Setting, Monitoring Medication, Monitoring Food Intake, Monitoring Exercise, and Monitoring Sleep.

Actors, use cases, and associations are interconnected and interact in one system (the mobile diabetes application), where each actor has different access rights in the system, and each use case will be associated with different actors or use cases according to the system that has been designed.

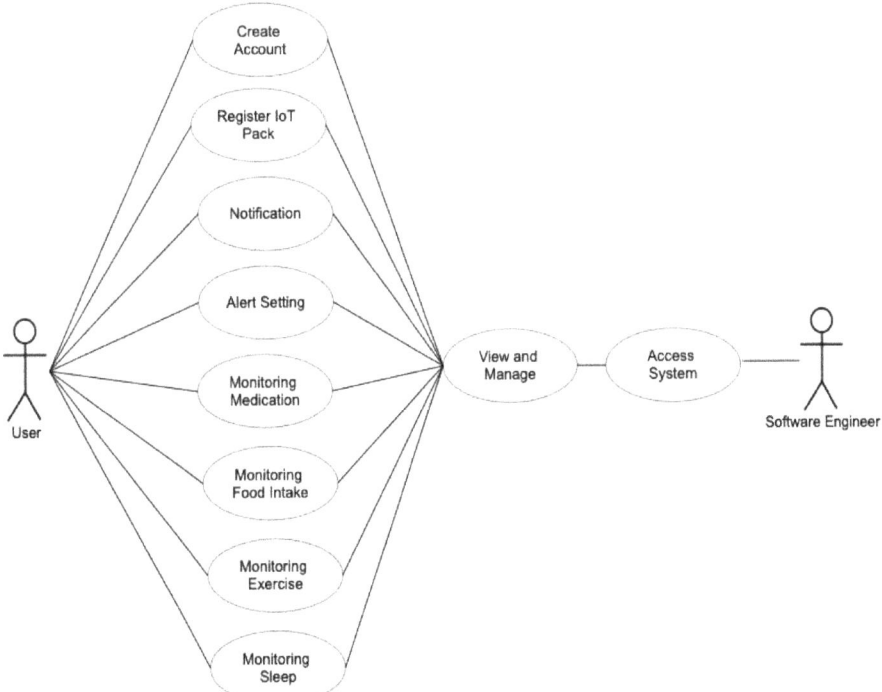

Figure 3. Use Case Diagram of User Activities.

- Activity Diagram

Activity diagrams in the system (diabetes mobile application) are sequentially described in an algorithm, where each process is carried out in parallel from the start to the finish point. In the design of the diabetes mobile application activity diagram, it consists of (Figure 4):

1. Start Point/Initial State;
2. Activity (13 activities): Authentication, Forgot Password/Register, Access and Evaluate Data, Report, Data Analytics, Register IoT Pack, Transfer Data, Receive Notification, Medication, Food Intake, Exercise, Sleep, and Recommendation;
3. Decision (two decisions): Decision After Activity (Authentication) and Decision after Activity (Recommendation);
4. Synchronization (two forks, one join): Fork after Decision of Activity (Authentication), Fork After Activity (Data Analytics), and 1 Join After Activities (Medication, Food Intake, Exercise and Sleep);
5. End state.

- Data Flow Diagram

The data flow diagram in the diabetes mobile application will describe the flow of data from the existing system in the application, where we can see the input and output of each process in the form of a design model consisting of (Figure 5):

1. Functions (two Functions): Username/Password and User ID Validation;
2. Input: User;
3. Output: Application;
4. File/Database: Database of User;
5. Flow (seven Flows): Input (User) to Function (Username/Password), Function (Username/Password) to File/Database (Database of User), File/Database (Database of User) to Function (Username/Password), Function (Username/Password) to Output (Application), Output (Application) to Function (User ID Validation), Function (User ID Validation) to Output (Application), and Function (User ID Validation) to Input (User).

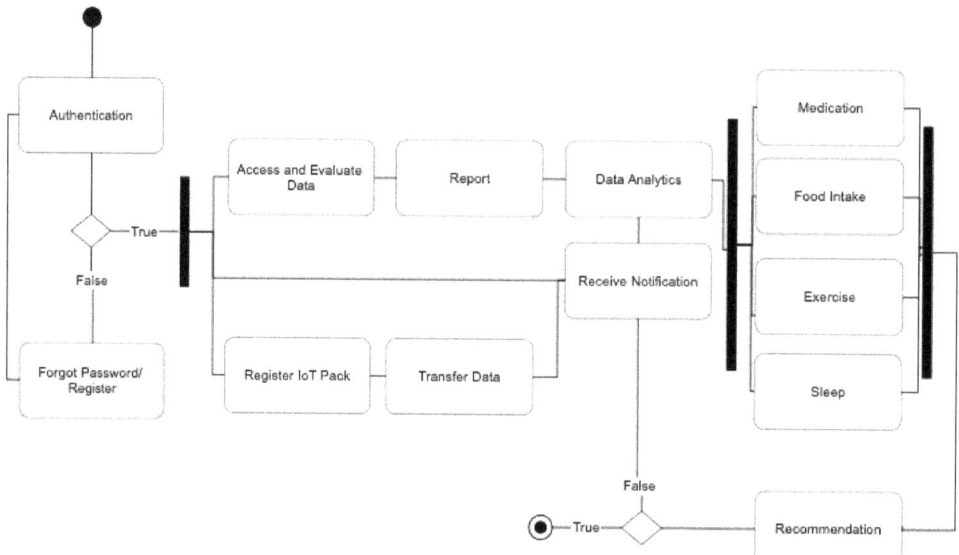

Figure 4. Activity Diagram of User Activities.

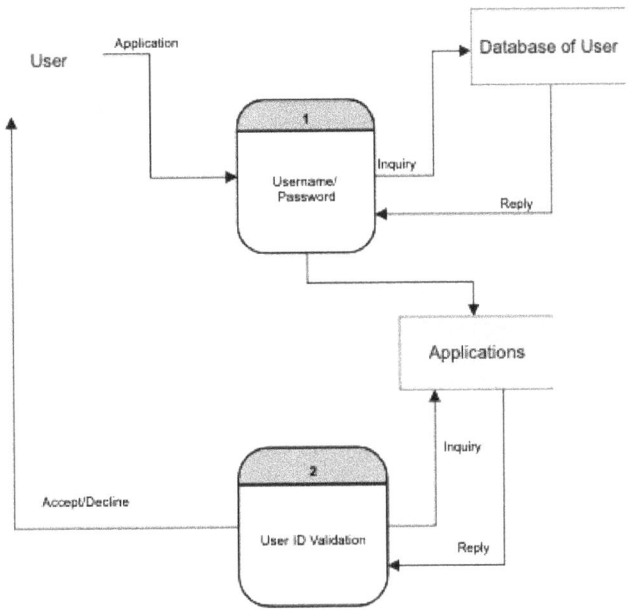

Figure 5. Data Flow Diagram of User Registration.

We analyze several factors that will be used as reference material for testing after the system (the diabetes mobile application) is implemented or used by the user after designing use case diagrams, activity diagrams, and data flow diagrams. We formulate five main trust factors (Table 10) in our proposed test, starting from the Functionality (Quality of Information, Core of Function, and Personalization), Ease of Use (User Interface Design and Efficiency), Usefulness, Security (Security and Privacy, Authentication) and Privacy and Costs. Figures 6 and 7 and Tables 11 and 12 show the results.

Table 10. Trust Factors.

No	Trust Factors	
	Factors	Variable
1	Functionality	• Quality of Information • Core of Function • Personalization
2	Ease of Use	• User Interface Design • Efficiency
3	Usefulness	• Usefulness
4	Security and Privacy	• Security and Privacy • Authentication
5	Cost	• Cost

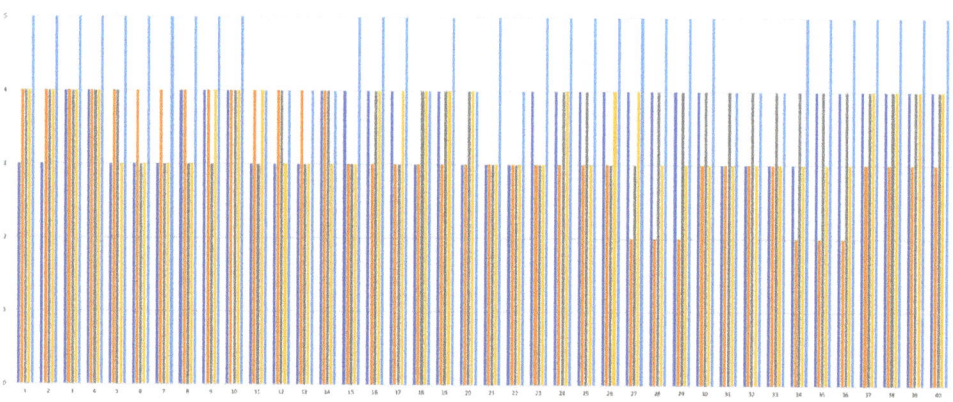

Figure 6. User Trust Evaluation for the Mobile application Version 1.

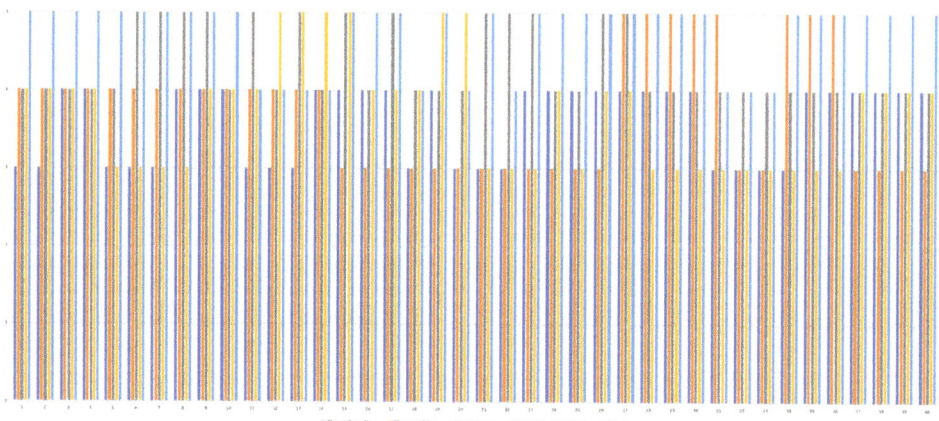

Figure 7. User Trust Evaluation for the Mobile application Version 2.

Table 11. Demographic Results for Trust Evaluation of the Mobile Application Version 1.

Demographics	Full (N = 40)		Mobile App (Version 1) (N = 40)			
	Frequency	%	High Trust Group		Low Trust Group	
			Frequency	%	Frequency	%
Sex						
Female	24	60	11	45.83	13	54.16
Male	16	40	5	31.25	11	68.75
Education						
High School	5	12.5	4	80	1	20
Undergraduate School	30	75	5	16.66	25	83.33
Graduate School	5	12.5	2	40	3	60

Table 12. Demographic Results for Trust Evaluation of the Mobile Application Version 2.

Demographics	Full (N = 40)		Mobile App (Version 2) (N = 40)			
			High Trust Group		Low Trust Group	
	Frequency	%	Frequency	%	Frequency	%
Sex						
Female	24	60	22	91.66	2	8.33
Male	16	40	13	81.25	3	23.07
Education						
High School	5	12.5	5	100%	0	0
Undergraduate School	30	75	28	93.33	3	7.14
Graduate School	5	12.5	4	80	1	30

Researchers conducted an evaluation stage on the development of a diabetes mobile application for 40 participants who were users of mobile-based diabetes applications (diabetic patients). The user's trust evaluation for mobile applications (Figure 7) adapts to five main trust factors (Table 10): functionality, ease of use, usefulness, security and privacy, and cost factors. The average value of each factor: functionality is 4.57; ease of use is 4.67; usefulness is 4.75; security and privacy are 5.0; cost is 4.70. The values as based on the results of the evaluation using a Likert scale of strongly agree, agree, neutral, disagree, and strongly disagree with an assessment weight of 5, 4, 3, 2, and 1, respectively. Based on the results of this evaluation, two indicators, namely the functionality and ease of use factors, have an evaluation with an input value of 3 (neutral). Table 13 describes the representations of the comparison between versions 1 and 2.

Table 13. Mobile Application's Feature Comparison.

No	Mobile Application		
	Feature	Version 1	Version 2
1	General		
1.1	Speed	x	✓
1.2	Navigation	✓	✓
1.3	Optimization	✓	✓
1.4	Internet Requirement	x	✓
1.4	File Storage and Sharing	x	✓
2	Services		
2.1	IoT Pack		
	a. Wearable Band	✓	✓
	b. Treadmill	✓	✓
	c. Gym Cycle	✓	✓
2.2	Medication		
	a. Morning	✓	✓
	b. Afternoon	✓	✓
	c. Night	✓	✓
2.3	Food Intake		
	a. Intake Recommendation (Breakfast, Lunch, and Dinner)	✓	✓
	b. Adjustmen Option	x	✓
2.4	Exercise		
	a. Monitoring Through IoT Pack	✓	✓
	b. Monitoring Through Steps Counter in the App	x	✓
2.5	Sleep		
	a. Evaluation/Result	✓	✓
	b. Suggestion	x	✓

5. Summary and Conclusions

The development of the type 2 diabetes mellitus mobile application at the development stage involves an operational feature that allows an application to run according to specified requirements. Testing is a very important stage and must be performed in software development. Tests must be carried out completely and thoroughly in order to cover all possibilities that may occur during the operation. Testing can demonstrate that the application meets the requirements and is error-free. If an error is found, it can be immediately corrected so that it can guarantee the quality of the software being developed. The testing design will boost application development success rates, allowing applications to be useful and optimally utilized by both patients and doctors involved in the treatment of type 2 diabetes mellitus (T2DM). Based on the trust evaluation results for mobile applications, we still need to update several indicators, specifically in terms of functionality and ease of use. Of course, this is a reference for us in developing this mobile-based diabetes application because the development of this application is still in the process of involving 40 participants who are diabetic patients. This study is also intended to serve as a reference for researchers who are currently conducting or will be conducting research in the field of developing type 2 diabetes mobile applications.

6. Future Work

Future work will aim to integrate our project mobile diabetes application with SmartPlate. In the future, through mobile diabetes applications and SmartPlate, patients and users with diabetes/non-diabetes can easily control their health through diet, activity, medication, and even control using a glucometer.

Supplementary Materials: The following supporting information about materials and previous work can be downloaded at: https://www.mdpi.com/2076-3417/11/5/2006, https://www.mdpi.com/2079-9292/10/15/1820, https://www.mdpi.com/2076-3417/13/1/8.

Author Contributions: S.R.J.: Evaluated project, methodology, investigation, resources, and supervision. W.A.: Developed software and evaluated functionality. J.-H.L.: Conceptualization, funding acquisition, resources, supervision, writing—original draft, review, and editing. All authors have read and agreed to the published version of the manuscript. S.K.K.: Evaluation, testing, and analysis.

Funding: This research was supported by the "Regional Innovation Strategy (RIS)" through the National Research Foundation of Korea (NRF), funded by the Ministry of Education (MOE) (2022RIS-005). This study was conducted with the support of the Samcheok Culture Understanding Platform Project operated by the Sampyo Cement Social Contribution Fund.

Institutional Review Board Statement: Not applicable.

Informed Consent Statement: Not applicable.

Data Availability Statement: All data is contained within the article or in the Supplementary Materials.

Conflicts of Interest: The authors declare no conflict of interest.

References

1. Sadhana, S.; Bandana, K.; Asgar, A.; Rajesh, Y.; Abhay, S.; Krishan, S.; Krishnan, H.; Girish, S. Mobile technology A tool for healthcare and a boon in pandemic. *J. Fam. Med. Prim. Care* **2022**, *11*, 37–43.
2. Żarnowski, A.; Jankowski, M.; Gujski, M. Use of Mobile Apps and Wearables to Monitor Diet, Weight, and Physical Activity: A CrossSectional Survey of Adults in Poland. *Med. Sci. Monit.* **2022**, 1–18. [CrossRef]
3. Pititto, B.D.A.; Eliaschewitz, F.G.; Paula, M.A.D.; Ferreira, G.C. BrazIliaN Type 1 & 2 DiabetEs Disease Registry (BINDER): Longitudinal, real-world study of diabetes mellitus control in Brazil. *Front. Clin. Diabetes Healthcare Diabetes Clin. Epidemol.* **2022**, 1–12. [CrossRef]
4. Naydenova, G. An overview of existing methods for evaluating mobile applications to change user behavior. *Int. Sci. J. Sci. Technol. Union Mech. Eng.* **2022**, *7*, 21–25.
5. Kirloskar, M.M.; Bhagat, V.V.; Kodilkar, J.V.; Ketkar, M.S.; Vankudre, A.J. Prevalence of Stress Induced Hyperglycemia and Its Contributing Factors in Patients with Post Covid Mucormycosis—A Retrolective Study. *Int. J. Recent Sci. Res.* **2022**, *13*, 926–931.
6. DiMeglio, L.A.; Molina, C.E.; Oram, R.A. Type 1 diabetes. *Lancet* **2019**, *391*, 2449–2462. [CrossRef] [PubMed]

7. Adu, M.D.; Malabu, U.H.; Malau-Aduli, A.E.; Malau-Aduli, B.S. Mobile application intervention to promote self-management in insulin-requiring type 1 and type 2 diabetes individuals: Protocol for a mixed methods study and non-blinded randomized controlled trial. *Diabetes Metab. Syndr. Obes.* **2019**, *12*, 789–800. [CrossRef] [PubMed]
8. Rachna, P.; Satish, R.K. Type 1 diabetes mellitus in pediatric age group A rising endemic. *J. Fam. Med. Prim. Care* **2022**, *11*, 2–31.
9. Assaad, M.; Hekmat-Joo, N.; Hosry, J.; Kassem, A.; Itani, A.; Dahabra, L.; Yassine, A.A.; Zaidan, J.; El Sayegh, D. Insulin use in Type 2 diabetic patients: A predictive of mortality in COVID-19 infection. *Diabetol. Metab. Syndr.* **2022**, *14*, 85. [CrossRef]
10. Mathur, P.; Leburu, S.; Kulothungan, V. Prevalence, Awareness, Treatment and Control of Diabetes in India from the Countrywide National NCD Monitoring Survey. *J. Front. Public Health* **2022**, *10*, 205. [CrossRef]
11. Nuland, E.V.; Dumitrescu, I.; Scheepmans, K.; Paquay, L.; Wandeler, E.D.; Vliegher, K.D. The Diabetes Team Dynamics Unraveled: A Qualitative Study. *Diabetology* **2022**, *3*, 246–257. [CrossRef]
12. Zajec, A.; Podkrajšek, K.; Tesovnik, T.; Šket, R.; Kern, B.; Bizjan, B.; Schweiger, D.; Kovac, J. Pathogenesis of Type 1 Diabetes: Established Facts and New Insights. *J. Genes* **2022**, *13*, 706. [CrossRef] [PubMed]
13. Więckowska, R.K.; Justyna, D.; Grażyna, D. The usefulness of the nutrition apps in self-control of diabetes mellitus—The review of literature and own experience. *Pediatr. Endocrinol. Diabetes Metab.* **2022**, *28*, 75–80. [CrossRef]
14. Apidechkul, T.; Chomchoei, C.; Upala, P. Epidemiology of undiagnosed type 2 diabetes mellitus among hill tribe adults in Thailand. *Sci. Rep.* **2022**, *12*, 1–9. [CrossRef] [PubMed]
15. Madan, A.; Dubey, S.K. Usability Evaluation Methods: A Literature Review. *Int. J. Eng. Sci. Technol.* **2012**, *4*, 590–599.
16. Christian Bastien, J.M. Usability testing: A review of some methodological andtechnical aspects of the method. *Int. J. Med. Inform.* **2010**, *79*, e18–e23. [CrossRef]
17. Georgsson, M.; Staggers, N.; Weir, C. A Modified User-Oriented Heuristic Evaluation of a Mobile Health System for Diabetes Self-Management Support. *Comput. Inform. Nurs.* **2016**, *34*, 78–84. [CrossRef]
18. Nasir, M.; Ikram, N.; Jallil, Z. Usability inspection: Novice crowd inspectors versus expert. *J. Sytstems Softw.* **2022**, *183*, 111122. [CrossRef]
19. Alqurni, J.; Alroobaea, R.; Alqahtani, M. Effect of User Sessions on the Heuristic Usability Method. *Int. J. Open Source Softw. Process.* **2018**, *9*, 62–81. [CrossRef]
20. Cho, H.; Keenan, G.; Madandola, O.O.; Santos, F.C.D.; Macieira, T.G.R.; Bjarnadottir, R.I.; Priola, K.J.B.; Lpoez, K.D. Assessing the Usability of a Clinical Decision Support System: Heuristic Evaluation. *JMIR Hum. Factors* **2022**, *10*, e31758. [CrossRef]
21. Johnson, S.G.; Potrebny, T.; Larun, L.; Ciliska, D.; Olsen, N.R. Usability Methods and Attributes Reported in Usability Studies of Mobile Apps for Health Care Education: Scoping Review. *JMIR Med. Educ.* **2022**, *8*, e38259. [CrossRef] [PubMed]
22. Banes, A. Development of App-Based E-Board Announcement System with SMS Support. *Indian J. Sci. Technol.* **2022**, *15*, 640–648. [CrossRef]
23. Sandesara, M.; Bodkhe, U.; Tanwar, S.; Alshehri, M.D.; Sharma, R.; Neagu, B.C.; Grigoras, G.; Raboaca, M.S. Design and Experience of Mobile Applications: A Pilot Survey. *J. Math.* **2022**, *10*, 2380. [CrossRef]
24. Maryam, S.; Purwono, A.; Syahril. Android application development for push notification feature for Indonesian space weather service based on Google Cloud Messaging. *J. Phys. Conf. Ser.* **2022**, 1–8. [CrossRef]
25. Hamid, K.; Iqbal, M.W.; Muhammad, H.A.B.; Fuzail, Z.; Ghafoor, Z.T.; Ahmad, S. Usability Evaluation of Mobile Banking Applications in Digital Business as Emerging Economy. *Int. J. Comput. Sci. Netw. Secur.* **2022**, *22*, 250–260.
26. Lee, J.-H.; Park, J.-C.; Kim, S.-B. Therapeutic Exercise Platform for Type-2 Diabetic Mellitus. *Electronics* **2021**, *10*, 1820. [CrossRef]
27. Park, J.C.; Kim, S.; Lee, J.-H. Self-Care IoT Platform for Diabetic Mellitus. *Appl. Sci.* **2021**, *11*, 2006. [CrossRef]
28. Kuria, J.; Peters, I.A.; Wabwoba, F. Determinants of University Students' Perceived Usefulness of Mobile Apps. *Int. J. Comput. Trends Technol.* **2022**, *7*, 10–19. [CrossRef]
29. Stocchi, L.; Pourazad, N.; Michaelidou, N.; Tanusondjaja, A.; Harrigan, P. Marketing research on Mobile apps: Past, present and future. *J. Acad. Mark. Sci.* **2022**, *50*, 195–225. [CrossRef]
30. Park, J.H.; Lee, Y.B.; Seo, Y.S.; Choi, J.H. Development and Effectiveness of a Smartphone Application for Clinical Practice Orientation. *Int. J. Internet Broadcast. Commun.* **2021**, *13*, 107–115.
31. Hinze, A.; Vanderschantz, N.; Timpany, C.; Cunningham, S.J.; Saravani, S.J.; Wilkinson, C. A Study of Mobile App Use for Teaching and Research in Higher Education. *Technol. Knowl. Learn.* **2022**, 1–29. [CrossRef]
32. Scarry, A.; Rice, J.; O'Connor, E.M.; Tierney, A.C. Usage of Mobile Applications or Mobile Health Technology to Improve Diet Quality in Adults. *J. Nutr.* **2022**, *14*, 2437. [CrossRef] [PubMed]
33. Totten, A.M.; Womack, D.M.; Eden, K.B.; McDonagh, M.S.; Griffin, J.C.; Grusing, S.; Hersh, W.R. Telehealth: Mapping the Evidence for Patient Outcomes from Systematic Reviews. In *AHRQ Comparative Effectiveness Technical Briefs*; Agency for Healthcare Research and Quality: Rockville, MD, USA, 2016; Volume 26.

34. Joshua, S.R.; Mogea, T. Analysis and Design of Service Oriented Architecture Based in Public Senior High School Academic Information System. In Proceedings of the 5th International Conference on Electrical, Electronics and Information Engineering, Malang, Indonesia, 6–8 October 2017; pp. 180–186.
35. Alshaheen, R.; Tang, R. User Experience and Information Architecture of Selected National Library Websites: A Comparative Content Inventory, Heuristic Evaluation, and Usability Investigation. *J. Web Librariansh.* **2022**, *16*, 31–67. [CrossRef]

Disclaimer/Publisher's Note: The statements, opinions and data contained in all publications are solely those of the individual author(s) and contributor(s) and not of MDPI and/or the editor(s). MDPI and/or the editor(s) disclaim responsibility for any injury to people or property resulting from any ideas, methods, instructions or products referred to in the content.

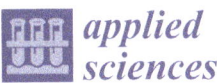

Article

M-Healthcare Model: An Architecture for a Type 2 Diabetes Mellitus Mobile Application

Salaki Reynaldo Joshua, Wasim Abbas and Je-Hoon Lee

Department of Electronics, Information and Communication Engineering, Kangwon National University, Samcheok-si 25913, Republic of Korea
* Correspondence: jehoon.lee@kangwon.ac.kr

Abstract: Type 2 diabetes mellitus (T2DM) is a metabolic disorder wherein the patients require DM management to keep their blood glucose under proper and regular control. Diabetes mellitus can be managed with the help of technologies, one of which is mobile health. Mobile health is an innovation in telemedicine that utilizes gadgets as a medium to access digitally based health information and services by utilizing electronic devices connected to the Internet. Mobile health services are distinguished based on interactions between users and medical personnel; namely, interactive and non-interactive services. The developed application can integrate Android mobile application software with supporting hardware, such as a glucometer, a wearable band, a heart rate sensor, a treadmill, and an exercise bike. The provided features in this mobile application include the monitoring of medication, food intake, exercise, and sleep. This study's goal was to create a mobile application architecture for type 2 diabetes mellitus mobile applications. This research focused on developing an architecture for mobile diabetes applications, a hardware block diagram design, and an architecture of sensors for a type 2 diabetes mellitus mobile application.

Keywords: mobile health; diabetes; architecture; mobile application; mobile operating system

1. Introduction

1.1. Smart Healthcare Systems

Smart healthcare systems enable users/patients and related parties in the healthcare sector, such as doctors and nurses, to access, collect, and manage medical data and information quickly and accurately, and to assist in recommending or supporting decisions in the healthcare sector. Still in their early stages of development, smart healthcare systems provide several focused service functions in which software and hardware are integrated to optimize the complete service of the smart healthcare system. Several technological developments in the field of smart healthcare systems help to treat patient illnesses and support the optimization of doctors' health services, whereas, in general, a smart healthcare system's architecture consists of software and hardware [1]. Challenges and supporting technology in a smart healthcare system are indicators that cannot be abandoned. The need (for various types of disease and services) is increasing every day in terms of both hardware and software technology. This, of course, requires appropriate integration so that service needs can be met, assisted by the development of adequate hardware and software technology. Several related studies apply the principles of smart healthcare systems in responding to existing challenges and needs [2].

1.2. Smart Healthcare Systems

Diabetes mellitus (DM) is a metabolic disorder that leads to high blood sugar levels. In addition to type 2 diabetes, there is also type 1 diabetes. Diabetes causes hyperglycemia because the pancreas cannot produce enough insulin. Under other conditions, the pancreas can produce insulin, but the insulin it produces cannot be used optimally. Both of these conditions can cause blood sugar spikes in diabetics [3].

Citation: Joshua, S.R.; Abbas, W.; Lee, J.-H. M-Healthcare Model: An Architecture for a Type 2 Diabetes Mellitus Mobile Application. *Appl. Sci.* **2023**, *13*, 8. https://doi.org/10.3390/app13010008

Academic Editors: Chien-Hung Yeh, Wenbin Shi, Xiaojuan Ban, Men-Tzung Lo and Shenghong He

Received: 6 October 2022
Revised: 12 November 2022
Accepted: 18 November 2022
Published: 20 December 2022

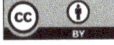

Copyright: © 2022 by the authors. Licensee MDPI, Basel, Switzerland. This article is an open access article distributed under the terms and conditions of the Creative Commons Attribution (CC BY) license (https://creativecommons.org/licenses/by/4.0/).

Diabetes (DM) is generally divided into type 1 diabetes, or insulin-dependent diabetes mellitus; type 2 diabetes, or non-insulin-dependent diabetes mellitus; other types of diabetes mellitus; and gestational diabetes mellitus (Table 1). Type 2 diabetes is a metabolic disorder characterized by hyperglycemia due to insulin resistance and/or deficiency. Patients with type 2 diabetes mellitus (T2DM) need DM management to properly and regularly control their blood glucose levels. Blood sugar levels can increase and decrease in an unstable manner if type 2 DM sufferers do not control their blood sugar levels properly, which can trigger complications [4]. Diabetes mellitus control is carried out using the basic principles of diabetes mellitus control management, including the modification of unhealthy lifestyles to become healthy in the form of diet, physical exercise, and adherence to antidiabetic drug consumption [5].

Table 1. Classification of diabetes mellitus.

No	Diabetes Mellitus	
	Type	Description
1	Type 1 [6]	Beta cell damage, generally leading to absolute insulin deficiency [3].
2	Type 2 [7]	It varies from dominant insulin resistance with relative insulin deficiency to dominant insulin secretion defect as a result of insulin resistance [7].
3	Other Types [8]	• Diabetes mellitus is caused by a disease of the exocrine pancreas. • Diabetes mellitus due to drugs (e.g., HIV and AIDS therapy or after kidney transplantation, etc.), chemicals, or infections. • Diabetes mellitus is caused by immunological disorders.
4	Gestational [9]	In gestational diabetes mellitus, the diagnosis of DM is made at the time that a patient's pregnancy is in progress.

Self-management is an integral part of diabetes control. Self-care management of diabetes can effectively reduce the risk of DM (Table 2) sufferers having coronary heart complications; in addition, self-care can control normal blood sugar levels, reduce the impact of DM problems, and reduce DM mortality [10,11]. Self-care performed by DM patients includes diet, eating habits, exercise, monitoring blood sugar levels, medication, and diabetic foot care. Efforts to overcome the weakness of self-care management of type 2 DM in controlling blood glucose levels that develop in the community to minimize DM complications can be assisted by utilizing technological developments [12].

Table 2. Risk factors.

No	Risk Factor [13,14]	
	Factor	Description
1	Obesity (overweight)	There is a significant link between obesity and blood sugar levels, and the degree of obesity with a body mass index (BMI) > 23, which can lead to an increase in blood glucose levels of up to 200 mg%.
2	Hypertension	An increase in blood pressure beyond the normal range of hypertensive patients is closely associated with the improper storage of salt and water, or increased pressure in the body of the peripheral vascular system.
3	Dyslipidemia	Dyslipidemia is a condition characterized by elevated blood fat levels (triglycerides > 250 mg/dl). There is a relationship between an increase in plasma insulin and low high-density lipoprotein (HDL) (<35 mg/dL).
4	Age	Individuals aged > 40 years are susceptible to DM, although it is possible for individuals aged < 40 years to avoid DM. The increase in blood glucose occurs at the age of about 45 years and the frequency increases with age.

Table 2. Cont.

No	Risk Factor [13,14]	
	Factor	Description
5	Genetic	Type 2 DM is thought to be associated with familial aggregation. The empirical risk in the event of Type 2 DM will increase two to six times if there are parents or family members suffering from type 2 DM.
6	Alcohol and Cigarettes	An individual's lifestyle is associated with an increase in the frequency of Type 2 DM. Most of this increase is associated with increased obesity and decreased physical activity; other factors associated with the shift from a traditional to a westernized environment, including changes in cigarette and alcohol consumption, also play a role in the increase. Alcohol will interfere with blood sugar metabolism, especially in people with Type 2 DM, so it will complicate regulation and increase blood sugar.

1.3. Development Mobile Application

ICT (Information and Communication Technology) is a tool that provides added value by generating high-speed, complete, accurate, transparent, and up-to-date information. The era of information and communication technology is being used to increase the provision of health information. Researchers are trying to innovate to develop diabetes care applications that take advantage of technological developments in providing information for self-care management in controlling blood glucose levels. The diabetes care application is expected to be able to answer the problem as a smart solution to minimize complications that arise in Type 2 diabetes mellitus (T2DM) patients [15].

Android is an operating system for Linux-based mobile devices that appears among other operating systems currently under development with a good set of supported features (Table 3). However, current development operating systems run in a way that prioritizes internally built core applications without taking into account the significant functionality of third-party applications [16]. Therefore, there are restrictions on third-party applications that can capture native mobile data and communicate between processes, and there are restrictions on distributing third-party applications to the platform. An application is a special set of instructions on a computer designed for us to complete certain tasks.

Table 3. Android features.

No	Android Features [17]	
	Features	Description
1	Storage	A data store, using SQLite, a lightweight database.
2	Connectivity	Android not only provides a standard network connection, but also an API that allows apps to connect and interact with other devices using protocols such as Bluetooth, NFC, Wi-Fi P2P, USB and SIP.
3	Messaging	Supports MMS and SMS
4	Media support	Media support for audio, video, images (MPEG4, H.264, MP3, AAC, AMR, JPG, PNG, GIF), and GSM telephony.
5	Hardware support	Camera, GPS, compass and accelerometer.
6	Play store	Online catalog application on smartphones, without using a PC (personal computer) that can download and install applications.

1.4. Previous Research

The Android mobile application's first development efforts were devoted to managing Type 2 diabetes. At this stage, the research team involved 20 people, consisting of 10 people with diabetes and 10 people without diabetes, in the use of diabetes mobile applications with supporting hardware, namely a wearable band, glucose meter, and treadmill [18]. The results of the initial research were used as reference material for the development of the second stage. At this stage, the researchers evaluated some of the functionality and accessibility of the application by conducting tests involving 40 people, consisting of

20 people with diabetes and 20 people without diabetes. The results of the second stage of research concluded that there was a need for changes and adaptation of applications for users, especially related to user registration for applications and glucometer and wearable band (smartwatch) connectivity with various versions [19]. Previous researchers have conducted preliminary research through two previous studies (Table 4).

Table 4. Comparison of our previous work.

No	Researcher	Features	IoT Devices	Participant
1	Lee, J.-H.	1. Blood glucose levels 2. Physical activities 3. Dosage or injection 4. Wake up and sleeping time	1. Glucometer 2. Wearable band and aerobic exercise equipment 3. Smart medication monitor 4. Wearable band	20
2	Park, J. C.	1. Blood glucose levels 2. Physical activities 3. Food intake 4. Dosage or injection 5. Wake up and sleeping time	1. Glucometer 2. Wearable band and aerobic exercise equipment 3. Smart food tray 4. Smart medication monitor 5. Wearable band	40

2. Analysis

2.1. Application in Healthcare

An application in healthcare is a program created by a user that aims to complete a specific task (Table 5). An application is the storage of data, problems, and work in a container or medium that can be used to implement or implement existing things or problems in a new form without losing the fundamental values of the data, problems, and work itself [20].

Table 5. Application classifications in healthcare.

No	Researcher	Classification	Description
1	I. Contreras	Disease Prediction	Disease prediction applications are applications that are used to help patients/application users to find out the prediction of diseases, along with the overall results of the diagnosis obtained based on the symptoms felt. This application was developed using certain methods according to the scope of the case study (disease) to be analyzed by calculating all parameters related to the symptoms of the disease. The development of this disease prediction application is useful to help doctors and also provide recommendations to patients/users who have difficulty knowing the disease they are suffering from but only know the symptoms they feel.
2	E. G. Spanakis	Clinical Communication	A clinical communication application is a development of technology in the health sector that helps achieve a state or health status as a whole, both physically, mentally, and socially. The focus of developing this application is the focus of communications related to health. The database in this application will store and process the existing data so that it can be useful for later use. Several clinical communication applications provide real-time communication services between patients/users and doctors to conduct health consultations. Doctors can collect information about the patient's health status, or they can access a database to view the patient's medical history.
3	Adu, U. H	Medication	The lack of information about treatment and about drugs is the basis for developing health applications in this field. If it is not handled properly, the patient/customer will self-regulate the drug therapy they receive, which will impact an increase in cases of drug administration errors that are not in accordance with the patient's needs. A medication health application focuses on education about drug information, assisting in health consultations on drug administration based on symptoms, and viewing the history of purchasing/using drugs stored in the database.
4	Lee, J.-H.	Exercise	Exercise health applications, also called health and fitness applications, are applications that can provide information to users related to health and fitness without limitations of place and time, and cam help users to achieve their health and fitness targets. Some exercise applications provide features to be able to connect applications with other supporting devices to collect health information more comprehensively; for example, connecting applications with treadmills, cycles, smartwatches, or other supporting devices used.

Table 5. Cont.

No	Researcher	Application Classification	
		Classification	Description
5	R. K Więckowska	Nutrition	A nutrition application is an application that helps patients/users to find out the number of nutritional needs and nutritional status by referring to nutrition and health sciences efficiently, cheaply, and accurately, where each country has different nutritional guidelines. This is very useful because food consumption affects a person's nutritional status. Good nutritional status or optimal nutritional status occurs when the body gets enough nutrients that are used efficiently, so as to support physical growth, brain development, workability, and general health as much as possible. A nutrition application already has a nutritional value based on a calculated formula (nutritional standards) by accessing the database; the application can find specific numbers (food/beverage) that will be or have been consumed.

The application can be categorized into three groups in its development, namely [21]:
(a) Desktop applications, namely applications that can only be run on a PC or laptop.
(b) Web applications, namely applications that are run using a computer or laptop and an internet connection.
(c) Mobile applications, namely applications that run on mobile devices.

2.2. Mobile Technology and Operating System

A mobile phone is a portable electronic device that functions like a regular phone and can be moved over a wide area. While mobile phones currently use a combination of wireless transmission and traditional telephone circuit switching, packet switching is used in parts of the mobile phone network, especially for Internet access and WAP services [22]. Mobile phones, or "cell phones", are electronic communication devices that have the same basic functionality as traditional landlines, but they can be carried anywhere (mobile) and do not need to be connected to a phone network using a cable (wireless) [23].

The mobile operating system is the primary software that directly manages and controls the hardware, and also manages and controls other software so that it can function (Table 6). Therefore, the mobile operating system is responsible for manipulating the various features and functions available on mobile devices. tasks, keyboards, WAPs, emails, text message scheduling, synchronization with other applications and devices, music playback, cameras, and control features [24]. In addition to the ability to control mobile phone hardware and software resources such as keyboards, screens, phonebooks, batteries, and network connections, the operating system controls all applications to run consistently and consistently. The operating system needs to be flexible so that software developers can easily create sophisticated new applications [25].

Table 6. Mobile operating systems.

No	Mobile Operating Systems	
	Operating System	Description
1	iOS	iOS is a software operating system developed by Apple specifically to support the operation of mobile or handheld devices. iOS is used not only on iPhone phones but also on other Apple handheld devices such as iPad tablets and iPod music players. As a handheld operating system, iOS works the same as Android, developed by Google. Basically, the function of iOS is to design the iPhone so that it can be operated by the user. iOS can create a bridge that connects the interaction between the user and the iPhone hardware. iOS is responsible for interpreting user commands for applications on the iPhone so that you can interact with, move, or activate hardware features. Conveniently, iPhone users can take pictures and videos, listen to music, and make phone calls. This is because the iOS feature successfully receives these commands and interprets them for the iPhone hardware. As *Lifewire* reports, without iOS, you cannot use the iPhone hardware or its functions. iOS features are generally the same as those on Android, but there are some differences.

Table 6. Cont.

No	Mobile Operating Systems	
	Operating System	Description
2	Android	Android is a mobile operating system based on a modified version of the Linux kernel and other open-source software designed primarily for touchscreen mobile devices, such as smartphones and tablets. Android was developed by a consortium of developers known as the Open Handset Alliance, with the participation of Google, a key contributor and commercial marketer. The core of the Android source code is called the Android Open Source Project (AOSP) and is primarily licensed under the Apache license. This allows Android variations to be developed for a variety of other electronic devices, including game consoles, digital cameras, PCs, and other user interface designs. Notable derivatives include Android TV for TV and Wear OS for wearables, both developed by Google. Android source code has been used as the basis for many different ecosystems in the context of its own software suite, Google Mobile Services (GMS), which includes applications such as Gmail, Google Play, and Google Chrome web browsers.
3	Windows Mobile	Windows Mobile is a mobile phone operating system developed by Microsoft but released only for specific markets. The kernel used by Windows Mobile is Windows CE. In the Indonesian market, Windows Mobile is still little known, and it seems that there is not much demand from the general public. At that time, the success of smartphones with Symbian operating systems, from brands such as Nokia, Samsung, and Sony Ericsson, was evident. Originally, Windows Mobile existed in 2000 after Pocket PC 2000, but Pocket PC at that time was not a mobile phone, as it is today, but was generally called a PDA (Personal Digital Assistant). Other than the development of smartphones at the time, the version of Windows Mobile at the time was far from the innovations that have appeared.
4	Blackberry OS	Blackberry OS is a proprietary cellular working device evolved via RIM (Research in Motion) for the company's Blackberry line of hand-held cellphone gadgets. This working device allows for multitasking and enables RIM-exclusive gadgets, such as the track wheel, trackball, and, more commonly these days, the trackpad and touchscreen, to be used in handhelds. The Blackberry platform is possibly well-known for its local support for business communications environments, which enable full Wi-Fi activation and synchronization of email, calendar, tasks, notes, and contacts. These operating system updates can be obtained automatically from Wi-Fi vendors that assist Blackberry in which software is loaded over the air (OTASL). Third-party builders can write software to program the use of the available Blackberry APIs (Application Programming Interface), but applications that use positive capability must be digitally signed.
5	Symbian OS	Symbian OS was created by Symbian Ltd. It is a descendant of Psion's EPOC and runs only on ARM processors, but it has x86 ports that are not officially exposed. Symbian OS can perform multithreading, multitasking, and memory-safe operations. Additionally, all programming in Symbian is event-based; that is, if there is no input in the form of a particular activity, the CPU hardware will be idle. Today, Symbian OS is widely used by suppliers of various mobile communication equipment products for different types of products. This operating system has an application programming interface (API) that allows this deviation from the hardware side on which Symbian OS is implemented. The API supports common hardware communication and behavior that can be used with other application objects. This is possible because the API is an application-level-defined interface object that contains procedures and functions (and variables and data structures) that manage or call the kernel and act as links between software and hardware. This API standard helps developers customize their applications so that they can be installed on a variety of mobile phone products.

2.3. Telehealth

Telecare is a part of telehealth. Telecare focuses on the therapeutic side, while telemedicine covers the prophylactic, preventive, and therapeutic aspects [26]. One of the functions of telehealth, and a major requirement in providing health services, is patient monitoring and scheduling. The coverage of telehealth, telemedicine, and electronic health (e-health), telecare, and m-health is described by Totten AM et al. [27].

3. Research Methodology

3.1. Research Method

The research was conducted at the Circuit and System Design Laboratory at Kangwon National University. The research was performed by carrying out several systematic stages (Figure 1) in order to produce research reports and products (Mobile Application) that were in accordance with the objectives of the research implementation. The research method included six stages, starting with identification of the problem, setting the research scope, data and information gathering, software development, analysis, and the final report.

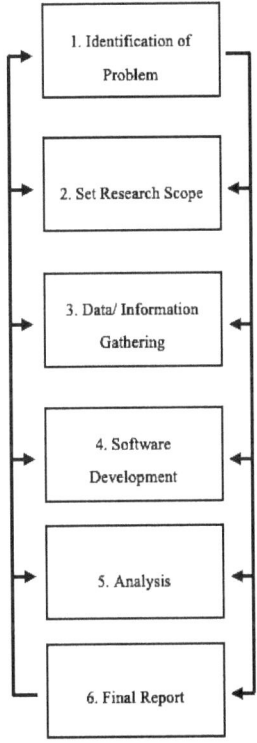

Figure 1. Research method.

3.2. Software Development Methodology

In developing this application, we used the prototype model [28] as an approach to mobile application development. We performed three stages: creating and revising the mockup, conducting customer test drives, and listening to customers. All steps in this prototype model were chosen because they were in accordance with the project being developed, which does not have many stages, and the parties or teams involved can also be maximized in the three existing stages [29,30].

4. Proposed Architecture

4.1. Mobile Application

The development of the architecture (Figure 2) for the Type 2 Diabetic Mellitus Mobile Application is broadly divided into three major parts:
- Medical Sensor and Exercise Equipment

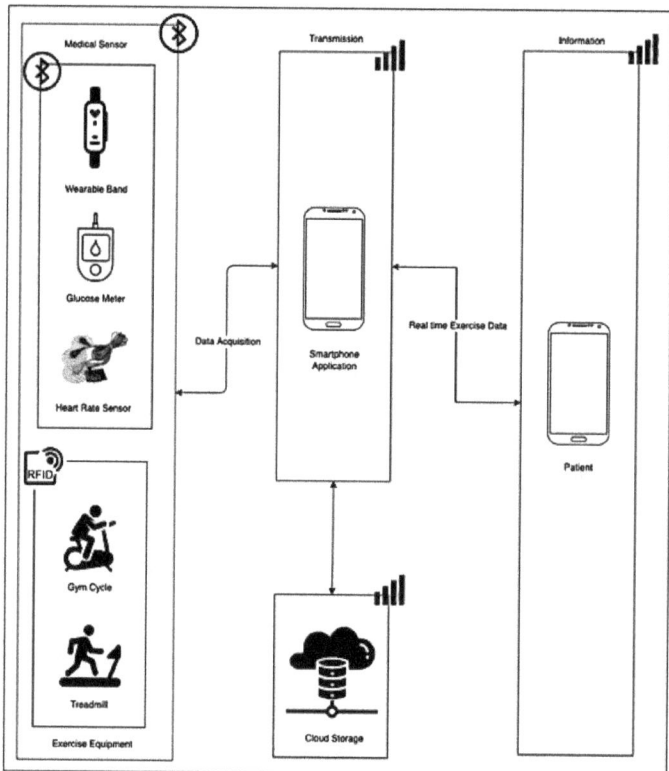

Figure 2. Proposed architecture for diabetic mobile application.

Medical sensors in the architecture section include supporting devices (inputs) in the form of wearable bands, glucose meters, and heart rate sensors. The exercise equipment consists of a gym cycle and a treadmill. In this section, the device is Bluetooth- and RFID-compatible. In this section, the device will work for the next stage of data acquisition before going to the transmission section.

- Transmission

Transmission in the architecture section consists of smartphone applications and cloud storage. In this section, the smartphone application receives input data from the Medical Sensor and Exercise Equipment section, which is referred to as the data acquisition process. The processed data are stored in cloud storage, and in this part of the process, the entire process is supported by the Internet network.

- Information

Information on the architecture is the final part (output), namely the process after the data are processed in the transmission section. The process at this stage is called "real-time exercise data", where the processed data can be received at the same time by the user (patient) with an Internet connection as network support.

4.2. Hardware Design and Implementation

The hardware design and implementation for the Type 2 Diabetes Mellitus Mobile Applications are written in block diagram format (Figure 3). Eight blocks (Figure 3) consist of RFID, DAQ for Treadmill and Gym Cycle, Heart Rate Sensor, Wearable Band, Glucometer, Signal Integration, Calculation and Memory, Smartphone Application, and Patient. The first five blocks consist of RFID, DAQ for Treadmill and Gym Cycle, Heart Rate Sensor, Wearable Band, and Glucometer, which interact with the Signal Integration, Calculation and Memory block, which in turn send User ID, Exercise Data, Heart Rate, Number of steps, Heart Rate and Blood Glucose Levels, where the data received in the Signal Integration, Calculation, and Memory block will interact with the smartphone application block to send Real-Time Exercise data. The last block is where the patient interacts with the smartphone application block, which is a process of real-time monitoring alerts.

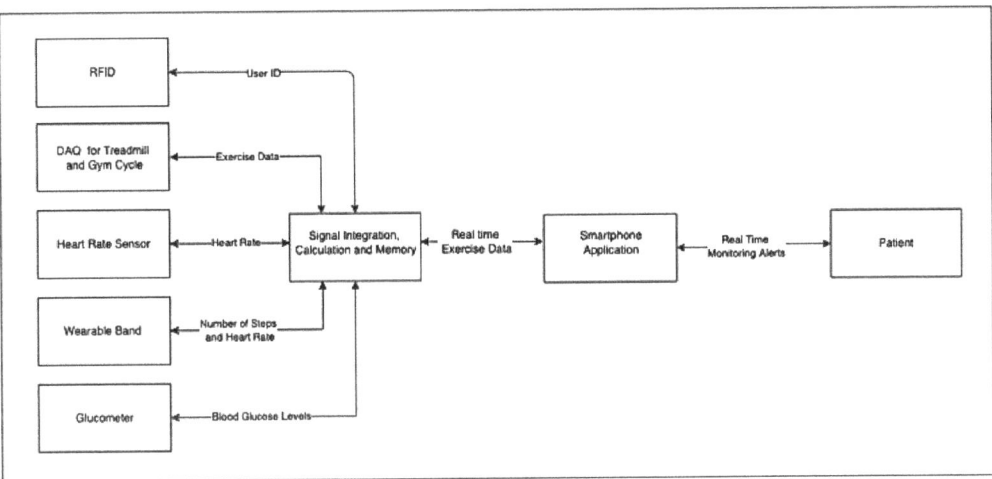

Figure 3. Hardware block diagram.

4.3. Sensor

The sensor is one part of the Type 2 Diabetes Mellitus Mobile Application. In Figure 4, the architecture of sensors is clearly described, starting from the deployment of sensors, active sensors taking measurements, reading RFID tags, and entering mobile applications. Then, in the stage of analyzing the measurement, there will be two choices: namely, updating details in storage with normal or above-normal conditions, or storing the updated data in the database and receiving real-time monitoring alerts.

4.4. Sensor User Interface

The user interface (UI) is what the user interacts with as part of an experience (Table 7). UI is not just about colors and shapes; it is about providing users with the right tools to achieve their goals. In addition, UI is more than just buttons, menus, and forms that the user must fill out. When the system and users can interact with each other through commands such as using content and entering data, this is referred to as a user interface. The user interface is one of the most important parts of application development because it relates to the user and can be seen, heard, and touched. At this stage, the researchers developed a user interface related to the appropriate needs and related to the development of the Type 2 Diabetes Mellitus Mobile Application.

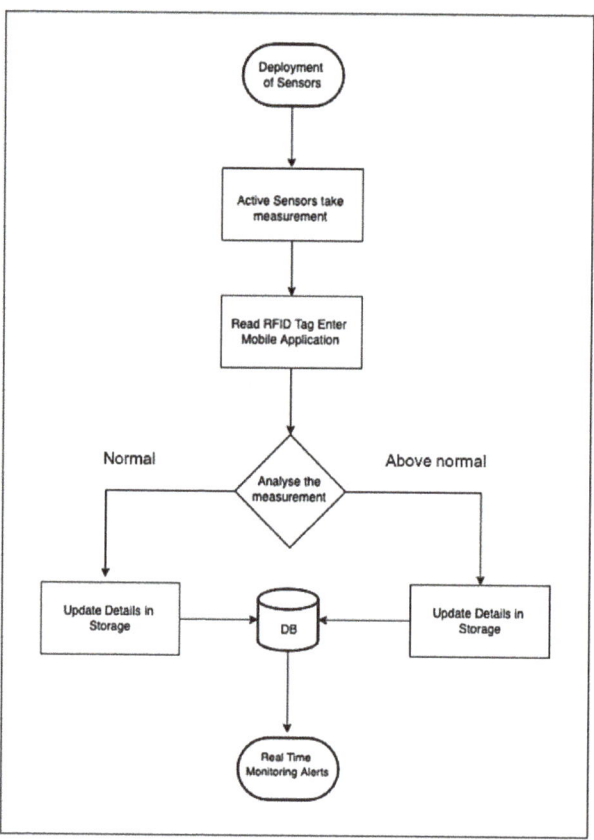

Figure 4. Architecture of sensor.

Table 7. Design user interface.

No	User Interface of Mobile Application		
	Page	User Interface	Description
1	Login	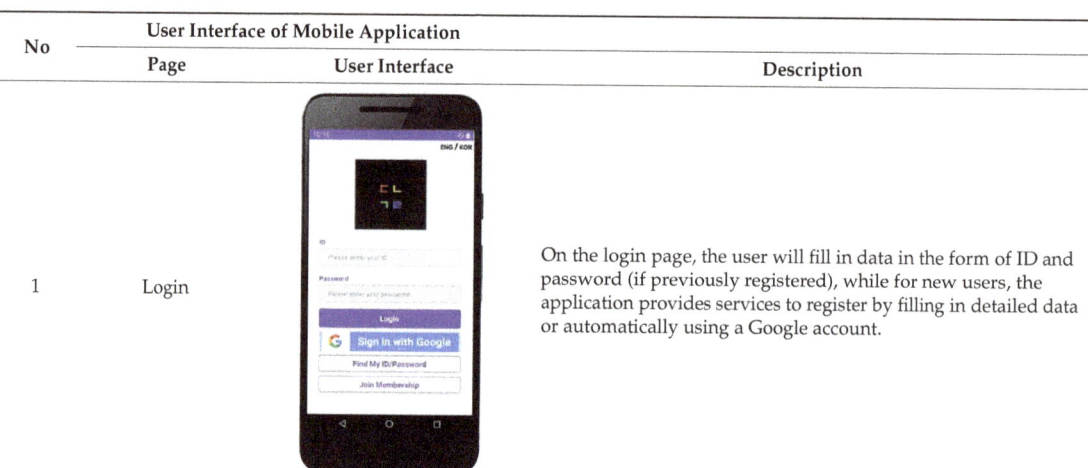	On the login page, the user will fill in data in the form of ID and password (if previously registered), while for new users, the application provides services to register by filling in detailed data or automatically using a Google account.

Table 7. *Cont.*

No	User Interface of Mobile Application		Description
	Page	User Interface	
2	Personal Information		Users are asked to enter information about their nickname, sex (male or female), date of birth, height, and weight on the personal information page.
3	Home		On the home page, the application briefly displays features that can be explored by users in the form of icon visualization, such as statistics to view the results of health data calculations, Bluetooth connections to devices, surveys, sugar levels, medicine, exercise, and a calendar.
4	Register Internet of Things Pack		Register for the Internet of Things Pack is a page used by users to connect applications used with devices owned by them, such as wearable bands, glucometers, treadmills, etc.

Table 7. *Cont.*

No	User Interface of Mobile Application		Description
	Page	User Interface	
5	Monitoring Medication		The medication monitoring page enables users to view or control the medication intake schedule as recommended, or it can be entered manually by the user.
6	Monitoring Food Intake		The food intake monitoring page allows users to directly control food intake by making direct adjustments at the specified time, which is divided into three parts, namely breakfast, lunch, and dinner.
7	Monitoring Exercise		The exercise monitoring page helps users see the exercise that has been done. The results of the exercise are in the form of current speed, average speed, distance, and heart rate.

Table 7. Cont.

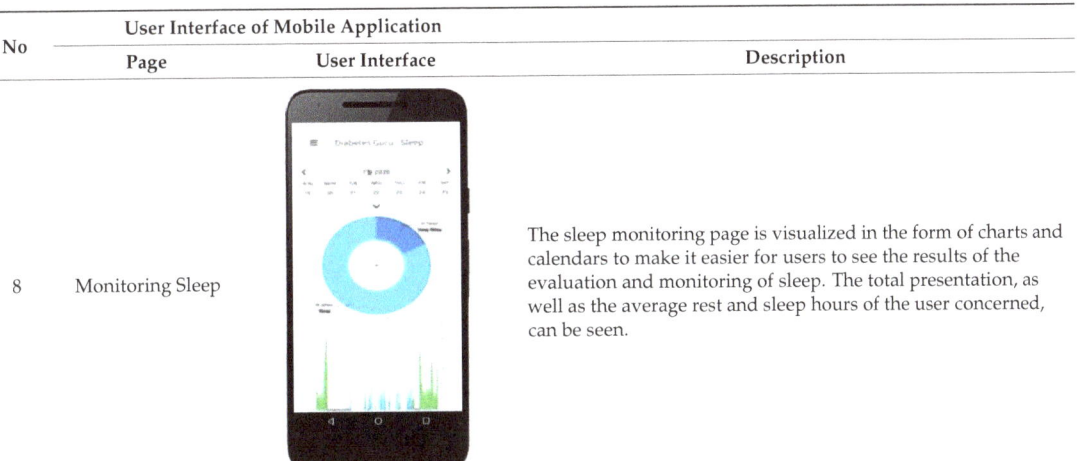

No	User Interface of Mobile Application		
	Page	User Interface	Description
8	Monitoring Sleep		The sleep monitoring page is visualized in the form of charts and calendars to make it easier for users to see the results of the evaluation and monitoring of sleep. The total presentation, as well as the average rest and sleep hours of the user concerned, can be seen.

5. Testing

Researchers conducted an evaluation stage on the development of a diabetes mobile application for 40 participants who were users of mobile-based diabetes applications (diabetic patients). Evaluation of user acceptance testing for mobile applications (Figure 5) adapted five main factors at the application testing stage (Table 8), which included functionality, ease of use, usefulness, security and privacy, and cost factors. Based on the results of the evaluation using a Likert scale (strongly agree, agree, neutral, disagree, strongly disagree) with an assessment weight of (5, 4, 3, 2, 1), the average value of factor functionality was 4.57, ease of use 4.67, usefulness 4.75, security and privacy 5.0, and cost 4.70. Based on the results of this evaluation, there are two indicators that have an evaluation value with an input value of 3 (neutral), namely the functionality and ease of use factors.

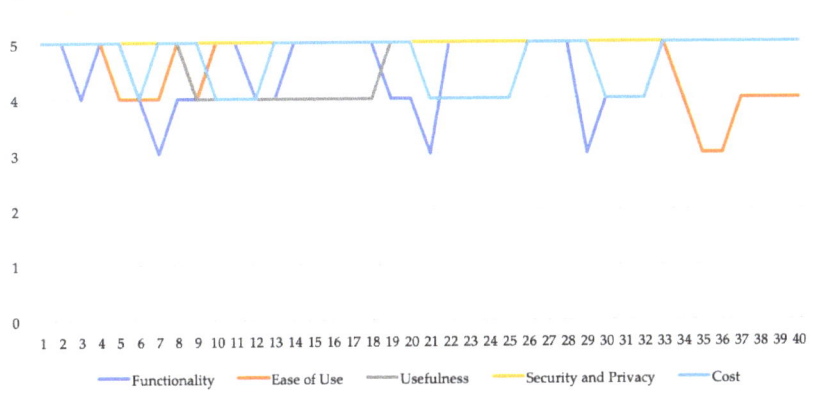

Figure 5. User acceptance testing for mobile application.

Table 8. Testing factors.

No	Testing Factors	
	Factors	Variable
1	Functionality	• Quality of Information • Core of Function • Personalization
2	Ease of Use	• User Interface Design • Efficiency
3	Usefulness	• Usefulness
4	Security and Privacy	• Security and Privacy • Authentication
5	Cost	• Cost

6. Summary and Conclusions

The development of the Type 2 Diabetes Mellitus Mobile Application involves an operational feature that allows an application to run according to specified requirements and can integrate an Android-based mobile application with supporting hardware such as a glucometer, wearable band, heart rate sensor, treadmill, and gym cycle. The provided features in this mobile application include monitoring medication, food intake, exercise, and sleep. Architectural Design for Diabetic Mobile Applications, Hardware Block Diagram Design, and Architecture of Sensors will be useful for the application development team as a benchmark or guideline for what kind of application or product will be produced. Based on the results of the analysis, this study resulted in three proposed architectures: namely, the architecture for mobile applications, the hardware block diagram, and the architecture of sensors, which clearly describe the operational functions that exist in the Type 2 Diabetes Mellitus Mobile Application. On the other hand, the architectural design will support the success rate of application development, so that applications can be useful and optimally utilized both by patients and doctors involved in the treatment of type 2 diabetes (T2DM). This study is also intended to serve as a reference for researchers who are currently conducting or will be conducting research in the field of developing type 2 diabetes mobile applications.

Author Contributions: S.R.J.: project evaluation, methodology, investigation, resources, supervision. W.A.: software developer, functionality evaluation. J.-H.L.: conceptualization, funding acquisition, resources, supervision, writing—original draft, writing—review and editing. All authors have read and agreed to the published version of the manuscript.

Funding: This research was supported by "Regional Innovation Strategy (RIS)" through the National Research Foundation of Korea (NRF), funded by the Ministry of Education (MOE) (2022RIS-005).

Institutional Review Board Statement: Not applicable.

Informed Consent Statement: Not applicable.

Data Availability Statement: Not applicable.

Conflicts of Interest: The authors declare no conflict of interest.

References

1. Abd-alrazaq, A.A.; Suleiman, N.; Baagar, K.; Jandali, N.; Alhuwail, D.; Abdalhakam, I.; Shahbal, S.; Abou-Samra, A.; Househ, M. Patients and healthcare workers experience with a mobile application for self-management of diabetes in Qatar: A qualitative study. *Comput. Methods Programs Biomed. Update* **2021**, *1*, 100002. [CrossRef]
2. Adu, M.D.; Malabu, U.H.; Malau-Aduli, A.E.; Malau-Aduli, B.S. Mobile application intervention to promote self-management in insulin-requiring type 1 and type 2 diabetes individuals: Protocol for a mixed methods study and non-blinded randomized controlled trial. *Diabetes Metab. Syndr. Obes.* **2019**, *12*, 789–800. [CrossRef] [PubMed]
3. Adu, M.D.; Malabu, U.H.; Malau-Aduli, A.E.; Malau-Aduli, B.S. The development of My Care Hub Mobile-Phone App to Support Self-Management in Australians with Type 1 or Type 2 Diabetes. *Sci. Rep.* **2020**, *10*, 7. [CrossRef] [PubMed]
4. Höll, B.; Spat, S.; Plank, J.; Schaupp, L.; Neubauer, K.; Beck, P.; Chiarugi, F.; Kontogiannis, V.; Pieber, T.R.; Holzinger, A. Design of a Mobile, Safety-Critical in-Patient Glucose Management System. *Stud. Health Technol. Inf.* **2011**, *169*, 950–954.
5. Jeffrey, B.; Bagala, M.; Creighton, A.; Leavey, A.; Nicholls, S.; Wood, C.; Longman, J.; Barker, J.; Pit, S. Mobile phone applications and their use in the self-management of Type 2 Diabetes Mellitus: A qualitative study among app users and non-app users. *Diabetol. Metab. Syndr.* **2019**, *11*, 84. [CrossRef]
6. Sultan, A.; Murtaza, K.; Mohammed, A. Mobile Health (m-Health) System in the Context of IoT. In Proceedings of the IEEE 4th International Conference on Future Internet of Things and Cloud Workshops (FiCloudW), Vienna, Austria, 22–24 August 2016; pp. 39–42.
7. Totten, A.M.; Womack, D.M.; Eden, K.B. *Telehealth: Mapping the Evidence for Patient Outcomes from Systematic Reviews*; Pacific Northwest Evidence-based Practice Center Portland, OR, Technical Briefs, No. 26; Agency for Healthcare Research and Quality: Rockville, MD, USA, 2016; pp. 1–125.
8. Hasan, A.M.Y.; Alina, S.; Nor, A. The Role of Different Types of Information Systems in Business Organizations: A Review. *Int. J. Res.* **2014**, *1*, 1270–1286.
9. Naseer, A.; Muhammad, B.W.; Abdul, H.M. Comparative Analysis of Operating System of Different Smart Phones. *J. Softw. Eng. Appl.* **2015**, *8*, 114.
10. Spanakis, E.G.; Chiarugi, F.; Kouroubali, A.; Spat, S.; Beck, P.; Asanin, S.; Rosengren, P.; Gergely, T.; Thestrup, J. Diabetes management using modern information and communication technologies and new care models. *Interact. J. Med. Res.* **2012**, *1*, e2193. [CrossRef]
11. Helen, F.N.C.; Jin, J.D.; Terrence, A.J. Content Analysis: First-Time Patient User Challenges with Top-Rated Commercial Diabetes Apps. *Telemed. E-Health* **2021**, *27*, 663–669.
12. Gunawardena, K.C.; Jackson, R.; Robinett, I.; Dhaniska, L.; Jayamanne, S.; Kalpani, S.; Muthukuda, D. The Influence of the Smart Glucose Manager Mobile Application on Diabetes Management. *J. Diabetes Sci. Technol.* **2019**, *13*, 75–81. [CrossRef]
13. Fernanda, C.F.; Thamiris, L.A.C.; Emerson, P.C.; Adriana, S.P.; Ilka, A.R.; Heloísa, C.T. Mobile applications for adolescents with type 1 diabetes mellitus: Integrative literature review. *Acta Paul Enferm.* **2017**, *30*, 565–572.
14. Kumar, D.S.; Prakash, B.; Chandra, B.J.S.; Shrinivas, K.P.; Vanishri, A.; Jom, T.J.; Praveen, K.; Arun, G.; Murthy, M.R.N. Technological innovations to improve health outcome in type 2 diabetes mellitus: A randomized controlled study. *Clin. Epidemiol. Glob. Health* **2021**, *9*, 53–56. [CrossRef]
15. Slagle, H.B.G.; Hoffman, M.K.; Caplan, R.; Shlossman, P.; Sciscione, A.C. Validation of a novel mobile phone application for type 2 diabetes screening following gestational diabetes mellitus. *mHealth* **2022**, *8*, 21–36.
16. Contreras, I.; Vehi, J. Artificial Intelligence for Diabetes Management and Decision Support: Literature Review. *J. Med. Internet Res.* **2018**, *20*, e10775. [CrossRef] [PubMed]
17. Maryam, J.; Asghar, E.; Shekoufeh, A. Developing "Aryan:" Diabetes self-care mobile application. *Int. J. Prev. Med.* **2019**, *10*, 59.
18. Lee, J.-H.; Park, J.-C.; Kim, S.-B. Therapeutic Exercise Platform for Type-2 Diabetic Mellitus. *Electronics* **2021**, *10*, 1820. [CrossRef]
19. Bults, M.; van Leersum, C.M.; Olthuis, T.J.J.; Bekhuis, R.E.M.; den Ouden, M.E.M. Barriers and Drivers Regarding the Use of Mobile Health Apps Among Patients With Type 2 Diabetes Mellitus in the Netherlands: Explanatory Sequential Design Study. *Jmir Diabetes* **2022**, *7*, e31451. [CrossRef]
20. Christian, M.; Isabel, S.; Stephan, M. User Experience Testing of My ePRO App in a Diabetes Mellitus Type 2 Focus Group. *Int. J. Clin. Exp. Med Sci.* **2022**, *11*, 8.
21. García, M.F.; Porras, Y.; Richmond, D.; Jensen, M.; Madrigal, M.; Zúñiga, G. Designing a Mobile Application to Support Type 2 Diabetes Mellitus Care in Costa Rica: A Qualitative Exploratory Study. *J. Acad. Nutr. Diabet.* **2016**, *116*, A75. [CrossRef]
22. Kebede, M.M.; Pischke, C.R. Popular Diabetes Apps and the Impact of Diabetes App Use on Self-Care Behaviour: A Survey Among the Digital Community of Persons with Diabetes on Social Media. *Front. Endocrinol.* **2019**, *10*, 135. [CrossRef]
23. Michael, O.A.; Taiwo, R.H.; Oluwabukola, A.A.; Joseph, F.O. Mobile phone ownership and willingness to receive mHealth services among patients with diabetes mellitus in South-West, Nigeria. *Panafrican Med. J.* **2020**, *37*, 29.
24. Park, J.C.; Kim, S.; Lee, J.-H. Self-Care IoT Platform for Diabetic Mellitus. *Appl. Sci.* **2021**, *11*, 5. [CrossRef]
25. Więckowska, R.K.; Justyna, D.; Grażyna, D. The usefulness of the nutrition apps in self-control of diabetes mellitus – the review of literature and own experience. *Pediatric Endocrinol. Diabetes Metab.* **2022**, *28*, 75–80. [CrossRef]
26. Joshua, S.R. Analysis and Design of Service Oriented Architecture Based in Public Senior High School Academic Information System. *IEEE Xplore* **2017**, 180–186.

27. Zeadally, S.; Siddiqui, F.; Baig, Z.; Ibrahim, A. Smart healthcare Challenges and potential solutions using internet of things (IoT) and big data analytics. *Psu Res. Rev.* **2020**, *4*, 93–109.
28. Chomutare, T.; Fernandez-Luque, L.; Årsand, E.; Hartvigsen, G. Features of Mobile Diabetes Applications: Review of the Literature and Analysis of Current Applications Compared Against Evidence-Based Guidelines. *J. Med. Internet Res.* **2011**, *13*, e1874. [CrossRef]
29. Pritee, U.S.; Rani, P.T.; Deepak, D.S.; Umesh, J.P. A Literature Review on Android—A Mobile Operating system. *Int. Res. J. Eng. Technol.* **2021**, *8*, 1–6.
30. Quy, V.K.; Hau, N.V.; Anh, D.V.; Ngoc, L.A. Smart healthcare IoT applications based on fog computing: Architecture, applications and challenges. *Complex Intell. Syst.* **2022**, *8*, 3805–3815. [CrossRef]

Disclaimer/Publisher's Note: The statements, opinions and data contained in all publications are solely those of the individual author(s) and contributor(s) and not of MDPI and/or the editor(s). MDPI and/or the editor(s) disclaim responsibility for any injury to people or property resulting from any ideas, methods, instructions or products referred to in the content.

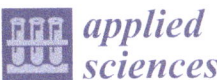

Review

Biomechanical, Healing and Therapeutic Effects of Stretching: A Comprehensive Review

Elissaveta Zvetkova [1,*], Eugeni Koytchev [2], Ivan Ivanov [3], Sergey Ranchev [2] and Antonio Antonov [3]

1. Bulgarian Society of Biorheology, 1113 Sofia, Bulgaria
2. Institute of Mechanics, Bulgarian Academy of Sciences, 1113 Sofia, Bulgaria; koytchev@imbm.bas.bg (E.K.); serg_ran@imbm.bas.bg (S.R.)
3. National Sports Academy "Vassil Levski", 1700 Sofia, Bulgaria; ivanmirchev@abv.bg (I.I.); antonio_hockey@yahoo.com (A.A.)
* Correspondence: elizvet@gmail.com

Abstract: Characterized in biomedical terms, stretching exercises have been defined as movements applied by external and/or internal forces to increase muscle and joint flexibility, decrease muscle stiffness, elevate the joint range of motion (ROM), increase the length of the "muscle–tendon" morpho-functional unit, and improve joint, muscle, and tendon movements, contraction, and relaxation. The present review examines and summarizes the initial and recent literature data related to the biomechanical, physiological, and therapeutic effects of static stretching (SS) on flexibility and other physiological characteristics of the main structure and the "joint–ligament–tendon–muscle" functional unit. The healing and therapeutic effects of SS, combined with other rehabilitation techniques (massage, foam rolling with and without vibrations, hot/cold therapy, etc.), are discussed in relation to the creation of individual (patient-specific) or group programs for the treatment and prevention of joint injuries, as well as for the improvement of performance in sports. From a theoretical point of view, the role of SS in positively affecting the composition of the connective tissue matrix is pointed out: types I–III collagen syntheses, hyaluronic acid, and glycosaminoglycan (GAG) turnover under the influence of the transforming growth factor beta-1 (TGF-β-1). Different variables, such as collagen type, biochemistry, elongation, and elasticity, are used as molecular biomarkers. Recent studies have indicated that static progressive stretching therapy can prevent/reduce the development of arthrogenic contractures, joint capsule fibrosis, and muscle stiffness and requires new clinical applications. Combined stretching techniques have been proposed and applied in medicine and sports, depending on their long- and short-term effects on variables, such as the ROM, EMG activity, and muscle stiffness. The results obtained are of theoretical and practical interest for the development of new experimental, mathematical, and computational models and the creation of efficient therapeutic programs. The healing effects of SS on the main structural and functional unit—"joint–ligament–tendon–muscle"—need further investigation, which can clarify and evaluate the benefits of SS in prophylaxis and the treatment of joint injuries in healthy and ill individuals and in older adults, compared to young, active, and well-trained persons, as well as compared to professional athletes.

Keywords: stretching; static stretching (SS); joint range of motion (ROM); muscle stiffness; joint–ligament–tendon–muscle unit; joint injuries—treatment and prophylaxis

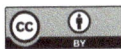

1. Introduction

In biomechanical terms, stretching has been characterized by Weerapong et al. as a movement applied by an external and/or internal force in order to increase muscle flexibility and to improve the joint range of motion (ROM) [1]. The aim of stretching in physical exercise is to increase the muscle–tendon unit length and to improve joint flexibility, as well as to decrease the risk of soft-tissue injuries [2–7].

For the purposes of the present review, the trusted and respected databases of PubMed and Web of Science were used. We aimed to prioritize the latest publications in the field of stretching over the last decade. We examined and summarized literature data related to the biomechanical characteristics and therapeutic effects of stretching on the main structural and functional unit, the "muscle–tendon–ligament–joint".

2. Topics and Results

2.1. Biomechanical Parameters, Healing, and Therapeutic Effects of Stretching

Interesting results arose from numerous recent investigations and various stretching programs applied in medical practice and sports. The biomechanical parameters and therapeutic effectiveness of stretching applications could modify joint, tendon, and muscle flexibility. For this purpose, different variables, such as collagen and elastin syntheses, fiber elongation and elasticity, energy absorption, etc., could be used as mechanobiological, cellular, and molecular biomarkers.

Many retrospective and prospective studies have been performed and stratified on the acute and chronic effects of stretching, both under physiological conditions and in pathological states. Progressive static stretching is effective during the prophylaxis of injuries in sports and exercise training [8–10]. The healing properties of stretching are of importance in the prophylaxis and treatment of joint injuries when also combined with other rehabilitation procedures (massage, heat/cold, warming up, etc.) [7,11–14]. Recent studies have reported a high effectiveness of stretching in the treatment and prevention of contractures and fasciitis, as well as useful methods for application in routine orthopedic and traumatological practice [5,15–19].

As a rehabilitation method, stretching has been applied to improve the biomechanical parameters of muscles, tendons, ligaments, fascia, and joints [4,6,7,9,20,21].

The viscoelastic responses of muscles, tendons, ligaments, fascia, and joints to slow stretching exercises could result in less passive tension, compared to faster procedures [22,23]. The faster the stretch, the higher the muscle stiffness will be [6]. Most stretching techniques (static, dynamic, ballistic, etc.) have been successfully implemented in clinical practice [2,4,24,25].

The effects of stretching on muscle and joint flexibility are closely related to the joint range of motion (ROM), whereby the increased range of motion induces the analgesic effects of stretching.

Various stretching techniques have been compared. Unfortunately, the current results of the chronic effects of static stretching (SS) exercises on the muscle strength, flexibility, joint ROM, and muscle power are still controversial [5,18,26].

2.2. Animal, Mathematical, and Computational Models of Stretching

More scientific information is needed for the creation of new, successful mathematical and computational models of stretching [27,28].

The mathematical and rheological models of the joint cavity capsule and intra-articular synovial fluid turnover (viscosity and permeation of hyaluronan, glycosaminoglycans (GAGs), and albumin) indicate cellular mechanisms of stretching and a role of the intercellular matrix as a selective molecular filter. The specific rheological properties of joint synovial fluid are altered in traumatic and post-traumatic pathological states (different arthroses, rheumatoid arthritis, osteoarthritis, etc.) [29].

In the treatment and prevention of sports injuries, as well as in the development of improved sports programs for injury prevention, static stretching (SS) is very important for the efficient rehabilitation of joints [3,30–34]. Based on the latest scientific findings, especially on the biomechanical contributions in this field, new preventive and therapeutic measures for avoiding stiffness and motion impairment in the joints can be adopted during the early stages of diseases [2,9,15].

The therapeutic effects of stretching have been established in a great number of experimental animal models (e.g., post-traumatic knee contractures in rat and rabbit models, which have significance for humans) [7,35–38]. Thus, it is possible to evaluate important data on cellular functions and the intracellular matrix components of joint cartilage, as well as information on the morphological structures and functions of joint capsules, both in healthy controls and in joints that have been modified in the processes of contractures (post-traumatic, myogenic, arthrogenic, etc.) [7,11,36–39]. Zhang et al. examined the effect of stretching combined with ultrashort wave diathermy on joint functions and clarified its cellular mechanisms in a rabbit knee contracture model [38]. Wang L. et al. [7] studied the effects of different static progressive stretching durations on the knee joint's range of motion, collagen- and alpha-actin expressions in fibroblasts, inflammatory cell number, and fibrotic changes in the joint capsule (as the result of different static progressive stretching durations applied to a post-traumatic knee contracture in a rat model). The authors concluded that static progressive stretching could improve post-traumatic knee contractures by increasing the knee joint mobility.

Numerous animal models that simulate a "knee flexion contracture" and a few models of a "knee extension contracture" have been proposed [11]. The authors determined that the "aggravation of contractures" was correlated with the degree of "fibrosis response" of the joints, which is related to the activation of type I and type III collagen syntheses, as well as to the stimulation of pro-fibrotic gene expression in fibroblasts and chondroblasts. A proteomic analysis of the muscles and joint capsule was performed by the same study group [11]. The expression of transforming growth factor beta-1 (TGF-β-1) was also examined as a significant biomarker of changes in the synthesis and distribution of different collagen types (I–III) in the intercellular matrix. An important fact of clinical relevance is that "extension contracture models" better mimic fractures and the bed-associated immobilization of patients in traumatology than "flexion contracture models".

The main question related to stretching biomechanics is: "Could chronic stretching change the joint–ligament–tendon–muscle mechanical properties?" The effects of stretching were reported for joint resistance and muscle and tendon stiffness, but a large heterogeneity was seen for most of the variables obtained [4]. The same authors analyzed 26 papers regarding longitudinal stretching (static, dynamic, and/or PNF) in humans of any age and with different health statuses. Structural and mechanical variables were evaluated for joints and muscle–tendon units: dynamic stretching, static stretching, flexibility, stiffness, mechanical joint properties, muscle morphology and functional activities, changes in the tendon characteristics, proprioceptive neuromuscular facilitation, etc. [6]. Adaptations to chronic stretching protocols shorter than 8 weeks seemed to occur mostly at the sensory level [6].

2.3. Biomechanical Effects of Static and Active Isometric Stretching Applied to the Human Knee Joint

The effects of stretching on muscle properties are clearly described in literature and depend on various factors, including stretching techniques, stretching time, retention time, rest time, and the time difference between the intervention and the measurement [28,40,41]. Most studies investigated the effects of static stretching on the passive properties of the muscle–tendon unit [42–46]. In a series of studies by Magnusson et al. [42,43,45–47], it was shown that static stretching for 90 s over five repetitions reduced muscle resistance, passive stiffness, peak torque, and stress relaxation. Another team of researchers [48,49] concluded that changes in the viscoelastic properties of the muscle–tendon unit depend more on the duration of stretching than on the number of stretches. An extension of static stretching time (from five to ten minutes) was shown to reduce tendon stiffness, as measured passively by ultrasonography [48,49]. The reduction in stiffness might be due to a change in the arrangement of collagen fibers in the tendon [48]. Stretching increased the range of motion of the femoral flexion and the outer rotation [21].

Isometric stretching is a type of static stretching associated with the resistance of muscle groups through isometric contractions of the stretched muscles. Due to the fact that this type of muscle stretching works in an isometric mode, the initiated muscle forces will affect the joints around which the muscles are located. The muscle forces produced by this type of stretching trigger processes within the joint itself. Cotofana et al. [50] demonstrated that the cartilage thickness decreased to 5.2% from a knee load with a force equal to 50% of the body weight. Herberthold et al. [51] evaluated the deformation at a force load equal to 150% of the body weight.

Our experimental model and working hypothesis estimated that, as the result of active isometric stretching of the adjacent locomotor muscles, changes in the distance between the femur and the corresponding end of the tibia could be observed [28]. The changes in the distance between the two bones would, in turn, be conditioned by several factors: the magnitude of the isometric muscle tension during stretching; the duration and direction of the tension applied; the tendon's biomechanical properties; and the biomechanical properties of the knee joint (shape, size, viscosity of the synovial fluid, and mechanical properties of the joint capsule elements).

Static investigations of knee joint stability are often directed to stretching exercises [28,52–56] and isometric back squats [55].

Our study group's quantitative estimation of the biomechanical processes in human knee joints during active isometric stretching was based on knee joint capsule ultrasound scanning during isometric stretching exercises [28,52,53,56]. During a right-lower-limb pose with a 140-degree femur–tibia angle, the distance between the tibia and femur bones forming the knee joint was measured using ultrasound scanning. Our experimental model included an ultrasound examination of the knee joint after the isometric stretching of healthy men (n = 10). The changes (in millimeters) in the distances between the femur and tibia were measured with a portable ultrasound system (Vinno 6, China; Figure 1). The apparatus was used for the purposes of our study in the musculoskeletal mode and in real time with a scanning frequency for the linear transducer of 8 to 10 MHz. The system was able to work in three different upright positions, all with a femur–tibia angle of 140 degrees at rest. In two of the three upright positions, extra loads of 4 and 8 kg were applied vertically down to the lower right limb to induce isometric stretching. Three quantitative parameters—distance up (Dup), distance down (Down), and area (A, cm^2)—were measured from the ultrasound pictures (Figure 1). They defined the two displacements (mm) and the area (cm^2) between the intra-articular femur and tibia cartilage surfaces.

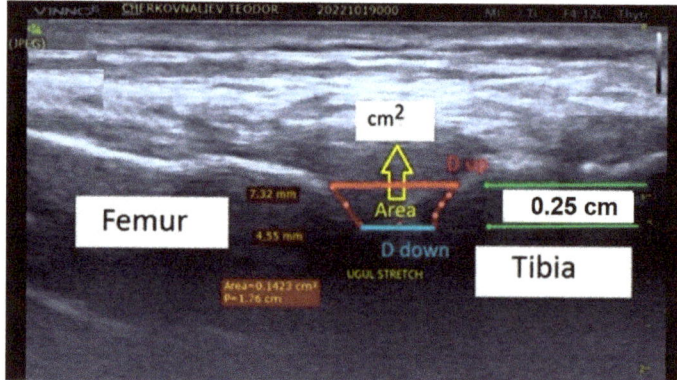

Figure 1. The screen view of the echography with measured distances between the femur and tibia bones in the knee joint of the participant. The distances Dup and Ddown between the femur and tibia for all participants at the reference position and at different loading levels were measured (in millimeters), with the depth space of the ultrasonographic scan equal to 0.25 cm. The next steps were used for improving the present experimental protocol with the addition of a "knee muff" for the stationary positioning of the ultrasound transducer toward the knee joint. The accuracy of the protocol was increased, with an error rate of less than 12%. The entire experimental approach will be published in another paper soon.

The results obtained for the change in the intra-articular geometry under a load and under stretching could serve as a quantitative assessment of the internal joint kinematics and might determine the joint mobility of individual participants in the stretching exercises [28,52,53,56].

The accuracy of the ultrasound pictures and measurements in our experimental model was limited by three main components (Figure 1) [56]. The first was related to the transducer accuracy characteristics. The second was the accuracy of the identity of the transducer–knee joint image position reproductions. The third component was the researcher's skill at obtaining scanning pictures. The present preliminary experimental model accuracy was defined as the sum of the three components cited and was lower than 30%.

2.4. Biomechanical and Biological (Cellular and Molecular) Mechanisms of Stretching

The cellular and molecular mechanisms underlying the changes in joint flexibility, muscle strength, and power are not well clarified in medicine and cell biology, and thus, further investigations are needed.

The additional effects of individual training status, age, sex, and different pathological states that moderate the influences of stretching exercises on the joints, muscles, tendons, and ligaments can be characterized as indirect [6,18,22,24,35].

Stretching modulates the synthesis, deposition, concentration, degradation, and distribution of collagen and glucosoaminoglycans (GAGs), affecting the remodeling of the extracellular matrix [57]. The data obtained encourage the therapeutic application of stretches and stretching physiotherapy at the cellular and molecular levels—preliminary in the treatment and management of arthritic joints [58].

The contributions of Bouffard et al. [59] and Wang et al. [7] demonstrate the importance of transforming growth factor β-1 (TGF β-1) in collagen synthesis and extracellular matrix remodeling after a brief static stretching (SS) application. Simultaneously, stretching also modulates the aggrecan concentrations in the matrix. Xiong et al. [60] examined the expression of TGF β-1 as a tissue inhibitor of metalloproteinases.

TGF β-1 is one of the more important cytokines regulating fibroblast responses in connective tissue. In health and diseases, collagen is a major protein in the extracellular matrix, and aggrecan is the main proteoglycan in articular cartilage. Stretching can be used to enhance and engineer the connective tissue's extracellular matrix with desirable collagen/elastin concentrations, improved elastic properties, and regular mesenchymal cell (fibroblast/chondroblast) functions [61].

Moreover, the biomechanical aspects underlying the different influences of active and passive stretches on joint, tendon, ligament, and muscle flexibility at rest are yet to be identified [5,26,62]. The recent results in medical and sports scientific literature indicate that chronic SS exercises have the potential to improve muscle strength and power [5,20]. Further investigations could examine the benefits of chronic SS exercises in old, healthy, and ill individuals, as compared to young, active, and well-trained persons, as well as compared to professional athletes [20,30,63–67].

2.5. Stretching Is an Integral Component of Mind–Body Exercises Such as Yoga (Mainly Hatha Yoga), Tai Chi, and Gingong

Gothe, McAuley et al. [65,67] compared the functional benefits of stretching and yoga exercises. Four standard fitness tests assessing balance, strength, flexibility, and mobility were administered [64,65]. The experimental stretching protocols varied with combinations of the functional parameters of exercise duration, intensity, frequency, and whole-body posture [66]. Patel and colleagues (2012) concluded that yoga practice and stretching exercises led to improvements in strength, flexibility, mobility, and quality of life in older adults [64]. Considering the benefits of stretching and yoga exercises, the special sports programs in functional fitness could be adapted for healthy individuals in the elderly population, as well as for people with socially important diseases (arthritis, diabetes mellitus, chronic inflammation, etc.). Gothe and co-authors [65,67] recommended the effects of stretching and/or yoga exercises for improving functional fitness outcomes in health and diseases, as well as for improving sports performance and health-related quality of life.

The potential preventive and therapeutic effects of static and yoga stretching (SS and YS) were examined in relation to different pathological states, such as chronic inflammation, wound healing, tumor growth, etc. [15,66,68–70].

The biological, cellular, and molecular mechanisms underlying the anti-inflammatory and anti-cancer properties of stretching, yoga, and TCC were very well summarized and presented in the review of Kròl et al. [16]. These physical exercises could enhance the immune state, change the IL-6 and IL-10 levels, and improve the health-related quality of life in older individuals [71–73]. On the other hand, chronic inflammation could contribute to the initiation, progression, and development of tumorigenesis [74]. In these and other pathological states, stretching exercises are recommended and included in programs for diabetes mellitus type 2 (DM-2) patients and in stroke and malignant disease rehabilitation and treatment [75,76]. Stretching may serve as a method of connective tissue healing [15,77]. Ferreti and colleagues (2006) [77] examined mechanical signals as having strong anti-inflammatory effects and recommended the use of mechanical forces of an appropriate intensity in the rehabilitation of knee meniscus cartilage. Further studies are required to understand the role of collagen and aggrecan in the remodeling and destruction of the articular cartilage's extracellular matrix (e.g., in osteoarthritis of various etiologies). Collagen and the impaired synthesis of proteoglycan/aggrecan is related to diseases such as local and systemic (disseminated) scleroses [16]. The same authors pointed out that daily stretching may be a part of therapy in patients with systemic sclerosis (SSc). Similar conclusions could be valid for a local Dupuytren contracture (Morbus Dupuytren) [25]. Guissard and Duchateau studied the effects of static stretching training on the characteristics of the plantar–flexor muscles in 12 subjects. An improved muscle flexibility was associated ($r^2 = 0.88$; $p < 0.001$) with a decrease in passive muscle stiffness. Although the changes in the flexibility and passive stiffness were partially maintained 1 month after the end of the training program, the reflex activities had already returned to control levels. It was concluded that the increased flexibility resulted mainly from the reduced passive stiffness of the muscle–tendon unit and the tonic reflex activity [25].

In only one study [78], a mouse breast cancer model was presented, and the results showed slower tumor growth (from 2–4 weeks) under the influence of stretching.

By comparing various stretching techniques to study their short- and long-term effects on different parameters (knee joint ROM, hamstring flexibility, muscle electromyographic activity, etc.), the researchers registered significant preliminary results for both the joint ROM and hamstring flexibility parameters [79]. The same authors applied static stretching (SS) as a variant of proprioceptive neuromuscular facilitation–contact–relax (PNF–CR) techniques. The knee range of motion (ROM), hamstring flexibility, and knee flexor muscle electromyographic (EMG) activity were also investigated [3,79]. The results obtained demonstrated an immediate, as well as a long-term, effect on the knee ROM and only a long-term effect on flexibility in the elderly. The aging human population exhibited an increase in muscle stiffness, as well as disturbances in the syntheses of types I–III collagens and an alteration in ROMs and EMG activities, due to the cellular and molecular processes in the elderly [3,25,30,31,63].

On the other hand, the PNF–CR and SS techniques were described as effective for increasing hamstring flexibility in young individuals [31,63,79].

Ferber R. et al. [3] applied three PNF stretching techniques: static stretching (SS), contact relaxation (CR), and agonist contact relaxation (ACR). The purposes of these studies were to characterize the effects of stretching on the ROM of joints and the EMG activity of muscles. The authors concluded that the PNF stretching technique increased the ROM in older adults. However, a paradoxical effect was also observed: PNF stretching might not induce muscular relaxation or reduce muscle stiffness in older adults due to age-related alterations in collagen synthesis and muscle elasticity [3,75,80,81].

Recent studies have examined the combined effects of static and/or dynamic stretching, followed by foam rolling (FR) and other techniques with or without local vibrations [12,32,34,38]. The combination of SS and FR is a very effective and frequently used method in sports programs and platforms to increase the ROM of joints and simultaneously decrease muscle stiffness. In this relationship, it has been reported [3,82] that the cell and tissue changes associated with aging are mainly related to the loss of the joint range of motion (ROM), increased muscle stiffness, and pathological changes in collagen and proteoglycan (GAG) synthesis and metabolism.

3. Conclusions

Stretching therapy and prophylaxis include passive and active stretching techniques and some partner-assisted methods precisely summarized in [5,53,83,84].

In this review paper, we briefly described the experiences of international researchers and our study group with the application of stretching as a very interesting field of theoretical and practical medicine, sports sciences, and biomechanics. The accuracy and limitations of therapeutic stretching techniques were also defined. We paid special attention to the simultaneous biomechanical and healing effects of static and/or active isometric stretching, which were also applied to our in vivo model of the human knee joint. The improvements to the knee joint range of motion (ROM) and flexibility were confirmed by ultrasound measurements. An accurately applied stretching treatment led to efficient short- and long-term results: a high movement quality and the reduced risk of further joint soft-tissue injuries in different pathological states, as well as in the elderly and those engaging in sports practice. Further investigations could continue to examine and compare the healing, therapeutic, and preventive effects of static stretching (SS) exercises in different study groups: ill adult patients, old healthy individuals, young persons (well-trained and physically active), and a group of professional athletes.

From a historical point of view and in the present day, the benefits and main components of mind–body exercises such as yoga (Hatha yoga) and stretching could be successfully applied in special sports platforms and programs for stretching management, prophylaxis, and treatment.

The therapeutic and preventive effects of stretching exercises have also been established in different experimental modeling systems, including animal, computational, and mathematical models, which have significance for human therapies and the prophylaxis of injuries.

In addition to static (passive) stretching, the authors characterized stretching therapy as the combined application of a wide range of techniques (e.g., stretching combined with foam rolling with or without vibration, massage, motion movements, etc.). The conclusions of prevalent studies suggest that when properly applied and combined with other techniques, stretching therapy could improve joint, muscle, fascia, tendon, and ligament health and flexibility and resolve problems associated with joint and muscle stiffness. The prevention of sports injuries in the morpho-functional unit of the joint–ligament–tendon–muscle could improve the health and sports performance of healthy persons and professional athletes. From a long-term perspective, increasing the flexibility and reducing the stiffness of muscles would lead to relaxation and muscle fiber elongation, which is also related to better sports performance.

The synthesis and localization of the main biomechanical variables and biomarkers in the extracellular matrix of the joints and cartilage at the cellular and molecular levels, such as collagen, elastin, hyaluronic acid, and other glucosaminoglycans (GAGs), specific genes, TgF-β1, etc., need further investigation.

The proposed combined stretching techniques could be applied in efficient therapeutic programs in medicine and sports, depending on their short- and long-term healing effects.

Recent studies have determined that static progressive stretching (SPS) therapy, alone or in a combined treatment, is the main way to improve the joint range of motion (ROM) and reduce or prevent the development of arthrogenic contractures, joint capsule fibrosis, and muscle stiffness, thus positively influencing the biological structures, functions, and biomechanics of the joint–ligament–capsule–tendon–muscle unit. The therapeutic and preventive effects of static stretching (SS) need new clinical and sports applications. Further successful retrospective and prospective studies could elucidate the cellular, molecular, and biomechanical mechanisms of the effects of stretching.

Static and/or dynamic stretching (SS and/or DS) applied in sports sciences could improve joint and muscle properties, which is of great importance in prophylaxis and the treatment of sports injuries.

However, the cellular and molecular mechanisms of stretching need further investigation.

Author Contributions: Conceptualization, S.R., E.Z., E.K. and I.I.; methodology, E.Z. and E.K.; software, E.K. and I.I.; validation, E.Z. and E.K.; formal analysis, E.Z.; investigation, E.Z., E.K. and I.I.; resources, E.Z., E.K. and I.I.; data curation, A.A.; writing—original draft preparation, E.Z.; writing—review and editing, E.Z. and E.K.; visualization, E.K., I.I. and A.A.; supervision, E.Z., E.K. and I.I.; project administration, I.I.; funding acquisition, S.R. and I.I. All authors have read and agreed to the published version of the manuscript.

Funding: This research was funded by the Bulgarian National Science Fund, grant number КП-06-H57/18, from 16.11.2021.

Institutional Review Board Statement: Not applicable.

Informed Consent Statement: Informed consent was obtained from all subjects involved in the study.

Data Availability Statement: Not applicable.

Conflicts of Interest: The authors declare no conflict of interest.

References

1. Weerapong, P.; Hume, P.A.; Kolt, G.S. Stretching: Mechanisms and benefits for sport performance and injury prevention. *Phys. Ther. Rev.* **2004**, *9*, 189–206. [CrossRef]
2. Taylor, D.C.; Dalton, J.D., Jr.; Seaber, A.V.; Garrett, W.E., Jr. Viscoelastic properties of muscle-tendon units: The biomechanical effects of stretching. *Am. J. Sports Med.* **1990**, *18*, 300–309. [CrossRef]
3. Ferber, R.; Osternig, L.R.; Gravelle, D.C. Effect of PNF stretch techniques on knee flexor muscle EMG activity in older adults. *J. Electromyogr. Kinesiol.* **2002**, *12*, 391–397. [CrossRef]
4. Freitas, S.R.; Mendes, B.; Le Sant, G.; Andrade, R.J.; Nordez, A.; Milanovic, Z. Can chronic stretching change the muscle-tendon mechanical properties? A review. *Scand. J. Med. Sci. Sports* **2018**, *28*, 794–806. [CrossRef] [PubMed]
5. Arntz, F.; Markov, A.; Behm, D.G.; Behrens, M.; Negra, Y.; Nakamura, M.; Chaabene, H. Chronic Effects of Static Stretching Exercises on Muscle Strength and Power in Healthy Individuals Across the Lifespan: A Systematic Review with Multi-level Meta-analysis. *Sports Med.* **2023**, *53*, 723–745. [CrossRef]
6. Knudson, D. The biomechanics of stretching. *J. Exerc. Sci. Physiother.* **2006**, *2*, 3–12.
7. Wang, L.; Cui, J.B.; Xie, H.M.; Zuo, X.Q.; He, J.L.; Jia, Z.S.; Zhang, L.N. Effects of Different Static Progressive Stretching Durations on Range of Motion, Myofibroblasts, and Collagen in a Posttraumatic Knee Contracture Rat Model. *Phys. Ther.* **2022**, *102*, pzab300. [CrossRef] [PubMed]
8. Salsich, G.B.; Mueller, M.J.; Sahrmann, S.A. Passive ankle stiffness in subjects with diabetes and peripheral neuropathy versus an age-matched comparison group. *Phys. Ther.* **2000**, *80*, 352–362. [CrossRef]
9. Sacco, I.C.; Sartor, C.D. From treatment to preventive actions: Improving function in patients with diabetic polyneuropathy. *Diabetes/Metab. Res. Rev.* **2016**, *32*, 206–212. [CrossRef]
10. Williams, D.B.; Brunt, D.; Tanenberg, R.J. Diabetic neuropathy is related to joint stiffness during late stance phase. *J. Appl. Biomech.* **2007**, *23*, 251–260. [CrossRef]
11. Zhang, R.; Zhang, Q.B.; Zhou, Y.; Zhang, R.; Wang, F. Possible mechanism of static progressive stretching combined with extracorporeal shock wave therapy in reducing knee joint contracture in rats based on MAPK/ERK pathway. *Biomol. Biomed.* **2023**, *23*, 277–286. [CrossRef]
12. Nakamura, M.; Konrad, A.; Kasahara, K.; Yoshida, R.; Murakami, Y.; Sato, S.; Wilke, J. The Combined Effect of Static Stretching and Foam Rolling With or Without Vibration on the Range of Motion, Muscle Performance, and Tissue Hardness of the Knee Extensor. *J. Strength Cond. Res.* **2022**, *37*, 322–327. [CrossRef]
13. Medeiros, D.M.; Cini, A.; Sbruzzi, G.; Lima, C.S. Influence of static stretching on hamstring flexibility in healthy young adults: Systematic review and meta-analysis. *Physiother. Theory Pract.* **2016**, *32*, 438–445. [CrossRef] [PubMed]
14. Fukaya, T.; Sato, S.; Yahata, K.; Yoshida, R.; Takeuchi, K.; Nakamura, M. Effects of stretching intensity on range of motion and muscle stiffness: A narrative review. *J. Bodyw. Mov. Ther.* **2022**, *32*, 68–76. [CrossRef] [PubMed]

15. Berrueta, L.; Muskaj, I.; Olenich, S.; Butler, T.; Badger, G.J.; Colas, R.A.; Spite, M.; Serhan, C.; Langevin, H.M. Stretching impacts inflammation resolution in connective tissue. *J. Cell. Physiol.* **2016**, *231*, 1621–1627. [CrossRef]
16. Król, M.; Kupnicka, P.; Bosiacki, M.; Chlubek, D. Mechanisms Underlying Anti-Inflammatory and Anti-Cancer Properties of Stretching—A Review. *Int. J. Mol. Sci.* **2022**, *23*, 10127. [CrossRef] [PubMed]
17. Su, H.; Chang, N.J.; Wu, W.L.; Guo, L.Y.; Chu, I.H. Acute effects of foam rolling, static stretching, and dynamic stretching during warm-ups on muscular flexibility and strength in young adults. *J. Sport Rehabil.* **2017**, *26*, 469–477. [CrossRef]
18. Cipriani, D.J.; Terry, M.E.; Haines, M.A.; Tabibnia, A.P.; Lyssanova, O. Effect of stretch frequency and sex on the rate of gain and rate of loss in muscle flexibility during a hamstring-stretching program: A randomized single-blind longitudinal study. *J. Strength Cond. Res.* **2012**, *26*, 2119–2129. [CrossRef] [PubMed]
19. Cramer, H.; Lauche, R.; Klose, P.; Lange, S.; Langhorst, J.; Dobos, G.J. Yoga for improving health-related quality of life, mental health and cancer-related symptoms in women diagnosed with breast cancer. *Cochrane Database Syst. Rev.* **2017**, *1*, CD010802. [CrossRef]
20. Taylor, D. Physical activity is medicine for older adults. *Postgrad. Med. J.* **2014**, *90*, 26–32. [CrossRef]
21. Copeland, J. Stretching: Mechanisms and benefits for sport performance and injury prevention. *New Zealand J. Physiother.* **2005**, *33*, 68–69.
22. Kataura, S.; Suzuki, S.; Matsuo, S.; Hatano, G.; Iwata, M.; Yokoi, K.; Tsuchida, W.; Banno, Y.; Asai, Y. Acute effects of the different intensity of static stretching on flexibility and isometric muscle force. *J. Strength Cond. Res.* **2017**, *31*, 3403–3410. [CrossRef] [PubMed]
23. Konrad, A.; Gad, M.; Tilp, M.J.S.J. Effect of PNF stretching training on the properties of human muscle and tendon structures. *Scand. J. Med. Sci. Sports* **2015**, *25*, 346–355. [CrossRef]
24. Hotta, K.; Behnke, B.J.; Arjmandi, B.; Ghosh, P.; Chen, B.; Brooks, R.; Maraj, J.J.; Elam, M.; Maher, P.; Kurien, D.; et al. Daily muscle stretching enhances blood flow, endothelial function, capillarity, vascular volume and connectivity in aged skeletal muscle. *J. Physiol.* **2018**, *596*, 1903–1917. [CrossRef]
25. Guissard, N.; Duchateau, J. Effect of static stretch training on neural and mechanical properties of the human plantar-flexor muscles. *Muscle Nerve Off. J. Am. Assoc. Electrodiagn. Med.* **2004**, *29*, 248–255. [CrossRef]
26. Middag, T.R.; Harmer, P. Active-isolated stretching is not more effective than static stretching for increasing hamstring ROM. *Med. Sci. Sports Exerc.* **2002**, *34*, S151. [CrossRef]
27. Stoichev, S.; Ivanov, I.; Ranchev, S.; Jotov, I. A review of the biomechanics of synovial joints with emphasize to static stretching exercise. *Ser. Biomech.* **2021**, *35*, 3–20.
28. Ranchev, S.; Ivanov, I.; Iotov, I.; Stoytchev, S. On the biomechanical processes in human knee joint during active isometric stretching. *Ser. Biomech.* **2019**, *33*, 56–61.
29. Davies, D.V. Synovial membrane and synovial fluid of joints. *Lancet* **1946**, *248*, 815–819. [CrossRef]
30. Bryanton, M.; Bilodeau, M. The role of thigh muscular efforts in limiting sit-to-stand capacity in healthy young and older adults. *Aging Clin. Exp. Res.* **2017**, *29*, 1211–1219. [CrossRef]
31. Hill, K.J.; Robinson, K.P.; Cuchna, J.W.; Hoch, M.C. Immediate effects of proprioceptive neuromuscular facilitation stretching programs compared with passive stretching programs for hamstring flexibility: A critically appraised topic. *J. Sport Rehabil.* **2017**, *26*, 567–572. [CrossRef]
32. Lin, W.C.; Lee, C.L.; Chang, N.J. Acute effects of dynamic stretching followed by vibration foam rolling on sports performance of badminton athletes. *J. Sports Sci. Med.* **2020**, *19*, 420. [PubMed]
33. Kokkonen, J.; Nelson, A.G.; Eldredge, C.; Winchester, J.B. Chronic static stretching improves exercise performance. *Med. Sci. Sports Exerc.* **2007**, *39*, 1825–1831. [CrossRef] [PubMed]
34. Konrad, A.; Nakamura, M.; Paternoster, F.K.; Tilp, M.; Behm, D.G. A comparison of a single bout of stretching or foam rolling on range of motion in healthy adults. *Eur. J. Appl. Physiol.* **2022**, *122*, 1545–1557. [CrossRef] [PubMed]
35. Hagiwara, Y.; Ando, A.; Chimoto, E.; Tsuchiya, M.; Takahashi, I.; Sasano, Y.; Onoda, Y.; Suda, H.; Itoi, E. Expression of collagen types I and II on articular cartilage in a rat knee contracture model. *Connect. Tissue Res.* **2010**, *51*, 22–30. [CrossRef]
36. Hildebrand, K.A.; Zhang, M.; Germscheid, N.M.; Wang, C.; Hart, D.A. Cellular, matrix, and growth factor components of the joint capsule are modified early in the process of posttraumatic contracture formation in a rabbit model. *Acta Orthop.* **2008**, *79*, 116–125. [CrossRef]
37. Tokuda, K.; Yamanaka, Y.; Kosugi, K.; Nishimura, H.; Okada, Y.; Tsukamoto, M.; Tajima, T.; Suzuki, H.; Kawasaki, M.; Uchida, S.; et al. Development of a novel knee contracture mouse model by immobilization using external fixation. *Connect. Tissue Res.* **2022**, *63*, 169–182. [CrossRef]
38. Zhang, Q.B.; Zhou, Y.; Zhong, H.Z.; Liu, Y. Effect of stretching combined with ultrashort wave diathermy on joint function and its possible mechanism in a rabbit knee contracture model. *Am. J. Phys. Med. Rehabil.* **2018**, *97*, 357–363. [CrossRef]
39. Stoytchev, S.; Nikolov, S. Effects of flow-dependent and flow-independent viscoelastic mechanisms on the stress relaxation of articular cartilage. *Ser. Biomech.* **2023**, *37*, 43–50. [CrossRef]
40. McNair, P.; Stanley, S. Effect of passive stretching and jogging on the series muscle stiffness and range of motion of the ankle joint. *Br. J. Sports Med.* **1996**, *30*, 313–318. [CrossRef]
41. Magnusson, S. Passive properties of human skeletal muscle during stretch manoeuvres. *MedSci. Sports Exerc.* **1998**, *8*, 65–77.

42. Magnusson, S.; Simonsen, E.; Aagaard, P.; Sorensen, H.; Kjaer, M. A mechanism for altered flexibility in human skeletal muscle. *J. Physiol.* **1996**, *497*, 291–298. [CrossRef] [PubMed]
43. Magnusson, S.; Simonsen, E.; Dyhre-Poulsen, P.; Aagaard, P.; Mohr, T.; Kjaer, M. Viscoelastic stressrelaxation during static stretch in human skeletal muscle in the absence of EMG activity. *MedSci. Sports Exerc.* **1996**, *6*, 323–328.
44. McNair, P.J.; Dombroski, E.W.; Hewson, D.J.; Stanley, S.N. Stretching at the ankle joint: Viscoelastic responses to holds and continuous passive motion. *Med. Sci. Sports Exerc.* **2001**, *33*, 354–358. [CrossRef]
45. Magnusson, S.; Simonsen, E.; Aagaard, P.; Gleim, G.; McHugh, M.; Kjaer, M. Viscoelastic response to repeated static stretching in the human hamstring muscle. *Scand. J. MedSci. Sports* **1995**, *5*, 342–347. [CrossRef]
46. Magnusson, S.; Aagaard, P.; Larsson, B.; Kjaer, M. Passive energy absorption by human muscle-tendon unit is unaffected by increase in intramuscular temperature. *J. Appl. Physiol.* **2000**, *88*, 1215–1220. [CrossRef]
47. Magnusson, S.; Simonsen, E.; Aagaard, P.; Kjaer, M. Biomechanical responses to repeated stretches in human hamstring muscle in vivo. *Am. J. Sports Med.* **1996**, *24*, 622–628. [CrossRef]
48. Kubo, K.; Kanehisa, H.; Fukunaga, T. Is passive stiffness in human muscles related to the elasticity of tendon structures? *Eur. J. Appl. Physiol.* **2001**, *85*, 226–232. [CrossRef]
49. Kubo, K.; Kanehisa, H.; Fukunaga, T. Effects of resistance and stretching training programs on the viscoelastic properties of human tendon structures in vivo. *J. Physiol.* **2002**, *538*, 219–226. [CrossRef]
50. Cotofana, S.; Eckstein, F.; Wirth, W.; Souza, R.B.; Li, X.; Wyman, B.; Graverand, M.-P.H.-L.; Link, T.; Majumdar, S. In vivo measures of cartilage deformation: Patterns in healthy and osteoarthritic female knees using 3T MR imaging. *Eur. Radiol.* **2011**, *21*, 1127–1135. [CrossRef]
51. Herberhold, C.; Faber, S.; Stammberger, T.; Steinlechner, M.; Putz, R.; Englmeier, K.H.; Reiser, M.; Eckstein, F. In situ measurement of articular cartilage deformation in intact femoropatellar joints under static loading. *J. Biomech.* **1999**, *32*, 1287–1295. [CrossRef]
52. Ranchev, S.; Ivanov, I.M.; Yotov, I.; Stoytchev, S. Studies on paradox in the work of musculoskeletal system in isometric stretching. *J. Appl. Sports Sci.* **2020**, *2*, 80–90. [CrossRef]
53. Behm, D.G.; Alizadeh, S.; Daneshjoo, A.; Konrad, A. Potential Effects of Dynamic Stretching on Injury Incidence of Athletes: A Narrative Review of Risk Factors. *Sports Med.* **2023**, *53*, 1359–1373. [CrossRef]
54. Kuntz, A.B.; Chopp-Hurley, J.N.; Brenneman, E.C.; Karampatos, S.; Wiebenga, E.G.; Adachi, J.D.; Noseworthy, M.; Maly, M.R. Efficacy of a biomechanically-based yoga exercise program in knee osteoarthritis: A randomized controlled trial. *PLoS ONE* **2018**, *13*, e0195653. [CrossRef]
55. Trindade, T.B.; de Medeiros, J.A.; Dantas, P.M.S.; de Oliveira Neto, L.; Schwade, D.; de Brito Vieira, W.H.; Oliveira-Dantas, F.F. A comparison of muscle electromyographic activity during different angles of the back and front squat. *Isokinet. Exerc. Sci.* **2020**, *28*, 1–8. [CrossRef]
56. Raikova, R.; Ivanov, I.; Hristov, O.; Markova, N.; Trenev, L.; Angelova, S. Detailed investigation of the knee biomechanics during posture maintenance applying different static loading on the spine. *Int. J. Bioautom.* **2023**, *27*, 83. [CrossRef]
57. Abusharkh, H.A.; Reynolds, O.M.; Mendenhall, J.; Gozen, B.A.; Tingstad, E.; Idone, V.; Abu-Lail, N.; Van Wie, B.J. Combining stretching and gallic acid to decrease inflammation indices and promote extracellular matrix production in osteoarthritic human articular chondrocytes. *Exp. Cell Res.* **2021**, *408*, 112841. [CrossRef]
58. Madhavan, S.; Anghelina, M.; Rath-Deschner, B.; Wypasek, E.; John, A.; Deschner, J.; Piesco, N.; Agarwal, S. Biomechanical signals exert sustained attenuation of proinflammatory gene induction in articular chondrocytes. *Osteoarthr. Cartil.* **2006**, *14*, 1023–1032. [CrossRef]
59. Bouffard, N.A.; Cutroneo, K.R.; Badger, G.J.; White, S.L.; Buttolph, T.R.; Ehrlich, H.P.; Stevens-Tuttle, D.; Langevin, H.M. Tissue stretch decreases soluble TGF-β1 and type-1 procollagen in mouse subcutaneous connective tissue: Evidence from ex vivo and in vivo models. *J. Cell. Physiol.* **2008**, *214*, 389–395. [CrossRef] [PubMed]
60. Xiong, Y.; Berrueta, L.; Urso, K.; Olenich, S.; Muskaj, I.; Badger, G.J.; Aliprantis, A.; Lafyatis, R.; Langevin, H.M. Stretching reduces skin thickness and improves subcutaneous tissue mobility in a murine model of systemic sclerosis. *Front. Immunol.* **2017**, *8*, 124. [CrossRef]
61. Syedain, Z.H.; Tranquillo, R.T. TGF-β1 diminishes collagen production during long-term cyclic stretching of engineered connective tissue: Implication of decreased ERK signaling. *J. Biomech.* **2011**, *44*, 848–855. [CrossRef] [PubMed]
62. Behm, D.G.; Blazevich, A.J.; Kay, A.D.; McHugh, M. Acute effects of muscle stretching on physical performance, range of motion, and injury incidence in healthy active individuals: A systematic review. *Appl. Physiol. Nutr. Metab.* **2016**, *41*, 1–11. [CrossRef] [PubMed]
63. Borges, M.O.; Medeiros, D.M.; Minotto, B.B.; Lima, C.S. Comparison between static stretching and proprioceptive neuromuscular facilitation on hamstring flexibility: Systematic review and meta-analysis. *Eur. J. Physiother.* **2018**, *20*, 12–19. [CrossRef]
64. Patel, N.K.; Newstead, A.H.; Ferrer, R.L. The effects of yoga on physical functioning and health related quality of life in older adults: A systematic review and meta-analysis. *J. Altern. Complement. Med.* **2012**, *18*, 902–917. [CrossRef]
65. Gothe, N.P.; Kramer, A.F.; McAuley, E. The effects of an 8-week Hatha yoga intervention on executive function in older adults. *J. Gerontol. Ser. A Biomed. Sci. Med. Sci.* **2014**, *69*, 1109–1116. [CrossRef] [PubMed]
66. Muñoz-Vergara, D.; Grabowska, W.; Yeh, G.Y.; Khalsa, S.B.; Schreiber, K.L.; Huang, C.A.; Zavacki, A.; Wayne, P.M. A systematic review of in vivo stretching regimens on inflammation and its relevance to translational yoga research. *PLoS ONE* **2022**, *17*, e0269300.

67. Gothe, N.P.; McAuley, E. Yoga is as good as stretching–strengthening exercises in improving functional fitness outcomes: Results from a randomized controlled trial. *J. Gerontol. Ser. A Biomed. Sci. Med. Sci.* **2016**, *71*, 406–411. [CrossRef]
68. Pizza, F.X.; Koh, T.J.; McGregor, S.J.; Brooks, S.V. Muscle inflammatory cells after passive stretches, isometric contractions, and lengthening contractions. *J. Appl. Physiol.* **2002**, *92*, 1873–1878. [CrossRef]
69. Chu, S.Y.; Chou, C.H.; Huang, H.D.; Yen, M.H.; Hong, H.C.; Chao, P.H.; Wang, Y.-H.; Chen, P.-Y.; Nian, S.-X.; Chen, Y.-R.; et al. Mechanical stretch induces hair regeneration through the alternative activation of macrophages. *Nat. Commun.* **2019**, *10*, 1524. [CrossRef]
70. Danhauer, S.C.; Addington, E.L.; Cohen, L.; Sohl, S.J.; Van Puymbroeck, M.; Albinati, N.K.; Culos-Reed, S.N. Yoga for symptom management in oncology: A review of the evidence base and future directions for research. *Cancer* **2019**, *125*, 1979–1989. [CrossRef]
71. Sumi, K.; Ashida, K.; Nakazato, K. Repeated stretch–shortening contraction of the triceps surae attenuates muscle atrophy and liver dysfunction in a rat model of inflammation. *Exp. Physiol.* **2019**, *105*, 1111–1123. [CrossRef] [PubMed]
72. Eda, N.; Ito, H.; Shimizu, K.; Suzuki, S.; Lee, E.; Akama, T. Yoga stretching for improving salivary immune function and mental stress in middle-aged and older adults. *J. Women Aging* **2018**, *30*, 227–241. [CrossRef] [PubMed]
73. Wang, C.; Collet, J.P.; Lau, J. The effect of Tai Chi on health outcomes in patients with chronic conditions: A systematic review. *Arch. Intern. Med.* **2004**, *164*, 493–501. [CrossRef]
74. Singh, N.; Baby, D.; Rajguru, J.P.; Patil, P.B.; Thakkannavar, S.S.; Pujari, V.B. Inflammation and cancer. *Ann. Afr. Med.* **2019**, *18*, 121. [CrossRef]
75. Ghasemi, E.; Khademi-Kalantari, K.; Khalkhali-Zavieh, M.; Rezasoltani, A.; Ghasemi, M.; Baghban, A.A.; Ghasemi, M. The effect of functional stretching exercises on functional outcomes in spastic stroke patients: A randomized controlled clinical trial. *J. Bodyw. Mov. Ther.* **2018**, *22*, 1004–1012. [CrossRef]
76. Park, S.H. Effects of passive static stretching on blood glucose levels in patients with type 2 diabetes mellitus. *J. Phys. Ther. Sci.* **2015**, *27*, 1463–1465. [CrossRef]
77. Ferretti, M.; Madhavan, S.; Deschner, J.; Rath-Deschner, B.; Wypasek, E.; Agarwal, S. Dynamic biophysical strain modulates proinflammatory gene induction in meniscal fibrochondrocytes. *Am. J. Physiol. Cell Physiol.* **2006**, *290*, C1610–C1615. [CrossRef] [PubMed]
78. Berrueta, L.; Bergholz, J.; Munoz, D.; Muskaj, I.; Badger, G.J.; Shukla, A.; Kim, H.J.; Zhao, J.J.; Langevin, H.M. Stretching reduces tumor growth in a mouse breast cancer model. *Sci. Rep.* **2018**, *8*, 7864. [CrossRef] [PubMed]
79. Zaidi, S.; Ahamad, A.; Fatima, A.; Ahmad, I.; Malhotra, D.; Al Muslem, W.H.; Abdulaziz, S.; Nuhmani, S. Immediate and Long-Term Effectiveness of Proprioceptive Neuromuscular Facilitation and Static Stretching on Joint Range of Motion, Flexibility, and Electromyographic Activity of Knee Muscles in Older Adults. *J. Clin. Med.* **2023**, *12*, 2610. [CrossRef] [PubMed]
80. Gautieri, A.; Passini, F.S.; Silván, U.; Guizar-Sicairos, M.; Carimati, G.; Volpi, P.; Moretti, M.; Schoenhuber, H.; Redaelli, A.; Berli, M.; et al. Advanced glycation end-products: Mechanics of aged collagen from molecule to tissue. *Matrix Biol.* **2017**, *59*, 95–108. [CrossRef]
81. Ferreira, J.P.; Araújo, V.L.; Leal, Â.M.; Serrão, P.R.; Perea, J.P.; Santune, A.H.; Sacco, I.; Aranha, G.A.; Fernandes, R.A.S.; Salvini, T.F.; et al. Diabetes and peripheral neuropathy are related to higher passive torque and stiffness of the knee and ankle joints. *Kinesiology* **2022**, *54*, 92–104. [CrossRef]
82. Smith, J.R.; Walker, J.M. Knee and elbow range of motion in healthy older individuals. *Phys. Occup. Ther. Geriatr.* **1983**, *2*, 31–38. [CrossRef]
83. Page, P. Current concepts in muscle stretching for exercise and rehabilitation. *Int. J. Sports Phys. Ther.* **2012**, *7*, 109. [PubMed]
84. Behm, D.G.; Aragão-Santos, J.C.; Korooshfard, N.; Anvar, S.H. Alternative Flexibility Training. *Int. J. Sports Phys. Ther.* **2023**, *18*, 285. [CrossRef]

Disclaimer/Publisher's Note: The statements, opinions and data contained in all publications are solely those of the individual author(s) and contributor(s) and not of MDPI and/or the editor(s). MDPI and/or the editor(s) disclaim responsibility for any injury to people or property resulting from any ideas, methods, instructions or products referred to in the content.

MDPI
St. Alban-Anlage 66
4052 Basel
Switzerland
www.mdpi.com

Applied Sciences Editorial Office
E-mail: applsci@mdpi.com
www.mdpi.com/journal/applsci

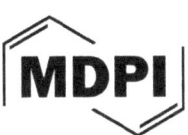

Disclaimer/Publisher's Note: The statements, opinions and data contained in all publications are solely those of the individual author(s) and contributor(s) and not of MDPI and/or the editor(s). MDPI and/or the editor(s) disclaim responsibility for any injury to people or property resulting from any ideas, methods, instructions or products referred to in the content.

www.ingramcontent.com/pod-product-compliance
Lightning Source LLC
LaVergne TN
LVHW070646100526
838202LV00013B/891